T0319459

The History of the Brain and Mind Sciences

Rochester Studies in Medical History

Senior Editor: Theodore M. Brown
Professor of History and Preventive Medicine
University of Rochester

Additional Titles of Interest

A complete list of titles in the Rochester Studies in Medical History
series may be found on our website, www.urpress.com.

The History of the Brain and Mind Sciences

Technique, Technology, Therapy

EDITED BY
STEPHEN T. CASPER AND DELIA GAVRUS

UNIVERSITY OF ROCHESTER PRESS

The University of Rochester Press gratefully acknowledges generous support from the University of Winnipeg.

First published 2017

University of Rochester Press
668 Mt. Hope Avenue, Rochester, NY 14620, USA
www.urpress.com
and Boydell & Brewer Limited
PO Box 9, Woodbridge, Suffolk IP12 3DF, UK
www.boydellandbrewer.com

ISBN-13: 978-1-58046-595-3
ISSN: 1526-2715

Library of Congress Cataloging-in-Publication Data

Names: Casper, Stephen T., editor. | Gavrus, Delia, editor.
Title: The history of the brain and mind sciences : technique, technology, therapy / edited by Stephen T. Casper and Delia Gavrus.
Other titles: Rochester studies in medical history ; v. 40. 1526–2715
Description: University of Rochester Press : Rochester, NY, 2017. | Series: Rochester studies in medical history, ISSN 1526-2715 ; v. 40. | Includes bibliographical references and index.
Identifiers: LCCN 2017011118 | ISBN 9781580465953 (hardcover : alk. paper)
Subjects: | MESH: Neurosciences—history | Neurology—history | Brain—physiology
Classification: LCC QP360 | NLM WL 11.1 | DDC 612.8—dc23 LC record available at https://lccn.loc.gov/2017011118

Contents

Acknowledgments

Many of the articles in this volume first found expression in a small workshop organized by Stephen at Clarkson University in Potsdam, New York, during the summer of 2012. Supported by generous grants from the Clarkson's Center for Canadian Studies, the David A. Walsh '67 Seminar Series, and the School of Arts and Sciences, the scholars from Canada and the United States gathered together in an Adirondack lodge to discuss numerous wide-ranging papers focusing on technique, technology, and therapy in the mind and brain sciences.

At the time, several participants commented that the experience seemed to them somewhat similar to the great science conferences that had taken place at Cold Spring Harbor or the Marine Biology Laboratory, and all hoped that such an experience might be replicated again in the future. While not all of the papers presented at the conference ultimately made their way into this volume, and while some additional chapters were subsequently solicited to fill out the range of techniques on display in the following pages, the overall frame that this volume asserts for the history of the mind and brain sciences first germinated in that bucolic setting.

During the planning stages of the workshop, Delia was funded by a Social Science and Humanities Research Council of Canada (SSHRC) postdoctoral fellowship, and she gratefully acknowledges SSHRC's vital financial support. She thanks the members of the Department of Social Studies of Medicine at McGill University (and especially George Weisz, Thomas Schlich, Tobias Rees, Susan Lamb, and Nick Whitfield) for the exceptionally rich intellectual environment they provided, as well as the members of the History Department at the University of Winnipeg, who have been extraordinarily supportive of her work and teaching during her first years as an assistant professor.

Finally, we extend our gratitude to all the participants of the workshop and all the contributors to the volume, who have not only produced outstanding intellectual work, but who have also demonstrated the importance of building a vibrant, stimulating, and—above all—a supportive community of scholars interested in the history of the mind and brain sciences.

Introduction

Technique, Technology, and Therapy in the Brain and Mind Sciences

DELIA GAVRUS AND STEPHEN T. CASPER

The essays in this volume visit episodes in the history of the mind and brain sciences through the historical looking glass of the broader concepts of technique, technology, and therapy. In the last three decades, technique and technology in particular have commanded increasing attention from scholars working on the history of science and medicine, but they have been less explored by historians of neuroscience.[1] Even therapy, which at first glance seems to have been widely discussed by scholars, has been explored only selectively; more marginal neurological therapies, for instance, have only recently captured historians' attention.[2] In putting together this volume, our first goal was to draw together more closely a community of scholars who study diverse topics pertaining to the history of the mind and brain sciences but who are also concerned about broader historiographical directions and who rely on similar conceptual styles. This volume was conceived as a meditation on the role that technique, technology, and therapy—as conceptual and rhetorical categories, as well as practical embodiments—have played in the constitution of the mind and brain sciences over the past one and a half centuries. Our second goal was to collect a series of papers able to provide a sophisticated and versatile teaching tool for graduate and senior undergraduate seminars.

Collectively, the papers contribute to and challenge some aspects of the current historiography of the neurosciences, which has broadly developed in a way that encourages constructing and thinking within grand narratives about progress in the studies of the mind and brain, and which tends to overemphasize the centrality of the human self within this history. In contrast, this volume makes a collective case for exploring the field through the lens of seemingly marginal stories—stories that appear, from a contemporary perspective—to be situated at the edges of history. By foregrounding these marginal stories, we hope to disrupt the standard narrative and to offer a competing view of the history of the mind and brain sciences. In place of a grand narrative, our volume offers a series of unconventional stories. In lieu of a linear history of progress, we suggest a congregation of fractured histories. Taken together, the essays in this volume offer a glimpse of the interrupted paths of scientists' and physicians' lives, their fragmented conversations, their globally influenced but locally crafted theories of mind and brain, and the work that led them at times directly into box canyons. Perhaps, too, this volume can shed some light on how once-perceived unshakeable sources of knowledge or practices became the forgotten foundations of the sciences and medicine of the mind and brain. In this introduction, we start by describing recent trends in scholarship in the humanities and social sciences that explore the mind and brain sciences. Thereafter, we consider the status of the historiography of the mind and brain sciences before looking more closely at the ways in which studies of technique, technology, and therapy have shaped that historical understanding. We end with an overview of the chapters and an analysis of the common themes that bind them together.

Big Histories of the Mind and Brain Sciences

It has become commonplace in academic scholarship to refer—with wonder and analytic urgency—to the increasing economic, social, and symbolic capital that the mind and brain sciences (or "the neurosciences" in their post-1960 incarnation) have secured within biomedicine, in policy and law, and in public culture at large over the past century and a half.[3] And indeed, the ubiquity of neuroscience at the beginning of the twenty-first century is remarkable: two vast initiatives in the United States and the European Union aim to "accelerate our understanding of the human brain, make advances in defining and diagnosing brain disorders, and develop new brain-like technologies,"[4] while the attention of the general public is continuously courted with neuroscience stories in the traditional and social media and in trendy TED talks that garner millions of views.[5] Neuroscience is everywhere, and overly optimistic stories about its power and its promise seem to both fascinate and sell. A recent issue of *Scientific American* claimed in a cover story titled "The Neuroscience of Habits" that "new techniques are finally allowing neuroscientists to decipher the neural mechanisms that underlie our rituals" and routines, and that this research could lead to "drugs, behavioral therapies and simple tricks to help us control habits, good and bad."[6]

As this quote suggests, the promises of neuroscience have often been cast by popularizers as mediating such interventions into the self. In fact, with the help of the mind and brain sciences—with their technologies of visualization, for instance[7]—the self itself has been read and reconstituted in different configurations. In the middle of the twentieth century, as sociologist Nikolas Rose has noted, a new "neurochemical self" was made possible, and assumed manifest by some educated individuals, by developments in basic science and in psychopharmacology. This was a self that invited specific ways of governance and intervention.[8] The neurochemical self may be, as anthropologist Tobias Rees has argued, just one iteration of the "neurological human," which is constantly undergoing conceptual change.[9] This project of making up humans in conjunction with their brains has been, of course, much older than the neurosciences themselves, which took shape in the middle of the twentieth century. As historian Fernando Vidal has argued, the "cerebral subject," the very idea that brain equals personhood, is a quintessentially modern one, traceable to the middle of the eighteenth century and predating the reductive neuroscientific techniques that eventually embraced it,[10] and one that has been actualized in the last four decades in formal medical practice through the elaboration of the brain-death criteria.[11]

Understanding the history of the mind and brain sciences has been deemed particularly critical because, at the end of the twentieth century, the neurosciences successfully left the laboratory and, as Rose and Abi-Rached put it, "gaine[d] traction in the world outside."[12] A host of neuro disciplines—social neuroscience, neuroethics, neuroeconomics, neuroesthetics, and neurohistory even[13]—have in recent decades incorporated neuroscientific principles as part of their methodologies.[14] This transition from the scientific world to the world at large was made possible, as Rose and Abi-Rached have shown, by a nexus of "conceptual, technological, economic and biopolitical" mutations,[15] including the advent of a new neuromolecular vision of the brain (reductive and material in nature) and politically strategic arguments about the economic burden of brain disorders. The claim that knowledge of the brain leads in an uncomplicated way to knowledge about such complex human affairs as education, ethics, the law, and so on, is in fact not new to this relatively recent "neuro-turn," as Stephen Casper has shown. Since the Victorian period, this rhetorical appeal has been a reliable tool for neurologists to deploy for the purpose of shoring up authority, advancing common professional interests, fashioning a shared professional identity, and claiming social and economic relevance.[16]

It is precisely a focus on these tendencies that have led some writers in both the natural sciences and the humanities to labor under a somewhat simplified conception of a unified neuroscience and to assert that "the neuro" brings nature, culture, and selfhood ever closer together. Some scholars find this growing authority of the mind and brain sciences and the neuro-turn itself truly alarming and in need of critical appraisal.[17] Others believe it to be a much more benign, even helpful development to both public culture generally, and the practice of history specifically.[18] Critics of the latter studies have argued, however, that current histories which create seemingly linear narratives and those that seek a too-close rapprochement with the various theories about the self currently fashionable in neuroscience can themselves become complicit in particular ideologies while failing to fulfill the role of public critic that befits historians,[19] a role that, others have observed, also befits scientists themselves.[20] Furthermore, the conflation of neuroscience with knowledge about the human self can erase the motley history of the brain sciences and the multiplicity of motives, interests, epistemologies, techniques, and questions that animate the various communities and individuals who were part of it or who labored at its margins. As the science itself shifts over time, a constant revision of the historical foundations of neuroscientific concepts creates the appearance of ever-greater epistemological unity for these sciences, an appearance which can be used to support various political and social ends. For while it is indeed important to excavate the history of the mind and brain sciences in order to understand the iterations of the human self that they make possible and the symbolic capital they marshal today, it is useful to remind ourselves constantly that, as historian Fabio de Sio has put it, the neurosciences represent "a contingent disciplinary and, later, historiographical umbrella-definition, which at once houses and shadows a number of relatively autonomous if historically related sets of issues, practices and models."[21] As such, it is often the case that the history of the mind and brain sciences contains many epistemic fractures and is more of a patchwork of loosely held together fragments than the sweeping narratives about the evolution of the understanding of the self might imply.

Neuroscience and Historical Scholarship

This volume was thus conceived at a moment when it appears that critical scholarship in a variety of fields of humanistic and social scientific writing on neuroscience and society/culture evinces a multiplicity of voices and perspectives. Scholars have offered a variety of *longue durée* studies, ranging from macro-level accounts of the birth of the neurosciences and the origins of neuroscientific concepts, to studies proclaiming the dawning of a neuroscientific, technocratic age or the now achievability of deep histories.[22]

At the same time, those big narrative histories have been supported by a host of rich case studies exploring, for instance, biographies of pioneering figures in the neurosciences, studies of the history of philosophically intriguing questions in the mind and brain sciences, or explorations of celebrated findings or procedures in the hands of particular individuals.[23] At times these historical works reciprocally augment the production of a vision of the history of the mind and brain sciences that takes as obvious the supposition that these sciences have as their end goal the transcendental and transhistorical re-making (neuro-making, one might say) of such topics as selfhood, environmental determinism, animal intelligence and ultimately that they articulate a means for transcending the limitations placed upon human flourishing by the structures and evolutionary inheritances that allegedly burden the brain, mind, and nervous system.[24]

Shades of such ambitious metaprojects have been visible for over a century in the writings of physicians and scientists writing the history of their disciplines. Among the countless scientific and medical papers focusing on the anatomy and physiology, physics and chemistry, developmental biology and genetics, and structure and function of the nervous system, behavior, and cognition, there existed a marked minority of polemical essays inquiring into the philosophical, sociological, and theological implications of studies of mind and brain.[25] While the bread and butter of "normal science" in the mind and brain sciences may have possessed markedly narrower ambitions, those humanistic essays now permit historical understanding of the ideological visions that guided the labor of those scientists and physicians through often-ornate, contradictory articulations. Thus, when illustrious figures such as Charles Sherrington, Francis Walshe, John C. Eccles, or Wilder Penfield took to writing philosophical and historical essays—or novels for that matter—they were seeking to build from often profoundly reductionist studies of nerve function or chemistry a deeper vision of mind and brain that robustly defended specific political or ideological visions.[26] Indeed, since the late eighteenth century, as historian Christopher Lawrence has shown, the nervous system and theories of mind and brain have formed (as it were) a crucible for such statements.[27]

When the work of charismatic figures in the past and present are supposed to reflect the views of a broader community of scientists and clinicians, scholarly focus is often directed to the content of the claims rather than the historical context in which the claims are embedded. Little thought, for example, is given to the questions of to whom the remarks were directed, in which professional communities the figure was situated, or even the paramount question of the precise importance of the figure in that historical moment. These tendencies are particularly pronounced in historical works that seek to trace the history of a given concept in the mind and brain sciences from the past through to the present. Many of these works build their argument through a chronologically organized family tree that identifies one or two key figures per generation across perhaps a century, claim for those figures certain canonical status within the scientific or medical tradition, and then articulate through their endeavors and theories the history of the concept. This characteristic form of internalist history of science (i.e., a reconstruction of the past of science in terms only of the scientific world) can at times appear as an externalist historical approach (i.e., judging the ways that social and cultural contexts guide sciences) because the programmatic incitements of specific figures appear to connect mind and brain science and medicine to society while placing those sciences directly into society.[28]

Such narratives are interesting, and they undoubtedly make an important contribution to the marketplace of ideas and historical interpretations, but at the same time such frames do raise questions for other scholars, especially those who are inclined to look for the messy alternatives lost to history. Trends in other related sciences may have transformed so completely within a generation the logic of the life sciences and biomedicine, and in ways so complete, that a linear account obscures some fascinating discontinuities.[29] Discoveries in other scientific and medical fields, too, may have been appropriated into the conceptual narrative of the mind and brain sciences, in the process ripping apart, in an arbitrary fashion, the inherent complex beauty of science in practice and in making. Political and cultural contexts of great importance in the construction of particular forms of knowledge can be stripped away, as the conceptual narrative is bent toward expounding upon a future desired rather than a past that occurred.[30] Local understandings of mind and brain (whether derived from working-class, religious, or ethnic identities and sensibilities, or, alternatively, carved out in universities placed in highly distinctive political and cultural contexts) become reduced in significance—are all unwittingly subordinated to an account of where something came from and where it is going, never mind that it came from many places and was originally very likely going toward no predestined future.[31]

Far from demanding capitulation in the face of such overwhelming complexity, this reality should hold the promise of rich projects for historians. One way in which that complexity can be ordered in some fashion is by showing how the broader historical context permeates the center and the periphery of these disciplines. The mind and brain sciences, for all of the antiquity of some threads of their conceptual foundations, are creations of modernity. This fact signals that in researching, writing, speaking, and thinking about the histories of these fields, it is essential to grapple with the emergence of particular forms of mass society that characterized, especially in the years following World War I, the Enlightenment project of modernity. Psychiatry, psychology, and neurology all emerged in modernity. Neuroscience, although rooted in research programs initiated in the 1950s and 1960s, by contrast, became a recognizable field of critical inquiry in the 1990s, that is, in a period most squarely associated with a time when many educated people thought they had become postmoderns.[32] Embedding, for instance, a particular therapy, whether marginal or mainstream, in its specific era reveals the ways in which the medicine of the mind and brain is co-produced with modernist or postmodernist structures.[33]

While we celebrate the diversity of historical methodologies, the optimism and exuberance that sometimes propagates—one might also say innervates—the historiography of neuroscience, thus, strikes us as imposing a purpose, directionality, and insularity on the mind and brain sciences that seems too selective to be the only significant approach for what ought to be a diligent and vibrant history of these sciences. There are great reasons for being particularly careful when attempting metanarratives about the mind and brain sciences that simplify those fields of inquiry to a few understandable, in vogue categories: by the close of the twentieth century, literally hundreds of thousands of people had published millions of pages of scientific and medical observations, hypotheses, experimental trials, consecutive hospital studies, retrospective studies, cultural and environmental analyses, public health inquires, technical papers, and reports on countless topics. Textbooks in a variety of disciplines and specialties had passed through myriad editions. Forms of objectivity, normative structures, practices of trust, technologies, therapeutic assumptions, social expectations, and the diversity of the fields (and the languages spoken and read as a matter of routine) had all undergone extraordinary changes. For these reasons and more, historians of science can set their sights on comparatively less ambitious aims, put their feet squarely on the ground, and focus historical attention on what the margins of the mind and brain sciences might tell us.

Technique, Technology, and Therapy in the Mind and Brain Sciences

This collection of essays joins the conversation exactly from this perspective. First, this volume attempts to go beyond a conceptual concern with the monolithic notion of the human self itself, exploring instead the heterogeneous, diverse, and ultimately exceptionally complex set of scientific and medical techniques, technologies, and therapies that allow their practitioners to claim expertise and license to intervene into some aspect of the nervous system and the mind. The chapters do so by offering empirical studies, some of which are in-depth microhistories while others are stories broader in scope. Second, the book showcases the heterogeneity of practices and intellectual aims; the epistemic breaks that occur for various historical reasons; and what appears to be, but only in retrospect, the marginal episodes that make up the complex and fractured history of the mind and brain sciences.

Collectively, the papers of this volume make two general arguments: that the marginal is itself a concept that needs to be historicized, and that the general (as embodied in broad narratives about the past) is easily destabilized by an attention to the techniques that constitute the marginal. As Katja Guenther puts it eloquently in the coda that closes this volume, for the scholar, technique can function as a key concept in "articulating that historical relationship between centrality and marginality." The authors of the essays suggest that historians should pay close attention to what appears to be (both from today's perspective and from past perspectives) obscure and peripheral, while at the same time striving not to (unwittingly and however subtly) rewrite the history of the mind and brain sciences from the presentist position that addles our perception of what the brain and mind sciences should encompass.

Historian Theodore Porter has argued that over the past century, science has come to be viewed as fundamentally technical in nature while moving away from an identification with an ideal of public reason.[34] To Porter and other historians, this shift is a key historical problem, and the essays in the volume both corroborate and complicate this story. The Greek *techne* is at the root of the English words *technical, technology,* and *technique*—ideas whose meaning, as historians have shown, has changed over time: *technical,* for instance, acquired in the twentieth century a connotation of expert knowledge, which it did not really have in the previous century.[35] The same is true of *technique:* this is a concept whose meaning is shifting both for the historical actors themselves as well as for scholars, who have employed it as a category of analysis in idiosyncratic ways. Michel Foucault, who at times used technique and technology interchangeably, wrote about the "specific techniques that human beings use to understand themselves," and he called "technologies of the self" those techniques that made it possible for individuals to intervene (in their minds or bodies) in order to effect a particular transformation.[36] Historians of science Lorraine Daston and Peter Galison have shown how scientific techniques and practices constitute different kinds of scientific selves and engender different kinds of objectivities.[37] More specifically in the broad history of the mind and brain sciences and medicine, historian Mical Raz has skillfully explored the history of the technique of lobotomy to dismantle facile binary divisions (such as somatic vs. dynamic approaches to mental illness) that exist only from an uninformed, presentist position.[38] For historian Otniel Dror, the brain itself became a technique for producing emotions more than an object of study in itself in the physiological laboratory of the 1920s,[39] and Delia Gavrus has shown how different kinds of performances constituted techniques of the self that allowed neurosurgeons to enact a shared professional identity.[40]

The essays in this volume use the concept of technique in many of its broad implications and connotations, but generally speaking they portray technique as a set of practices that are performed to particular ends by specific individuals. As categories of analysis, technique and technology are useful because they focus the attention of the historian on practice—whether this practice is itself material or rhetorical, as with literary techniques and technologies of persuasion and illusion. For the authors of this volume, technique performs this function by being inextricably linked to the intentionality of specific historical actors—even though this intentionality can have different effects from the ones that are originally intended (as it does, for instance, in the case of Stephen Casper's exhibit architects) and even if technique itself limits as well as expands the scientist's gaze in particular directions (as it does for Penfield and Dockrill's work on the vaso-motor reflex as a mechanism for epilepsy, in Gavrus's chapter).

Other scholars—in particular science studies scholars who write from a theoretical commitment to actor-network theory (ANT)—have used the concept of technique to erase the traditional boundaries between the human and the object, arguing that techniques function as mediators that allow nonhuman actors to act.[41] This interest in techniques has certainly allowed ANT scholars to focus on the material, but they have done so by displacing humans and by muddling the notion of subjectivity and intentionality—an enterprise that has drawn criticism from social and cultural historians in particular.[42] The essays in this volume demonstrate that technique (and the material) can occupy a privileged role of analysis without decentralizing human agency.

Where technique has perhaps been undervalued as a means for analyzing the emergent assumptions and practices of the mind and brain sciences, the opposite case could be made for technologies, albeit with the caveat that the technologies which receive attention are often highly circumscribed in the sense that they are more often captivating in their claims and products. This attention on the more spectacular components of mind and brain technology often visibly contributes to the further overdetermination seen in historical scholarship on the neurosciences.[43] In general, scholarly attention has been placed on those technologies that trick invisible processes in the nervous system into becoming visible ones, whether through illuminating metaphors of electricity in the nervous system or the actual imaging technologies that came to the fore in the 1980s.[44] Similarly, scholarly attention on intelligence testing, personality inventories, psychoanalytic technologies, psychometrics, and psychotechnics all promised within particular historical cultural paradigms to make normal and abnormal minds knowable, trainable, and controllable.[45]

Scholarship in this area has reached a very high level of sophistication, one all too rarely replicated. The instruments, apparatuses, and technology designed to visualize the brain in action hold incredible power to constitute contemporary notions of personhood.[46] As Katja Guenther and Volker Hess argue in a special issue of *Medical History*, "The instruments and material culture of the modern mind and brain sciences function like soul catchers because they are grappling with the same problem: how to make the invisible visible, to capture and study that which seems fleeting and ethereal."[47] Moreover, foregrounding technology allows historians to draw connections between the social body and the human body—such as was the case with the simultaneous "electrification" of society and the brain in the 1920s, as historian Cornelius Borck has shown.[48]

It is altogether too rare, however, to find works of scholarship that follow the pattern of Guenther, Hess, and Borck and place these technologies into deeper cultural contexts in the periods in which they emerged, a practice much more common in the wider history of medicine and science. In the historical scholarship on medicine, for instance, numerous historians have analyzed the role of technology in constructing medical diagnoses, transforming patient care in hospitals and clinics; creating disputes and competition among specialists; and opening up ethical and economic questions about access to, and informed consent about, procedures and treatments.[49] By contrast, works like that by Elizabeth Green Musselman, which center on overlaps between technological metaphors, industrial and engineering science, and the cultural construction of nervous conditions are rare, and those that do exist almost invariably focus on past nervous diseases or forms of technologically made objectivity in particular schools of psychology.[50]

Beyond these limited and exemplary examples, studies of technology in the history of the mind and brain science tend to follow a commonplace script. Missing from that conversation are, as Max Stadler puts it in his contribution in this volume, narratives of technology in the mind and brain sciences that "defamiliarize us from a neuroscientific past" that is all too familiar. Or as he also puts it more adroitly, missing is a fractious narrative that explains that beyond "soup and sparks," a reference to the discovery of the mechanism of nerve cell firing, there is also a story to be examined about "algae and whipped cream" that connects reductionist mind, brain, and behavior science to such seemingly removed industrial corners as the material science of food production.[51]

Such observations are not to say that historians examining, for example, the practices of imaging science are wrong to do so, but rather to confront an observable tendency to ignore contexts that unsettle the object of study. Returning to Stadler's point, one might rightly ponder whether a story about nerve membrane functioning that features whipped cream has identified a subject of cultural significance worthy of historical exploration in ways that the precise discovery of the mechanism of action potentials might not. While there is no real dichotomy between the two historical inquiries, it is the claim of this volume that the former approach takes us further and explains more.

These observations about technique and technology hold true for therapy as well, although therapy is arguably the most extensively studied topic in the history of the mind and brain sciences. There are specific studies of neurological diseases, injuries, and patients, and these are complemented by a broad literature focused particularly on talking therapies and pharmaceutical interventions.[52] Yet even in this more richly established literature, historical scholarship gravitates to a selection of procedures and interventions. Neurosurgery is almost always brain surgery and only rarely involves spinal cord injuries.[53] Lobotomy figures more extensively in studies of neurosurgery than do other forms of "heroic" brain interventions that had similar aims, as Delia Gavrus has shown.[54] Procedures involving convulsive therapies have received extensive commentary. It is again the more familiar procedures that enjoy attention, while the marginal therapies, as for example stretching or electrology, that fade into the background, often even wrongly pilloried as quackish remedies from the "dark ages" of medicine. Also less studied are the narratives about therapy—or the lack thereof—that are sometimes crafted to particular ends by historical actors themselves.[55]

By focusing on the margins, on the rich diversity of therapies available at one time, on the failed interventions that only briefly light up the therapeutic scene, historians can articulate the complexity of the mind and brain sciences. The fact that this history is a complex and fractured assemblage of techniques, technologies, models, and therapies does not mean that all of our stories should be limited in time and scope. Coherence and explanatory impact are not necessarily lost if we accept the heterogeneous history of these disciplines.[56] An attention to the marginal does not necessarily mean that richly detailed microhistories are the only type of studies that historians ought to produce.[57] As we outlined above, we recognize and celebrate the plurality of authorial voices and historical methodologies.

At the same time, however, the authors of these papers do demonstrate the value of finely detailed, temporally bounded studies. Some branches of history—most notably intellectual history—have recently been animated by an embrace of "big history" that privileges the long time frame.[58] "Across the historical profession, the telescope rather than the microscope is increasingly the preferred instrument of examination; the long-shot not the close-up is becoming an ever-more prevalent picture of the past,"[59] writes historian David Armitage. *Longue durée* historians see this methodology as particularly fruitful and necessary in a world in which "short-termism" has been undermining the ability to respond wisely to long-term challenges such as global warming or environmental degradation.[60] The historian, these authors argue, has lost authority in the public sphere—both in terms of policy setting and in terms of public consumption of history—because of the profession's recent focus on narrow time frames.[61]

Together, the papers in this volume span nearly two centuries,[62] but even in their individual shorter time-bound focus, they aim to be a powerful corrective against the ubiquitous and wildly overstated claims in popular discourse about the explanatory power of neuroscientific studies; against the overly optimistic rhetoric about the practical and symbolic impact of contemporary neuroscientific techniques (as it is embodied, for instance, in the claims of the "brain training industry"); and against any illusion that the history of the mind and brain sciences is a linear and coherent one of progress and unity of technique, goals, and object of study. In fact, a conceptual focus on the marginal shares the aims, if not always the practice, of *longue durée* history at its best: to be socially relevant, to draw attention to the historical context of contemporary claims about neuroscience, to lay out the inescapable and fascinating messiness of the history of scientific research, and to give voice to all historical actors.

Certainly, there are many different ways to accomplish such a task; this collection of essays offers a few suggestions. First, the focus on the marginal, in all the possible meanings of the word—that which (from today's perspective or a past perspective) appears unusual, unimportant, insufficient, minor, insignificant, on the edge, on the sidelines, flat-out wrong—may offer such openings. The strange spaces, unusual materials, discarded models, forgotten medical conditions, and less prominent people whose stories the authors explore in this volume, offer a much richer, much more fragmented view of the history of the mind and brain sciences. What and who appears to be marginal to us may have been central at some moment in time. What may have been considered marginal became, for good historical reasons, central later on. When exposed, this shifting category of *the marginal* reveals the ways in which science is constantly constructing teleologies—narratives that reach back into the past and reconstitute themselves to give us the illusion of direct paths of discovery, invention, and ultimately progress.

At the same time, focusing on historical actors who occupied a decentralized role in the scientific milieu is equally important for the aim of historians to be socially relevant. Social and cultural historians have long argued for the importance of rescuing the voices of marginalized groups (like the Menagerie keepers in Stephen Jacyna's chapter in this volume or, in Delia Gavrus's essay, the laboratory technicians) and exploring the ways in which they make meaning from their marginal position.[63] Likewise, rescuing places that appear marginal in retrospect enriches historical scholarship by grounding the understanding of the past in its own terms and by exposing its multidimensionality.

Second, an analytical focus on technique, technology, and therapy is a good way to unveil and theorize marginality. Technique and technology are used here in a broad and nuanced sense—there are laboratory techniques, bibliographic techniques, technologies of exhibition, techniques of the self, narrative techniques—that at any moment in time work to shape scientific knowledge and the identities of practitioners. These techniques often become invisible, especially in retrospect, as the field moves on in new directions, and therefore the very nature of technique binds it closely to the historical construction of marginality. A close reading of technique in its own context, following the reasoning and justification with which it was applied at the time, will uncover the manner in which models and therapies were built and demolished over time, will train the historian's gaze on the material and the rhetorical alike, and will do so without decentralizing human agency.

Overview of Volume

The essays in this volume accomplish just that. In their richness and diversity, they are not meant to be an exhaustive or representative guide to the diversity of the mind and brain sciences in history. Indeed, it is problematic (and, given the very arguments raised in this volume, evidently self-defeating) to attempt to piece together a "representative" slice of the history of the mind and brain sciences;[64] our volume does not cover, for instance, such a central topic as psychoanalysis, which has received extensive and well deserved scholarly attention elsewhere. Furthermore, while two of the authors (Jacyna and Schlich) engage with the long nineteenth century, most of the essays are grounded in the twentieth century. Although the papers are arranged in chronological order for easier consultation, chronology itself is not an important aspect of the story we want to tell. Rather, the essays make the collective point that the brain and mind sciences do not have a unitary and seamless history, even as their historians are guided by similar historiographical concerns. As Alison Winter showed so elegantly in a book about memory, understanding expansive historical developments related to many-sided concepts is sometimes best served by focusing on well chosen fragments of that history.[65]

The volume opens in postrevolutionary France. The Menagerie (or, as we see later in Casper's chapter, the Great Exhibition) doesn't generally come to mind as the kind of space where the brain and mind sciences are constituted and thrive. And yet, as Stephen Jacyna shows, the naturalists and the keepers of the Menagerie of the Jardin des Plantes animated a powerful "truth machine" that made pronouncements about the nature of animals and humans. Operating under a novel utilitarian ethos, the Menagerie fulfilled practical economic objectives such as the breeding and domestication of exotic animals, but it was also used as a resource to investigate the question of animal intelligence and its contentious and ultimately unresolved relationship to human intelligence. Techniques of observation, along with comparative anatomical techniques supported by the Museum of Natural History's collection, provided a foundation from which correlations were made between animal *moeurs* and underlying nervous structures. Jacyna argues that ultimately this work constituted "a contribution to the creation of 'Man' as an object of study for the emergent human sciences," whose practical purpose was to serve the new social order by helping to better govern its subjects. The human subjects were constituted at the same time in conjunction with and in contrast to the animals of the Menagerie, and thus the animals, like their keepers, became central players in this unusual space that produced truths about intelligence, *moeurs*, and minds.

In the next chapter, Thomas Schlich describes how nineteenth-century "physiological surgery" became the epistemic basis of neurosurgery, as this branch of surgery developed into a bona fide medical specialty at the beginning of the twentieth century. Neurosurgery naturally began by privileging the practical issue of alleviating suffering over the philosophical quest for understanding human nature. By noting the surgeons' attitudes not only to particular forms of practice, but also to the notion of specialization itself, Schlich shows how this history can be written in a sophisticated, non-anachronistic way. He documents the increasing attempts of European and American surgeons in the late nineteenth century to rely on "experimental physiology as an important practical, epistemological, and rhetorical resource" which shaped the techniques that were employed in the operating room, as well as influenced the trust accorded by the public to the profession as a whole. One practice that emerged from the surgeons' use of the physiological laboratory and the development of cellular pathology was called radical surgery, in which a resective approach was pushed to the limits of completeness and which demanded "radical" techniques. Thus Halstead, in his radical mastectomy, removed a large area of the affected breast without touching the actual tumor itself and developed surgical techniques that allowed the surgeon to handle the tissue in a gentle fashion over a prolonged period of time. Along similar lines, experimental physiology provided the rationale for transplant surgery, and the laboratory became an important locus of expertise that allowed surgeons to argue that "a real surgeon is above all a natural scientist." The experimental science of the laboratory, Schlich argues, offered to modern neurosurgery a reassuring image of technicality and objectivity, and in turn neurosurgery was seen to reciprocally expand scientific knowledge in the mind and brain sciences.

Complicating assumptions that may seem unproblematic from a contemporary perspective, Kenton Kroker argues that the history of encephalitis lethargica "offers a profound challenge to any assumption that, in the early twentieth century, pathologies of the nervous system were somehow the exclusive province of a systematic body of specialized knowledge known as 'neurology.'" Thus, the techniques and the epistemological practices that helped establish encephalitis lethargica as an epidemic were much more diverse than the "neurological armamentarium" of the time. In addition, Kroker identifies significant epistemological fractures between local

(American) and international efforts to engage with this mysterious condition, and he highlights one novel technique in particular: the technique of the bibliographic surveillance project that the Matheson Commission mobilized to produce in 1929 a tome that eschewed expert judgment and synthesis while claiming impartiality and comprehensiveness. This technique, Kroker shows, was borne out of a contemporary ethos that cast cooperative bibliography as an essential buttress to American medicine—both as progressive practice and as business.

Max Stadler rereads the production of electrophysiological knowledge in the radio age of the 1920s and 1930s by focusing on the surprising materials—the "electrical things"—that were marshaled by a range of scientists to various practical ends. He shows that familiar concepts such as circuits and nerves participated in the effort, but at the same time, center stage was also occupied by items that appear misplaced to the presentist eye—things such as algae and whipped cream. Stadler argues that in the age that preceded the microelectrodes necessary for recording the electrical activity of single cells, "a great many disparate things went into the electrical fabrication of the nerve impulse": from sea urchins and plants to the electronic arts and medical physics. The diversity of materials reflected a diversity of techniques as well as a diversity of scientists. This diversity, Stadler argues, would remain opaque if the historian approached the question of the nervous impulse from the narrow standpoint of nerve physiology. Here again, seemingly marginal materials, like marginal spaces and people, deepen and re-enchant the past, reconceptualizing the very nature of the sciences that contribute to the history of a particular concept, while demonstrating that the idea of marginality exists in a constantly shifting context.

In the 1920s, for the second generation of neurosurgeons, the laboratory fulfilled an important epistemic and rhetorical function in the crafting of novel therapies, just like "physiological surgery" had in Schlich's example of the first generation of brain surgeons. The laboratory is where Wilder Penfield anchored his argument that epilepsy therapy ought to be in some cases surgical. Gavrus approaches this story through the perspective of a laboratory technician who labored in Penfield's neurocytology laboratory, perfecting histological techniques and taking care of the experimental animals. In this chapter, too, an analytical focus on technique sheds light on a story that at first glance may appear marginal to the history of brain science in the first half of the twentieth century. Dockrill's neurohistological work, despite the fact that it was done by an "invisible technician,"[66] and despite the fact that it was used to justify a surgical therapy that "failed" and is now obscure,[67] constituted work that was central to the aims of the sciences and medicine of the brain during the interwar period. Dockrill's case, Gavrus argues, throws into sharp relief "the relationship between early twentieth-century neurohistological techniques; new epistemological commitments to an ideal of bench science in medicine; and the urgent, if unfulfilled, hope of devising radical and rational therapies for a serious neurological condition." At the same time, Dockrill's aspirations as a technician whose symbolic and economic capital were equally limited found an unusual outlet in the writing of a novel that embodied his hope for recognition and fashioned an identity rooted in a romantic ideal of science.

Materials and techniques that were incorporated into the sciences of the brain and mind in the postwar era migrated to North America with their displaced owners, as Frank Stahnisch shows in a chapter that places "luggage" at the forefront of historical analysis. In the wake of the Nazis' rise to power, thousands of medical doctors and scientists of Jewish descent in Central Europe saw their professional and personal worlds destroyed. Some of these men and women escaped Europe with an assortment of books, instruments, and technologies that they attempted to reintegrate into the conceptual frameworks and the social networks of North American mind and brain specialists. Stahnisch shows that things such as "histo-anatomical microscopy in neuro-oncology, the holist neurological therapies, or the neurophysiological synapse research based on electrical stimulation devices," in addition to numerous other belongings such as datasets and photographs were mobilized in the transatlantic journey, allowing their owners to claim expertise in their search for new jobs, but also grounding the professional and personal identity of the scientists in very material things that connoted the home they had left behind. Highlighting the stories of those scientists who did not find professional positions comparable to the ones left behind, Stahnisch argues that the brain-gain theory (which emphasizes North America's great gain as a result of the scientists' forced migration) obscures the enormous difficulties that these scientists experienced. Here, too, a gaze directed away from the central stories of the elites and the historically successful brings into focus a much more complex historical tableau.

In the next chapter, Stephen Casper shows how the Committee for Science and Technology of the 1951 Festival of Britain provided a powerful platform for British scientists to communicate a particular view of the world to a general audience. Seeking to boost the morale of the public after a devastating war, the Festival entertained, instructed, and celebrated national ingenuity and achievement. Science, technology, and medicine took center stage in this celebration, and the brain sciences in particular were put on stage in dramatic exhibits that explored the function of the brain and nervous system in humans and animals. Casper argues that the British scientists who at midcentury aimed to introduce a particularly materialist, reductionist, and unitary view of nature—from subatomic particles to human conduct—were unwittingly introducing dualisms in the imagined architecture of their exhibits. Casper shows that "the techniques of persuasion the organizers used to convey their reductionist and materialistic story to the public ironically relied upon intentionally engineered psychotechnic illusions in assembling the physical space of the exhibit." Since the scientists did not explain the structure of psychic phenomena, through their techniques of illusion they inadvertently "created a participatory space filled by an invisible reaction formation, a dualism to haunt their materialist claim." The visitors, caught between a material world and a world of illusion, may have very well subverted and reappropriated those techniques of persuasion to their own idiosyncratic aims.

Justin Garson looks at the rise and fall of a particular reductionist enterprise: the dopamine hypothesis of schizophrenia. He reconstructs the historical process by which in the early 1970s a host of scientific and cultural elements—from a reconceptualization of stereotypy to the late 1960s countercultural revolution—led to the establishment of amphetamine psychosis as a biochemical model of schizophrenia. By painstakingly following the techniques, observations, and assumptions that allowed a handful of scientists to reframe amphetamine psychosis as a mirror of the broad range of schizophrenia symptoms, Garson shows that the architects of the dopamine hypothesis contributed to and greatly shaped the psychiatric reductionism of the late twentieth century, "putatively demonstrating that a major mental disorder could be successfully reduced to neurotransmitter abnormalities." Garson argues that complex mental illnesses such as schizophrenia, characterized as they are by a multitude of clinical manifestations, force the researcher to classify the symptoms into two broad categories: the essential and the secondary. It is only once this has been sorted out that the researchers conceive of techniques to build a model that explains the underlying mechanism. Because all these variables can change with time, research in the sciences of the mind and brain, Garson argues, "gives us a window on the way that madness is being collectively imagined" at any given historical moment.

In his essay, Brian Casey analyzes the ways in which the National Institute of Mental Health (NIMH) influenced academic psychiatry by promoting technologies and techniques that led to the "re-biologization of psychiatry" and steered it away from psychosocial approaches. This movement was influenced by certain scientific developments, to be sure, but it was also constrained, Casey argues, by internal and external forces such as economic and bureaucratic pressures. NIMH, Casey shows, was originally a great supporter of psychoanalysis, but over the course of the second half of the twentieth century, the institution "bolstered all five pillars of the biological revolution: drugs, genetics, nosology, brain imaging, and informatics." The powerful rhetoric of biological reductionism that the institution sanctioned was undiminished by failures, such as the fact that the first generation of antidepressant drugs did not seem to perform much better than placebo. One of the benefits of reductionism, Casey shows, was its ability to help NIMH mount a defense of the psychiatric profession as a whole, whose diagnostic variability and uncertainty in the 1970s and 1980s was raising doubts about the reality of mental illness. Such reductionist rhetoric, disseminated through press releases, radio and television programs, and more recently through websites, helped foster the faith in and the popularity of biological psychiatry in America. As Casey argues, rhetoric "can serve as a placeholder, sustaining belief until science fills in knowledge gaps." This rhetoric not only sheds light on what the NIMH wants to marginalize—sociological and psychological approaches—but it also performs the work of biomedicine on the margins by guiding and defending its research agenda.

As Katja Guenther reminds us in the coda, historians must remember that history itself is a technique, and that they must therefore work under the burden of continuous reflexivity. Collectively, the essays in this book show that the history of the mind and brain sciences is fractured in the sense that straight lines of historical narrative do not always exist to connect the present with the past; on the contrary, over the past century and a half, these sciences have consisted of a heterogeneous assortment of practices and disciplines, models and therapies. These essays, we hope, will inspire other scholars and students of the mind and brain sciences to be reflexive and vigilant, to find openings for other (future) histories of the brain, and to re-enchant the past. This is a task well worth doing in an era when there appears to be a lot at stake when it comes to matters of the brain and the mind.

Notes

1. For broader explorations on the role of technique in the history of science, see, for instance, Lorraine Daston and Peter Galison, *Objectivity* (New York: Zone Books, 2007); Otniel E. Dror, "Techniques of the Brain and the Paradox of Emotions, 1880–1930," *Science in Context* 14, no. 4 (2001): 643–60; and Theodore M. Porter, "How Science Became Technical," *Isis* 100, no. 2 (2009): 292–309.

2. See Katja Guenther, *Localization and Its Discontents: A Genealogy of Psychoanalysis and the Neuro Disciplines* (Chicago: University of Chicago Press, 2015); Katja Guenther, "Exercises in Therapy—Neurological Gymnastics between Kurort and Hospital Medicine, 1880–1945," *Bulletin of the History of Medicine* 88, no. 1 (2014): 102–31.

3. Martyn Pickersgill and Ira van Keulen, *Sociological Reflections on the Neurosciences* (Bingley, UK: Emerald Group, 2011); Nita A. Farahany, *The Impact of Behavioral Sciences on Criminal Law* (New York: Oxford University Press, 2009); Suparna Choudhury and Jan Slaby, *Critical Neuroscience: A Handbook of the Social and Cultural Contexts of Neuroscience* (Chichester, UK: Wiley-Blackwell, 2012); Davi Johnson Thornton, *Brain Culture: Neuroscience and Popular Media* (New Brunswick, NJ: Rutgers University Press, 2011); Michael Hagner and Cornelius Borck, "Mindful Practices: On the Neurosciences in the Twentieth Century," *Science in Context* 14, no. 4 (2001): 507–10.

4. The Brain Research through Advancing Innovative Neurotechnologies Initiative (part of the White House Neuroscience Initiative) and the Human Brain Project (established in 2013 and conceived to last a decade), respectively. The quote comes from the description of the latter project; see Human Brain Project, https://www.humanbrainproject.eu/discover/the-project/overview.

5. See "Neuroscience," *TED*, accessed December 15, 2016, https://www.ted.com/topics/neuroscience. To give just one example, as of July 6, 2016, neuroscientist Antonio Damasio's TED talk, "The Quest to Understand Consciousness," has been viewed 1,436,883 times, https://www.ted.com/talks/antonio_damasio_the_quest_to_understand_consciousness.

6. Ann M. Graybiel and Kyle S. Smith, "Good Habits, Bad Habits," *Scientific American* 310, no. 6 (2014): 39–40.

7. Joseph Dumit, *Picturing Personhood: Brain Scans and Biomedical Identity* (Princeton, NJ: Princeton University Press, 2004).

8. Nikolas Rose, "The Neurochemical Self and Its Anomalies," in *Risk and Morality*, ed. R. Ericson (Toronto: University of Toronto Press, 2003).

9. Tobias Rees, "Being Neurologically Human Today: Life, Science, and Adult Cerebral Plasticity (an Ethical Analysis)," *American Ethnologist* 37, no. 1 (2010): 150–66; Tobias Rees, *Plastic Reason: An Anthropology of Brain Science in Embryogenetic Terms* (Berkley: University of California Press, 2016).

10. F. Vidal, "Brainhood, Anthropological Figure of Modernity," *History of Human Science* 22, no. 1 (2009).

11. Stephen T. Casper, *The Neurologists: A History of a Medical Specialty in Modern Britain, c. 1789–2000* (Oxford: Oxford University Press, 2014), 155.

12. Nikolas S. Rose and Joelle M. Abi-Rached, *Neuro: The New Brain Sciences and the Management of the Mind* (Princeton, NJ: Princeton University Press, 2013), 9. See also older studies that make similar points about the impact of the science of the brain on broader cultural developments of earlier periods: Anne Harrington, *Medicine, Mind, and the Double Brain: A Study in Nineteenth-Century Thought* (Princeton, NJ: Princeton University Press, 1987), and Robert Maxwell Young, *Mind, Brain and Adaptation in the Nineteenth Century: Cerebral Localization and Its Biological Context from Gall to Ferrier* (Oxford: Clarendon Press, 1970).

13. On neurohistory and the history of science, see the recent Isis Focus section: D. L. Smail, "Neurohistory in Action: Hoarding and the Human Past," *Isis* 105, no. 1 (2014): 110–22; Steve Fuller, "Neuroscience, Neurohistory, and the History of Science: A Tale of Two Brain Images," *Isis* 105, no. 1 (2014): 100–109.

14. For a transdisciplinary engagement with and a contextualization of the neuro-turn, see Jenell M. Johnson and Melissa M. Littlefield, eds., *The Neuroscientific Turn: Transdisciplinarity in the Age of the Brain* (Ann Arbor: University of Michigan Press, 2012).

15. Rose and Abi-Rached, *Neuro*, 9.

16. Stephen T. Casper, "History and Neuroscience: An Integrative Legacy," *Isis* 105, no. 1 (2014): 123–32; S. T. Casper, *The Neurologists* (Manchester, UK: University of Manchester Press, 2014).

17. Choudhury and Slaby, *Critical Neuroscience*; Roger Cooter, "Neural Veils and the Will to Historical Critique: Why Historians of Science Need to Take the Neuro-Turn

Seriously," *Isis* 105, no. 1 (2014): 145–54; Ruth Leys, "The Turn to Affect: A Critique," *Critical Inquiry* 37 (2011): 434–72.

18. Rose and Abi-Rached, *Neuro*; Smail, "Neurohistory in Action"; Anne Harrington, *The Cure Within: A History of Mind-Body Medicine* (New York: W. W. Norton, 2008); Fuller, "Neuroscience, Neurohistory, and the History of Science: A Tale of Two Brain Images."

19. See Stephen T. Casper, Review of "Neuro: The New Brain Sciences and the Management of the Mind," by Nikolas S. Rose and Joelle M. Abi-Rached, *Journal of the History of the Behavioral Sciences* 51, no. 1 (2015): 95–98, and Stephen T. Casper, "Of Means and Ends: Mind and Brain Science in the Twentieth Century," *Science in Context* 28, no. 1 (2015): 1–7. For a critique of the ways in which some humanities and social sciences scholars have borrowed from contemporary theories in the neurosciences of emotions, see Leys, "The Turn to Affect."

20. See the example of David Healy, a psychiatrist and historian who has written extensively on the enormous influence that the pharmaceutical industry exerts on psychiatry. David Healy, *Pharmageddon* (Berkeley: University of California Press, 2012); *Let Them Eat Prozac: The Unhealthy Relationship between the Pharmaceutical Industry and Depression* (New York: New York University Press, 2004).

21. F. De Sio, "Leviathan and the Soft Animal: Medical Humanism and the Invertebrate Models for Higher Nervous Functions, 1950s–90s," *Medical History* 55, no. 3 (2011): 370.

22. See, for examples, Stanley Finger, *Origins of Neuroscience: A History of Explorations into Brain Function* (New York: Oxford University Press, 1994); Michel Anctil, *Dawn of the Neuron: The Early Struggles to Trace the Origin of Nervous Systems* (Montreal: McGill-Queen's University Press, 2015); Steve Fuller, *Preparing for Life in Humanity 2.0* (Basingstoke, UK: Palgrave MacMillan, 2013), and Daniel Lord Smail, *On Deep History and the Brain* (Berkeley: University of California Press, 2008).

23. The biographies are too numerous to cite, but see the Oxford University Press series, which has released several noteworthy studies of key figures in the history of neurology over the last two decades. For historical essays on philosophically interesting problems and questions in the neurosciences, see Charles G. Gross, *Brain, Vision, Memory: Tales in the History of Neuroscience* (Cambridge: MIT Press, 1998), and Charles G. Gross, *A Hole in the Head: More Tales in the History of Neuroscience* (Cambridge, MA: MIT Press, 2009).

24. The leading critic of such works is Ruth Leys. See her essay, "The Turn to Affect: A Critique," *Critical Inquiry* 37 (2011): 434–72.

25. Casper, "History and Neuroscience."

26. Delia Gavrus, "Mind over Matter: Sherrington, Penfield, Eccles, Walshe and the Dualist Movement in Neuroscience," in *Comparative Program on Health and Society Lupina Foundation Working Paper Series 2005–2006* (Toronto: Munk Centre for International Studies, University of Toronto, 2006).

27. Christopher Lawrence, "The Nervous System and Society in the Scottish Enlightenment," In *Natural Order: Historical Studies of Scientific Culture*, ed. Barry Barnes and Steven Shapin, 19–40 (Beverly Hills, CA, and London: Sage, 1979). On this point, also see Elizabeth Green Musselman, *Nervous Conditions: Science and the Body Politic in Early Industrial Britain* (Albany: State University of New York, 2006),

and G. S. Rousseau, *Nervous Acts: Essays on Literature, Culture, and Sensibility* (New York: Palgrave Macmillan, 2004).

28. This critique was developed with characteristic clarity by Ellen Dwyer. See her essay, "Toward New Narratives of Twentieth-Century Medicine," *Bulletin of the History of Medicine* 74, no. 4 (2000): 786–93.

29. The centrality, for example, of the mind and brain sciences in the emergence of statistics has been little acknowledged. See, for a discussion, Theodore M. Porter, *The Rise of Statistical Thinking, 1820–1900* (Princeton, NJ: Princeton University Press, 1986). Similarly, while numerous authors working on the history of eugenics have commented on the ways that mental disability and psychiatry (though less neurology) were dominant considerations in the politics of eugenics, few historians of the mind and brain sciences have placed their narratives within that obviously significant context. Mathew Thompson, "Disability, Psychiatry, and Eugenics," in *The Oxford Handbook of the History of Eugenics*, ed. Alison Bashford and Philippa Levine, 116–33 (Oxford: Oxford University Press, 2010).

30. Consider as one example Piers J. Hale, *Political Descent: Malthus, Mutualism, and the Politics of Evolution in Victorian England* (Chicago: University of Chicago Press, 2014). Hale's deeply researched book appears on the surface to be a long consideration of the conflict between competitive and cooperative visions of evolutionary biology. But upon a close examination, his study appears as well to inform about the centrality of mind, habits, and personality, and the sciences of mind in the formulation and subsequent controversies at stake in the evolutionary sciences. Yet the evolutionary biology context for the study of mind and brain has been broadly ignored in the historiography of the neurosciences, and (ironically), seemingly as a consequence, the historiography of the mind and brain sciences have done little to shape the history of biology. For further background, see the classic philosophical study by Robert J. Richards, *Darwin and the Emergence of Evolutionary Theories of Mind and Behavior* (Chicago: University of Chicago Press, 1989).

31. It seems somehow surprising that the agenda for exploring the body, mind, and brain in ways that explore the collision of lived experience with professional discourses that construct and articulate limitations to mind and brain has only been identified by medical anthropologists and not taken up as a call to urgently stand against historical constructions of universal neurological/psychiatric selves. See, for a study of local biologies that could (and should) spawn imitation in the studies of the mind and brain sciences, Margaret Lock, *Encounters with Aging: Mythologies of Menopause in Japan and North America* (Berkeley: University of California Press, 1993).

32. For a discussion, see Casper, ed., "Of Means and Ends," *Science in Context* 28, no. 1 (2015): 1–170.

33. See, for instance, a particular neurosurgical therapy that was developed in conjunction with broader social changes in the Progressive Era: Delia Gavrus, "'Making Bad Boys Good': Brain Surgery and the Juvenile Court in Progressive Era America," in *Beyond Innovation: Historical Perspectives of Technological Change in Modern Surgery*, ed. Thomas Schlich and Christopher Crenner (Rochester, NY: University of Rochester Press, 2017).

34. Porter, "How Science Became Technical."

35. Ibid., 293–94.

36. Michel Foucault et al., *Technologies of the Self: A Seminar with Michel Foucault* (Amherst: University of Massachusetts Press, 1988), 18.

37. Daston and Galison, *Objectivity*.

38. Mical Raz, *The Lobotomy Letters: The Making of American Psychosurgery* (Rochester, NY: University of Rochester Press, 2013).

39. Dror, "Techniques of the Brain and the Paradox of Emotions, 1880–1930."

40. Delia Gavrus, "Men of Strong Opinions: Identity, Self-Representation, and the Performance of Neurosurgery, 1919–1950" (PhD diss., University of Toronto, 2011), and Delia Gavrus, "Skill, Judgement and Conduct for the First Generation of Neurosurgeons, 1900–1930," *Medical History* 59, no. 3 (2015): 361–78.

41. Bruno Latour, "On Technical Mediation—Philosophy, Sociology, Geenalogy," *Common Knowledge* 3, no. 2 (1994): 29–64.

42. Some point out that in its commitment to dissolving such boundaries, ANT reflects the values of neoliberalism. See Roger Cooter and Claudia Stein, "The New Poverty of Theory: Material Turns in a Latourian World," in *Writing History in the Age of Biomedicine*, ed. Roger Cooter and Claudia Stein (New Haven, CT: Yale University Press, 2013).

43. Again the limits of this approach are most obvious in Rose and Abi-Rached *Neuro*.

44. The classic study was Edwin Clarke, Kenneth Dewhurst, and Michael Jeffrey Aminoff, *An Illustrated History of Brain Function: Imaging the Brain from Antiquity to the Present* (San Francisco: Norman Publishing, 1996).

45. Ellen Herman, *The Romance of American Psychology: Political Culture in the Age of Experts* (Berkeley: University of California Press, 1995); Michael M. Sokal, ed., *Psychological Testing and American Society 1890–1930* (Newark, NJ: Rutgers University Press, 1987; Kurt Danziger, *Constructing the Subject: Historical Origins of Psychological Research* (Cambridge: Cambridge University Press, 1994).

46. Dumit, *Picturing Personhood.*

47. Katja Guenther and Volker Hess, "Soul Catchers: The Material Culture of the Mind Sciences," *Medical History* 60, no. 3 (2016): 301–7.

48. Cornelius Borck, "Electrifying the Brain in the 1920s: Electrical Technology as a Mediator in Brain Research," in *Electric Bodies: Episodes in the History of Medical Electricity*, ed. Paola Bertucci and Giuliano Pancaldi (Bologna, Italy: University of Bologna, 2001).

49. George Rosen, *The Specialization of Medicine with Particular Reference to Ophthalmology* (New York: Froben Press, 1944) was the classic study. Other classics include Stanley Joel Reiser, *Medicine and the Reign of Technology* (Cambridge: Cambridge University Press, 1981); Joel D. Howell, *Technology in the Hospital: Transforming Patient Care in the Early Twentieth Century* (Baltimore: Johns Hopkins University Press, 1995); and Keith Keith Wailoo, *Drawing Blood: Technology and Disease Identity in Twentieth-Century America* (Baltimore: Johns Hopkins University Press, 1999.

50. Elizabeth Green Musselman, *Nervous Conditions: Science and the Body Politic in Early Industrial Britain* (Albany, NY: SUNY Press, 2012; Christopher D. Green, "Scientific Objectivity and E. B. Titchener's Experimental Psychology," *Isis* 101, no. 4 (2010): 697–721.

51. Elliot S Valenstein, *The War of the Soups and the Sparks: The Discovery of Neurotransmitters and the Dispute over How Nerves Communicate* (New York: Columbia University Press, 2005).

52. The literature is vast, from classics such as Owsei Temkin, *The Falling Sickness: A History of Epilepsy from the Greeks to the Beginnings of Modern Neurology*, 2nd ed. (Baltimore: Johns Hopkins University Press, 1971), to newer contributions such as Edward Shorter and David Healy, *Shock Therapy: A History of Electroconvulsive Treatment in Mental Illness* (New Brunswick, NJ: Rutgers University Press, 2007); Healy, *Pharmageddon*; and Jan Goldstein, *Hysteria Complicated by Ecstasy: The Case of Nanette Leroux* (Princeton, NJ: Princeton University Press, 2010).

53. On spinal cord injuries, see John R. Silver, *History of the Treatment of Spinal Injuries* (New York: Kluwer Academic/Plenum Publishers, 2003).

54. Gavrus, "'Making Bad Boys Good.'"

55. For an example of how neurosurgeons in the 1920s and 1930s claimed that neurologists had not been interested in therapy, see Delia Gavrus, "Men of Dreams and Men of Action: Neurologists, Neurosurgeons, and the Performance of Professional Identity, 1920–1950," *Bulletin of the History of Medicine* 85, no. 1 (2011): 57–92.

56. For a call to inclusiveness and coherence beyond a simple internalist/externalist division in the history of the neurosciences, see Samuel H. Greenblatt, "Inclusiveness and Coherency in the History of the Neurosciences," *Journal of the History of the Neurosciences* 11, no. 2 (2002): 185–93.

57. This volume contains several essays that are broad in scope. More generally in the history of mind and brain literature, here are just a few excellent examples: Ellen Dwyer, *Homes for the Mad: Life Inside Two Nineteenth-Century Asylums* (New Brunswick, NJ: Rutgers University Press, 1987); Jack Pressman, *Last Resort: Psychosurgery and the Limits of Medicine* (Cambridge: Cambridge University Press, 1998); L. S. Jacyna, *Lost Words: Narratives of Language and the Brain, 1825–1926* (Princeton, NJ: Princeton University Press, 2000); John C. Burnham, *Accident Prone: A History of Technology, Psychology, and Misfits of the Machine Age* (Chicago: University of Chicago Press, 2009); and Elizabeth Lunbeck, *The Americanization of Narcissism* (Cambridge, MA: Harvard University Press, 2014).

58. And on an even longer time frame, "deep history": Daniel Lord Smail, *On Deep History and the Brain* (Berkeley: University of California Press, 2008).

59. David Armitage, "What's the Big Idea? Intellectual History and the Longue Durée," *History of European Ideas* 38, no. 4 (2012): 493–507. For a recent engagement with this methodology, see the special issue on "big history" in the *Journal of the Philosophy of History* 9, no. 2 (2015).

60. Jo Guldi and David Armitage, *The History Manifesto* (Cambridge: Cambridge University Press, 2014).

61. On a recent discussion about the *longue durée* approach vis-à-vis the history of science, see the focus section of *Isis* 107, no. 2 (2016).

62. In fact, the *longue durée* approach provides an excellent rationale for collaborative history and for edited volumes such as this one.

63. As far as the cultural history of medicine is concerned, see the programmatic message of Mary E. Fissell, "Making Meaning from the Margins: The New Cultural

History of Medicine," in *Locating Medical History: The Stories and Their Meanings*, ed. Frank Huisman and John Harley Warner (Baltimore: Johns Hopkins University Press, 2004).

64. On this point see Anne Harrington, "Towards a History of the Brain and Behavioral Sciences: Themes and Provocations," in *The Cambridge History of Science*, vol. 6, *Modern Biological and Earth Sciences*, ed. Peter J. Bowler and John V. Pickstone (Cambridge: Cambridge University Press, 2008).

65. Alison Winter, *Memory: Fragments of a Modern History* (Chicago: University of Chicago Press, 2011).

66. See Steven Shapin, "The Invisible Technician," *American Scientist* 77 (1989): 554–63.

67. The reference here is not to the surgical therapy for traumatic epilepsy, but rather to Penfield's surgical therapy for idiopathic epilepsy—the cervicothoracic sympathetic ganglionectomy and the periarterial sympathectomy of internal carotid arteries and vertebral arteries.

Chapter One

"We Are Veritable Animals"

The Nineteenth-Century Paris Menagerie as a Site for the Science of Intelligence

L. STEPHEN JACYNA

Introduction

In his paper "The Mental Hospital and the Zoological Garden" (1965), the psychiatrist and historian Henry E. Ellenberger drew a provocative parallel between the histories of these two institutions.[1] He pointed out a chronological synchronicity in the emergence of the appearance of a recognizable modern version of the asylum and the zoo: both were products of the era of the French Revolution and its aftermath. There was even a certain overlap in the personnel who oversaw these developments. Philippe Pinel (1745–1826), best known as an alienist famed for striking off the chains of the inmates at Bicêtre, was a member of the commission that in 1792 drew up a blueprint for a new Menagerie in the Jardin des Plantes in Paris.[2]

Ellenberger, moreover, discerned a certain structural homology between the asylum and the zoo. One shared feature was a category that Ellenberger designates "Authorities." In the case of the asylum, these Authorities were the alienists who provided medical direction of the establishment. In the Paris Menagerie, the zoologist possessed a comparable status. Corresponding to the asylum patients were the animals housed in the Menagerie. Both may be seen as subject to—perhaps even constituted by—the gaze of the presiding Authority. The asylum and menagerie also shared a third, often overlooked yet significant, category: the lay staff who were responsible for the daily running of these institutions. The care and control of asylum patients was largely delegated to attendants drawn from a variety of backgrounds but with little or any in the way of specialist training.[3] Still less is known about the keepers who performed a similar indispensable role in the menagerie, seeing to the daily needs of the animals.

Ellenberger also parenthetically notes that in respect of the role of the public there is, however, a divergence. While the public was largely excluded from the nineteenth-century asylum—in contrast to the voyeurism of earlier epochs—part of the rationale for the reformed post-revolutionary Menagerie was that it should be open to the citizenry. Such a populist ethos was in explicit contrast to the elitism of the old royal menagerie at Versailles.

Moreover, while the pre-revolutionary zoo was tainted with its associations with "luxury" and idleness, the new Menagerie possessed a more austere and serious function. As well as edifying and instructing the people, it was to be a center for scientific research. In the words of the 1792 commission, "A menagerie like those that princes and kings are accustomed to maintain is nothing but a costly and unnecessary imitation of Asiatic pomp; but we think that a menagerie without frills could be extremely useful to natural history, to physiology and to the economy."[4] The modern asylum was similarly conceived as an institution not only for the accommodation, care, and treatment of the patients, but as one in which the varieties of insanity could be classified and better understood.[5] All three homologous components of the two institutions cooperated to generate this knowledge, albeit with varying degrees of agency.

There are of course points of divergence between the two institutions at which Ehrenberg's comparison becomes at best tenuous. The asylum, for instance, possessed a therapeutic role that distinguishes it from the menagerie. The analogy between the two nonetheless offers considerable historiographic potential.

Both the post-revolutionary asylum and menagerie may be viewed as "truth machines"—as a "machinery of forces, spaces and subjects which bring into existence and configure the space which truths inhabit, and for which truths themselves provide the fuel."[6] They were, in other words, sites at which power of the Foucauldian variety was exerted in order to generate knowledge. As we shall see, the menagerie was also enmeshed in a nexus of power of a different order: that exerted by the armies, fleets, and diplomats of the revolutionary and post-revolutionary French state.

The report of the 1792 commission hinted at the kinds of knowledge that the newly constituted Menagerie was expected to generate. It formed part of a wider set of institutions comprising the Jardin des Plantes. Another component of this grouping was the Museum of Natural History where, especially under the direction of Georges Cuvier (1769–1832), a monumental collection of specimens illuminating the comparative anatomy of the animal kingdom was in train.[7] Much as the bodies of deceased asylum patients made their way to the dissecting room to cast further posthumous light on the nature of their condition, so the bodies of animals that died in the Menagerie were expected to help fill the cabinets of the Museum.

But the Menagerie was intended not merely to facilitate, but also to complement the work of the Museum. While the latter institution was devoted to the study of what could be learned of the animal body after death, the Menagerie was the site where the living animal was the subject of scrutiny. It would be too crude to draw a simple structure/function contrast between the foci of the Museum and the Menagerie because Georges Cuvier's comparative anatomy possessed a distinct functional bias. Nonetheless, the Menagerie was conceived as the site at which aspects of animal life that escaped the anatomist's knife could be subjected to scientific scrutiny.

More generally, the research program of the Menagerie was concerned with the *moeurs* of the animal inhabitants of the institution. *Moeurs* was a comprehensive term, which included such topics as breeding and susceptibility to domestication that were seen to have practical economic implications. But another important focus of attention was animal "intelligence." This was a term that was habitually deployed without any attempt at definition; its meaning was deemed self-evident. But it was through the exploration of the nature of animal intelligence—and in particular through the comparison of animal and human intelligence—that the work of the Menagerie was to draw from and contribute to the contemporary sciences of mind and brain.

L'utilité des ménageries

The inauguration of this ambitious research program is usually ascribed to the appointment in 1804 of Frédéric Cuvier (1773–1838) to the post of Garde de la menagerie.[8] This was envisaged as a subordinate role, with the younger Cuvier undertaking investigations at the direction of the professors of the Museum. In the event, Cuvier showed himself capable of undertaking and promulgating research on his own initiative. He also presided over an extensive publishing enterprise designed to propagate knowledge of the specimens housed in the Menagerie to a wide audience. Cuvier insisted on the need to accompany each verbal description of an animal with a colored plate displaying its most definitive characteristics.[9]

However, particularly in his early publications, Cuvier displayed a concern to convince a potentially skeptical audience of the value of the modern menagerie as a site for the generation of scientifically and socially valuable knowledge. In the preamble to the *Notice des animaux vivans de la Ménagerie*, an attempt was made to place the issue in broader historical context. A sharp distinction was drawn between the new post-revolutionary menagerie and institutions that had borne that label in the past. The latter were mere "establishments of luxury rather than establishments of utility."[10] In the ancient world, menageries served the frivolous purpose of ostentation or to show the power of wealth of their possessors; the science of natural history was left to languish. Even with the revival of learning at the Renaissance, natural history was disadvantaged because of its almost exclusive reliance upon travelers' tales as a source of information. These accounts, however, were unreliable. Nor could the claims found in the texts written by even those who professed to be devotees of natural history be taken at face value.[11]

It was against this background that the true utility of the modern menagerie became apparent. These were "establishments where the diverse species from all the continents are placed side by side, compared in all their relations, in all periods of their life, and by men who are dedicated to the study of nature."[12] It was only upon the foundations furnished by this felicitous combination of circumstances that natural history could attain scientific certainty.

Despite his professed confidence in the self-evidence of the value of the menagerie as a site for the production of reliable scientific knowledge, Cuvier felt the need to elaborate his case in later publications. The simplicity of his previous argument was replaced by a considerably more elaborate rhetoric, one that moreover alluded to some of the great ideological motifs of the day.

Thus, his "Essai sur la domesticité des mammifères" (1825) is characterized by a dialectic between the concepts of "liberty" and "servitude." *Liberté* was the prime of the triad of virtues proclaimed by the defunct but far from forgotten Republic. Cuvier's text suggested that some of his critics ascribed an epistemic as well as political and moral value to this quality. They maintained that "because the most complete form of servitude [*esclavage*] is the situation the least favourable to the exercise of the faculties, total independence, in a word, the state of nature, is most appropriate to their exercise and development."[13] Whereas in 1804 Cuvier had been chiefly concerned with how the Menagerie could facilitate the reliable classification of species in zoology, it is noteworthy that by 1825 he was more concerned with the best way in which to study the *moeurs* of animals: of how they exercised the "faculties" with which they were endowed.

He set himself against those who seemed to wish to transfer the ideals of the Revolution to the study of animal behavior. In particular, he set out to refute the Rousseau-inspired view that the animal, as well as the human, essence was displayed in its most authentic form in "an imaginary state of nature, the only state in which man is supposedly capable of revealing himself in all his glory and beauty."[14]

Just as the chains of *esclavage* could only deform the human spirit, so could servitude of any kind—including that suffered in an institution such as the Menagerie—only distort the exercise of animal faculties. The best place to study their *moeurs*, on this reasoning, was therefore when they lived in a state of "complete independence."[15] Only "animals at liberty reveal themselves to us as they are . . . with the [full] complement of their faculties."[16]

This romanticized philosophy of science did not, however, bear serious scrutiny. Cuvier had no doubt of the source of such fallacies: they arose from a mistaken application to animals of insights that had been derived from the study of human nature. *Esclavage*, defined as "an absolute submission to the will of another," was indeed "the situation the most contrary to the moral and intellectual development of the human species, of which one of the most essential qualities is liberty."[17]

Whatever value the notion that humanity only revealed itself fully in the savage state might have, Cuvier maintained that it was inadmissible to apply the same principle to animals for the simple reason that, whether in the wild or captivity, they were *never* free—they never possessed "this imaginary absolute independence called the state of nature."[18] Unlike humans, animals were endowed with an immutable essence that manifested itself in whatever circumstances they found themselves: "these conditions may change, the nature of animals does not change at all."[19]

Even in their state of "natural independence," animals were subject to "the yoke of these preponderant forces." It was possible to learn something of their place in the economy of nature when animals were studied in their natural state. But under these circumstances, "they can usually provide us with only very restricted and always questionable notions of their general faculties."[20] This was because in the wild, it was impossible to carry out the "experiments" that might cast further light on an animal's faculties.

It was in fact only in a state of captivity when it was feasible to undertake a more "exact and complete study" of the faculties with which an animal was truly endowed. Cuvier maintained that in terms of technique, there were no distinctions between the various branches of natural science: all should aspire to the methodology of the laboratory scientist. What, he asked, "would be known in physics if we kept to the phenomena that present themselves in the actual state of the world, if we had not acted on them with apparatus, with instruments designed to modify them? And did it ever enter anyone's head that the results the chemist obtains by artifice are not natural, and cannot reveal to him the laws that are the object of his researches?"[21]

Cuvier was thus ascribing to the Menagerie the status of a laboratory in which the rigorous experimental investigation of animal faculties could be undertaken. Thereby, zoology could transcend the limits of mere "empiricism" and attain the status of a true science thanks to the "general truths with which it is enriched."[22] In some ways his argument anticipated aspects of Claude Bernard's later assertion of the superiority of experimental over clinical medicine.[23] Intervention and manipulation in an artificial setting afforded a more potent methodology than the passive observation of phenomena whether it was in an animal's natural habitat or at the patient's bedside.

Moreover, like medicine, the new experimental study of animal faculties was to be an applied science. Cuvier's particular focus was on the domestication of animals, a topic with obvious economic implications. He claimed to have done no more than scratch the surface of a topic that demanded the creation of "the science of one of the most important branches of our industry, the behaviour [*couduite*] of animals: that is, to subject to basic laws the blind practices and empirical rules from which we today generally take direction."[24] Cuvier professed that he had shown that "if animals at liberty are amenable to showing us the role that they play upon the earth, they do little to reveal the general causes of their actions, their intellectual faculties, and that it is only with the aid of captive animals that we can attain to that."[25] On this reasoning, an institution such as the Paris Menagerie became the premier site for the pursuit of knowledge of animal "intelligence." From whatever direction the problem was approached, "we arrive constantly at this truth: that the rational observation of animals in captivity [*esclavage*] is one of the most certain ways available to us to study and understand them as they should be by the naturalist."[26]

In arriving at this conclusion, Cuvier had touched upon some of the most delicate themes of contemporary political discourse. Ultimately, however, he concluded that the attempt to transfer terms from the human sciences to the study of animals was profoundly misleading: the analogy between slavery and animal domestication, for instance, was false. Cuvier insisted that "there is an infinite distance between the domestic animal and the human slave."[27] Questions of the relations and boundaries between humans and animals were, however, to loom large in the psychological inquiries of the time. The Menagerie was seen as a resource especially equipped to provide material with which to address these issues.

Configuring the Menagerie

Writing in 1851, the physiologist Pierre Flourens (1794–1867) asserted that the "positive" science of animal intelligence was the invention of such eighteenth-century naturalists as Buffon and Leroy. Flourens insisted that at the time this was an "entirely new" science. The question of animal intelligence (if such existed) had, he conceded, been extensively debated since the time of Descartes. But these discussions had all been "metaphysical" in character: "for positive study and observation, for the study of facts, [animal psychology] commenced with Reamur, Buffon, and G. Leroy." A number of other able observers had continued this line of work, culminating "in our days, in a certain collection of works by F. Cuvier."[28] Flourens thus ascribed a canonical status to the body of work that Cuvier had accumulated, a corpus that constituted an archive upon which later investigators could draw for information and direction.

Flourens's contrast between the "metaphysical" and "positive" stages of the development of a field of study has Comtean overtones. However, he maintained that further important development had occurred in the recent history of the study of animal intelligence. Whereas eighteenth-century workers such as Leroy had seen the "forest" as the premier site to pursue their researches, Cuvier had shown that the most propitious site for the positive science of animal psychology was the menagerie: "He did in the middle of Paris what Leroy [did] amid the forests."[29] Rather than the naturalist having to go out into the world, with all the inconveniences that entailed, the animal world came to the naturalist ensconced within the walls of the Jardin des Plantes.

The Paris Menagerie can thus be viewed as one of many of what Bruno Latour has called "centres of calculation" that arose in western metropolitan centers in the course of the eighteenth and nineteenth centuries.[30] That is, it constituted a focal point for the collection of material resources for the generation of new bodies of knowledge. As already intimated, this scientific activity was predicated upon the power and reach of the French state, and it sought legitimation through claims to further the aims of that polity. In its early years, the collection of the Menagerie had been augmented by the appropriation of zoological collections of other European cities by the conquering armies of the Republic. In later years, foreign potentates such as the Bey of Algeria and Pasha of Egypt would send exotic specimens to Paris as a token of their obeisance to the power of France. Moreover, the French government launched a number of expeditions to distant parts of the world, the primary goals of which may have been military and political, but which also afforded the opportunity for the collection of animals for eventual transportation to the metropole.[31]

The sum of these activities provided Cuvier and other naturalists with the raw materials upon which self-consciously to experiment in order to create a science of animal intelligence. He was scrupulous in recording the—often convoluted—provenance of the creatures upon which he conducted his experiments. One, a panther—an animal "almost entirely unknown to naturalists"—for instance, was derived from "the eastern coast of Java; it was purchased by General Decan at l'Isle de France [i.e., Mauritius], and sent to Mme Bonaparte who donated it to the Menagerie."[32] The explorer Nicolas Baudin (1754–1803) was a particularly prolific provider of specimens.

In order to make these raw materials serviceable to science, other resources were required: most notably, the buildings and grounds that comprised the physical plant of the Menagerie. An 1839 guide to Paris declared that "the great establishment of the *Jardin des Plantes* lies out of the noise and traffic of the town, and is a world within itself." The ambitious plans devised at the founding of the establishment had taken time to realize. Thanks to a government grant in 1835–36, however, the Menagerie now possessed impressive facilities:

> The space appropriated to tame animals is divided into numerous parks or enclosures. These parks, round which the public can walk, are subdivided into converging compartments, each terminated by one side of a central building, into which the animals retire at will in the day-time, and are shut up during the night. At the extremity of these parks, and near the river, is the building for wild beasts. The dens, 24 in number, are sufficiently large for the animals to gambol and show themselves with advantage to the public, who are separated from them by a space of four feet and a strong iron railing. The collection of wild animals includes lions, varieties of the bear, tigers, leopards, hyaenas, wolves, etc. Among the parks appropriated to the tamer animals is one called the rotunda, from a large building erected in the middle. Here are an elephant, a giraffe, a North American bison, etc. The other parks contain a great variety of the deer and antelope species; numerous individuals of the various tribes of goats and sheep from Asia, Corsica, etc.; camels, zebras, and their related species; ostriches, cassowaries, and a large collection of waterbirds. The pheasant-house contains numerous varieties of that tribe of birds: it is a pretty semicircular building, and is divided into ample and airy cages.[33]

This design was intended primarily to make the Menagerie attractive to the casual visitor; Galignani's guide listed the establishment among the sites that every tourist in Paris should visit. But by seeking to make the animals as visible as possible, the layout of the Menagerie also constituted a veritable panopticon that served the needs of the naturalist. This was especially the case with the simian inhabitants: "The monkeys are kept in a stone building of much elegance, with a large circular space in front covered with iron wire, where they have ample room for exercise and their amusing gambols. They form a very large family, comprising a great proportion of all the species at present known."[34] These apes and monkeys were to be the subject of particular scrutiny.

A final component in the configuration of the Menagerie as a truth machine was the keepers. Like asylum attendants, these figures are often overlooked. In this regard, they may also be compared to the technician whose contribution to laboratory work is usually invisible.[35] The keepers were, of course, indispensable to the daily maintenance of the Menagerie animals. However, the fact that they had regular and intimate contact with the nonhuman denizens of the institution meant that they were also a valuable source of the "observations" that the naturalist craved.

By the early decades of the nineteenth century, the Paris Menagerie had thus been fashioned as a formidable device for the generation of truths:

substantial material resources had been invested to create a space in which human and nonhuman actors could collaborate in the production of knowledge. A tool must, however, be put to a purpose.

Agendas

Cuvier and his associates had, as we have seen, sought to legitimate the existence of the Menagerie by contrasting the relative certainty to be derived from the considered study of animal *mouers* by expert naturalists undertaken within its confines with the unreliability of the accounts of "voyagers" that had previously been the sole source of information on these matters.[36] The 1804 *Notice* of animals living in the Menagerie gave an extensive list of errors and misconceptions that had already been corrected by this method.

Voyagers had, for example, always represented the polar bear as being "an extremely ferocious and very voracious animal." It had, however, taken but brief observation of the specimen housed in the Menagerie to overturn this received view: "In fact, the animal we had under our observation [*sous les yeux*] has always shown a gentle enough character, and is content with bread as nourishment."[37] The fact that the bear was housed in the Menagerie allowed it to be moreover *sous les yeux* for an extended period. During this time, she had "never shown the least ferocity, her keeper [*maître*] has always lived very familiarly with her."[38] The testimony of the ancillary staff of the Menagerie was thus afforded a credibility denied to other witnesses precisely because of the role the keepers played in the daily running of the institution.

Rather than relying upon passive observation, Cuvier sometimes resorted to direct experiment in order to corroborate received knowledge of an animal's behavior. He noted that "several authors have reported the error that the lion fears the crow of the cock and the grunting of the pig." In fact, whenever unlucky specimens of these animals were placed within the lion's reach, they were promptly devoured.[39]

It was an error, however, to believe that the lion was necessarily ferocious and intractable in its character. One of the specimens that Félix Cassal had brought to Paris from Africa in 1798 had always shown signs of aggression in his presence as long as Cassal remained its *maître*.[40] But the same animal manifested far less ferocity when it saw its current keepers [*gardiens*], especially when they spoke to it "with gentleness." One could conclude "from these observations that ferociousness is not at all natural to him." The animal would in fact have been very friendly had it been previously treated "more gently."[41]

There are perhaps intimations here of another parallel between the menagerie and the lunatic asylum. In the latter institution, contemporary alienists, rather than viewing the insane as incorrigible raging beasts, sought to restore them to reason through a regime of "moral therapy."[42] Observations undertaken in the Paris Menagerie had shown that the behavior of even the most reputedly fierce animal could similarly be mollified if the creature was shown kindness by the guardians of the institution in which it was housed. This was yet another instance of the advantages accruing from the opportunity for extended surveillance.

However, Cuvier and others who made use of the facilities offered by the Menagerie were not concerned merely to correct existing misconceptions. They had embarked upon the more formidable task of creating a science of animal intelligence. In the first volume of the *Histoire naturelle des mammifères* (1833) the place and scope of this field of study within the science of zoology was formally defined. Alongside the anatomical and physiological investigation of the animal body was a "Psychology" that concerned itself with "the intellectual functions."[43] This was, of course, to extend to the study of animals issues previously addressed solely in relation to humans.

As Flourens had intimated, in the post-Cartesian era there had been some uncertainty about whether animals possessed a mind to study. While acknowledging these controversies, Cuvier was, however, in no doubt that animals were motivated in their actions by two principles. The first, "instinct," was entirely "organic" in nature; the other, "reason," was, however, "entirely independent of the organs." While instinctual actions were governed by necessity, those derived from an animal's reason presupposed "liberty" of a sort.[44] Thus, "reason" as well as "instinct" were ascribed to animals. In this regard, animal psychology was further assimilated to human psychology. Some human behavior was acknowledged to be instinctual in character. The human species was unique only in respect of being most generously endowed with "intelligence"—an attribute that explained its ability to spread across the globe and thrive in a wide range of climates and environments.[45]

Having, however, established that animals possessed *some* intelligence, the question then became the extent of that faculty in a range of species. This on Cuvier's view was a purely empirical question to be addressed through the multiplication of observations and experiments, an exercise for which the Paris Menagerie provided the ideal setting. But what lent the quest for these unadorned "facts" and "observations" their significance was their import for certain fundamental issues. In particular, the Menagerie proved to be a tool well suited to the exploration of the boundaries between the human and the animal.

The Limits of Animal Intelligence

At the outset of an 1825 discussion titled Animal Sociability, Cuvier declared that "when Buffon said that if animals did not exist the nature of man would be still more incomprehensible, he was far from perceiving the full extent and truth of this thought."[46] Guided by Descartes, the animal was for Buffon no more than a mindless mechanism; humans and brutes could therefore only be compared in respect of their physical organization. Once some degree of intelligence was allowed to animals, however, an entirely new range of comparisons and contrasts became possible.

The question of how far humans were unique in their intellectual endowments, whether the mind was a property of matter or of some immaterial substance, and of whether man could himself be considered as a mere machine had been among the most fraught issues contested during the Enlightenment.[47] In the period of reaction following the Revolution, these highly charged topics had to be approached with caution. Nonetheless, for Cuvier and his colleagues, the rewards attached to such an inquiry outweighed any risks. There was, however, a more pragmatic obstacle: psychology at the time scarcely possessed the linguistic tools necessary for the task.

While repudiating the Cartesian denial of intelligence to animals, Cuvier made it clear that he was not aiming to assimilate the human to the animal mind. He took care to insist that humans were distinguished from animals by virtue of their possession of "reason." But he added that "in every respect except those introduced in us by reason, we are veritable animals."[48]

Cuvier's particular concern in this paper was to discern the points of similarity and difference between human and animal societies. Sociability was a primitive instinct that humans shared with animals; yet human societies had been modified by the exercise of rational powers that other living beings lacked. Reason and liberty were, moreover, closely associated. Animals possessed no real agency in forming social ties; these were determined by necessity. Human social arrangements were, in contrast, complicated through the exercise of freedom and rationality. An animal society, on the other hand, possessed "nothing of the intellectual and nothing moral; it is determined [fatale] and necessary as is its immediate cause."[49]

This made animal societies of considerable heuristic value in distinguishing between aspects of human associations. Cuvier drew a direct comparison with comparative anatomy where it was possible to gain insights through the study in lower beings of simple structures that were considerably more complex and therefore obscure in humans.

While seeking to establish clear lines of distinction between human and animal, however, Cuvier's text immediately began to blur these distinctions. Some aspects of human sociability were *not* the result of the free exercise of reason, but were the outcome of the play of "necessary causes." To some extent, therefore, human societies and animal societies arose from the same sources—hence the possibility of making comparisons between the two. Moreover, rather than there being a categorical difference between human and animal society, Cuvier posited a continuum. He maintained that animals possessed no true agency in the creation of their societies; they were "blind instruments that an all-powerful and hidden hand directs and makes act." But "the more that humans approach this passive state, the more their society resembles that of brutes." Thus, the aboriginal inhabitants of Australia were "men for whom the qualities that distinguish them essentially from animals have received almost no development."[50]

It is worth noting that this societal hierarchy was not fixed. As the "activity of man" developed, as "he came to realize that he can exercise free will because his thought is independent," then the forms of sociability would evolve to a higher, less animalistic, level. A society that had been "instinctive and material, transforms itself into an intellectual and moral society."[51] Cuvier suggested that, given sufficient understanding of the circumstances most favorable to this transition, it might be possible to intervene in order to facilitate this evolution from a primitive instinctual to a truly human society—techniques that would be of special value to an enlightened imperial administrator. Cuvier modestly disavowed, however, any aspiration to generate knowledge that might enable such social engineering. His task, he declared, "is complete if I have fixed the limit, with regards to the social, between animal nature and human nature."[52] The net effect of his argument was in fact to show just how problematic was any attempt to establish that limit.

If the "lowest" human might approximate to the animal, so the highest of animals could be remarkably close to human. This assimilation was particularly apparent in the account of the *moeurs* of the female orangutan detailed in the first volume of the *Histoire naturelle des mammifères*.

As usual, Cuvier provided a scrupulous account of the provenance of this specimen. It had been captured in Borneo and conveyed to Paris via Mauritius in March 1808 by Decaen, who had presented it to Mme Bonaparte "whose enlightened taste for natural history was so favorable to the progress of this science."[53] The health of this animal had suffered so much in the course of this long journey—which included a winter crossing of the Pyrenees—that, despite the care devoted to the orangutan, it died only five months after its arrival at the Menagerie. While this limited the opportunity to study its *moeurs*, Cuvier was able to supplement his own observations with those made by Decaen during the voyage, thus allowing for a fuller appreciation of the animal's capacities and propensities.

Cuvier was anxious to stress the pristine nature of this animal. He pointed out that it had "never been subject to any particular training [éducation], and had received no other influence than that of the milieu it inhabited." It was this unspoiled character that endowed this specimen with its particular scientific values: "it owed nothing to habit, all its actions were independent and the simple effects of its will."[54] The actions of the orangutan were thus deemed to be volitional in nature rather than automatic or instinctual.

The ape's status as a simulacrum for humanity had been noted previously. Cuvier remarked that "this animal employs its hands as we generally employ ours, and it was observed that it only needed experience to make the same use of them that we do in a very large number of particulars."[55] It was also capable of "cunning [*ruse*]" and "caution": Cuvier, for instance, detailed the stratagems the orang had developed to try to insure that it was undisturbed in its favorite perch—a sign that it possessed "judgment." Cuvier noted that the "experiment" that revealed this capacity had been repeated several times. These observations sufficed, he concluded, "to convince that these animals can compensate for their feeble bodily organization with the resources of their intelligence"[56]—a further characteristic that they shared with humans.

The intelligence of apes was, moreover, capable of adaptation to novel surroundings. Whereas in the wild it was mostly directed to avoiding danger, in captivity, where the animal was relatively safe, this astuteness found other employment. The ape developed affectionate ties with those humans who had shown it kindness—and in particular with its *maître*, Decaen. When it was frustrated in satisfying its desires, the orang demonstrated its feelings by striking its head, a trait that Cuvier had himself witnessed on a number of occasions. While this might seem a purely emotional response, Cuvier wondered whether "this orang-utan was led to behave in this way by a sort of calculation? It is tempting to believe so; because in his rage he lifted his head from time to time and suspended his cries in order to look at those around him to see if it had produced any effect on them, and if they were disposed to give way to it."[57] Cuvier provided further examples of how the ape "employed its intelligence in a most remarkable fashion."[58]

The overall import of these observations was to highlight the ways in which simian intelligence approximated that of humans. Even when he noted particulars in which the orang's capacities fell short, ways were found to bridge the gap. Thus, the orang had difficulty using cutlery, preferring to use its fingers or lips to take food. But in this regard, it was "was like [*dans le cas*] savages who have tried to eat with forks and knives." Moreover, in a further demonstration of its "intelligence," the ape had found a means to circumvent this impediment by enlisting the aid of the person seated next to it at table when a morsel needed cutting.[59]

There were exceptions to this tendency to erase any sharp categorical distinction between human and animal intelligence. One basic point of divergence, Cuvier maintained, was that the intellectual faculties of animals were strongest in youth and subsequently became more feeble. The converse was true in humans. This was therefore "a new demonstration of the fundamental difference that distinguishes [animals] from man."[60]

Moreover, even when at its peak, the intelligence of the ape was more akin to that of a child or a savage than that of a civilized man. The illustration of the ape that accompanied his account is indeed childlike in aspect. This was especially so in the case of the most refined forms of sensibility. The ape, Cuvier noted, had no appreciation of music, which was "for us indeed a need that we owe to our refinement [*perfectionnement*]: it never has any effect on savages than that of noise."[61]

Competing threads within the texts that were the main output of the scientific work undertaken at the Paris Menagerie seem therefore to subvert one another. A steadfast insistence on the existence of a "fundamental difference" between human and animal intelligence risks erasure by a growing body of "observations" that appear to prove the contrary. There was thus a conflict between an imperative to insist on categorical distinctions and a seemingly irresistible urge to discern continuity between human and non-human—especially when the humans concerned were "savages" who lay beyond the pale of civilization.[62]

Faits matériels et faits psychiques

Cuvier's main concern was with the *moeurs* of the animals under his surveillance at the Menagerie. He had little to say about what forms of material organization might underlie and perhaps explain the varying intellectual capacities that they displayed. In his account of the anatomy of the orangutan to which he devoted such close attention, he did however note that "the head resembles, much more than that of any other animal, the human head; the forehead is elevated and protruding, and the capacity of the cranium markedly enlarged."[63] Elsewhere, the suggestion of a correlation between cranial capacity—and therefore the size of the brain—and intelligence is made explicit.

When young, the langur, for instance, possessed a prominent forehead and the skull contained "a brain possessing the same dimensions as itself." Conjoined to these "organic traits" were "very extensive intellectual qualities." As the animal matured, however, the size of the skull and therefore brain diminished as did the monkey's mental capabilities: "Apathy replaces penetration; the need for solitude succeeds confidence, and force supplants in large part dexterity." So great was this contrast that "in the perverse [*vicieuse*] practice of judging the actions of animals by our own, we take the young langur for an individual of an age where the most late-stage developments are attained, where the entire moral perfection of the species is attained, and where physical forces begin to weaken; and the adult langur for an individual that possesses nothing but physical forces."[64] This reduction of brain size as the animal matured was the material basis of the one of the fundamental differences between humans and animals that Cuvier had discovered. While young, all the apes "almost rival man in respect of penetration and confidence."[65] They required this degree of intelligence to survive while they were still relatively physically feeble. Once they grew stronger, however, this need for guile diminished *pari passu* with the shrinking of their skull. In effect, with age, muscle power supplanted brain power.

Elsewhere, Cuvier in a casual aside declared that an animal's *moeurs* "depend more exclusively upon the structure of the brain than on that of the intestines and teeth."[66] He made no systematic attempt to develop this principle, which he appeared to regard as self-evident. Underlying the extensive observations that he undertook in the course of his career at the Paris Menagerie was, however, the tacit assumption of the existence of a material substrate for animal intelligence, an intelligence that was at times almost human.

Other investigators whose interest was primarily in the nature of this substrate also made use of the resources afforded by the Menagerie. Pierre Flourens, best known for his ablation experiments designed to test the degree to which function could be said to be localized in the brain, also took an interest in the question of how animal "intelligence" compared to that of humans. Flourens argued for the existence of a graduated scale of intelligence in mammals—a fact that was confirmed "on the one hand, by direct observation [and] confirmed on the other, by anatomy showing that the part of the brain, [which is] the particular seat of intelligence in animals, more and more developed, from the rodents to the ruminants, and from the ruminants to the pachyderms, to the carnivores and to the quadrumana."[67] Flourens sought support for this assertion by reference to Cuvier's works and also from information he seems to have gleaned from keepers at the Menagerie. He also made some observations of animal *moeurs* at the Jardin des Plantes personally, including some of an "experimental" nature.[68]

Flourens's object in recording these observations was similar to Cuvier's. He too wished to determine the extent of animal intelligence and to establish to what degree it was comparable to that of humans. He was less equivocal on this question than Cuvier had been. While admitting, contra Descartes and Buffon, that animals *did* possess intelligence of a sort, Flourens was determined to safeguard the superiority of the human intellect. "Everything in animals that is *intelligence*, does not approximate in any respect to the intelligence of man."[69] There was a "profound line of demarcation" between animals and human intelligence.[70]

Flourens strenuously denied, for example, that animals possessed a language in any proper use of the term. The various sounds that animals made were at most "a language of the body." Human language, in contrast, was distinguished by its artificial, conventional character. Its source was incorporeal: "the mind [*esprit*] also has a language that is artificial, created, conventional, volitional."[71]

Flourens was thus intent on reserving certain aspects of human intelligence to *l'esprit* rather than deriving them from the properties of the *corps*. Here a certain tension is visible in his text. While he saw the growth of intelligence in animals as correlated with the emergence of ever more sophisticated nervous structures, he balked at Franz Joseph Gall's attempt to "explain our faculties by his [Gall's] little *brains*."[72] Flourens had indeed published an entire book devoted to refuting Gall's attempt at a system of cerebral localization.[73] Gall's organology was fundamentally flawed both because it lacked physiological foundation, but also on "philosophical grounds." The system was an affront to "the *unity of the self* [*moi*], *the unity of the soul* [âme]."[74]

A more systematic attempt at correlating intelligence with its cerebral basis was found in the work of François Leuret (1797–1851) and Louis Pierre Gratiolet (1815–65), the joint authors of the *Anatomie comparée du système nerveux considéré dans ses rapports avec l'intelligence* (1839–57). Leuret was the author of the first volume of this work. At the time of Leuret's sudden death, Gratiolet had been commissioned to complete the projected second volume.

The book was largely, though not exclusively, concerned with an account of the organization of the nervous system throughout the animal kingdom. It is recognized as a milestone in understanding the unity underlying the apparent diversity of cerebral structure in the vertebrate subphylum. In particular, Leuret and Gratiolet's "lasting and seminal contribution was to show the fixed pattern of the brain's convolutions and to systematize the study of the cortex in man and lower animals."[75]

One can go further and assert that the cerebral cortex was a construct of the early decades of the nineteenth century. Previously, the received view had been that there was no regularity in the form of the cerebral convolutions even when the two hemispheres in the same individual were compared. Nor was any such uniformity to be expected when the brains of different individuals were compared. Any identity in structure between species was out of the question. When anatomists looked at the surface of the brain they saw only chaos: it was conventional to compare the surface of the cerebral hemispheres to the random tangle of the intestines. By 1861 Paul Broca was able to dismiss this view as an "old prejudice."[76] But it was a prejudice that had prevailed until the very recent past—and one that had been finally dispelled by the efforts of Leuret and Gratiolet.

Leuret's professed aim was to complement this anatomical text with a second volume devoted exclusively to the human brain in conjunction with an account of the human mind in both a normal and in a pathological state. He was himself an alienist who had published on the topic of the moral treatment of insanity.[77] However, just as the structure of the human brain was only intelligible when placed in a comparative perspective, so the mind was to be understood in conjunction with an inquiry into the mental faculties of animals.

Leuret found a variety of sites readily available in Paris to undertake the necessary researches. The accomplishments of the elephants that performed in theatrical productions and the displays of the horses at the Écoles d'equitation were among the locations where he sought insights into the extent of animal intelligence.[78] But for both Leuret and Gratiolet, the Paris Menagerie of the Jardin des Plantes remained the most eligible place in which to pursue these inquiries.

Leuret made many personal observations of the *moeurs* of the animals housed in the Menagerie. Thus, he noted that he had seen "only one living civet; it is at the Menagerie of the Jardin des Plantes." The behavior of this specimen inclined him to the view that "this is a transitional animal, in regard to instincts and external form, between the fox and the cat." Cerebral anatomy provided corroboration of this view: the brain of the civet manifested "characteristics of the brain of the fox and of the weasel."[79] The Museum of Comparative Anatomy that also formed part of the Jardin des Plantes provided a ready resource for drawing such parallels.

Like Cuvier, however, he also relied on facts avowed by the keepers and other staff at the Menagerie to supplement the data that he himself gathered. Thus "M. Sénéchal, Assistant Naturalist at the Museum," provided an example of how it was possible for a human to play safely with a lion, while one of the current keepers at the Menagerie testified to the animal's ability to remember previous mistreatment.[80] Leuret also reported aspects of the behavior of the bears housed in the Menagerie reported to him by "M. [Charles] Laurillard before whose eyes they had occurred."[81] Laurillard held the post of conservator of the Museum of Comparative Anatomy at the Jardin des Plantes.

The primates housed in the Menagerie were a special focus of Leuret's attention. Leuret recognized that observations of this kind were not new. But he pointed out that

> because they had always lived in isolation in menageries, until now one had been unable to study at close quarters the way of life of monkeys when they are joined together in great numbers. Since the construction of the vast enclosure at the Botanical Garden of Paris where they are free to live together, one can make new and very extensive observations about them. The keeper of these animals . . . , [an] intelligent man who discharges his duties with much zeal, collected curious details on the life of the monkeys, which he communicated to me, and the accuracy of which I was able to corroborate, for the most part, in the visits that I made to the Menagerie.[82]

Here, once more, the value of the observations communicated by an "intelligent" keeper are acknowledged.

On occasion, the usually invisible attendant was afforded the compliment of being named: "Keeper Daboncourt reported to me that a sajou at the

Menagerie, having managed to get out of its cage, had closed the latches of the door leading to a corridor, and nestled in a cabinet after removing the key." This particular *fait*, along with a number of similar observations, was particularly significant because it gave reason to conclude that primates possessed intellectual powers of some sophistication. An action of this complexity required a mind capable of a performing a "combination of ideas."[83]

The "intelligence" of the simian inhabitants of the Menagerie was not the only focus of Leuret's observations. He also studied their dietary preferences, how they reared their young, and their social interactions. A persistent thread among his interests was, however, the degree to which the faculties of the animal mind might be assimilated to that of humans.

Gratiolet, for his part, maintained that "there is no doubt that animals imagine"; the "chimpanzees that lived in the Jardin des Plantes often provided the most striking proofs of this." When their keeper was absent, for instance, they would climb to the top of their cage in order to look for his return. This behavior proved, Gratiolet maintained, that the apes possessed "an idea of their absent master" that could not be ascribed to immediate sensory experience.[84] Nor was this faculty unique to primates. He recounted some observations made of one of the elephants housed in the Menagerie that seemed to show a capacity to possess "an idea of food in the absence of any actual sensation of its presence."[85] The animal mind thus appeared capable of employing abstract concepts. Like Cuvier and Leuret, Gratiolet derived his information both from his own observations at the Menagerie and from those of the staff employed there.

Conclusion

The postrevolutionary Menagerie of the Jardin des Plantes thus served as a versatile and productive "truth machine." The components of this machine comprised the physical site that, especially after it had been improved in the 1830s, provided a set of spaces peculiarly amenable to the operations of a scientific gaze. The mechanism also relied on its human parts. These included naturalists dedicated to the study of animal *moeurs*. Some of these were employed within the precincts of the Museum of Natural History; others visited in pursuit of materials pertinent to their researches. There were also the keepers whose labor was indispensable to the workings of the establishment, but who also possessed an intimate knowledge of the behavior of the animals based on daily contact that could be put to the service of science. Lastly were the animals themselves, often brought with great difficulty and considerable expense from the far corners of the world to satisfy a felt need for enlightenment.

The chief output of the interactions of these components were the "observations" inscribed in a stream of publications that issued from the studies undertaken in the Menagerie. As well as text, these works included a significant iconographic element. The sum of these products supplied an archive on which later investigators such as Flourens, Leuret, and Gratiolet could draw and supplement.

The Menagerie may moreover be viewed as but one part of a larger truth machine comprised by the Museum. In particular, the collection of comparative anatomy housed there permitted inference about correlations between animal *moeurs* and the nervous structures that might underlie and explain these traits. The Museum was in turn but one part of a complex of scientific, clinical and veterinary institutions in Paris that served from the outset of the nineteenth century to provide a torrent of data to be analyzed and put to use.

The ethos of the new Menagerie was explicitly utilitarian—this is what distinguished it from the decadent "luxury" of the animal collections of the ancien régime. Thus, Cuvier stressed the value of his observations to such economically significant issues as animal breeding and domestication especially when Europeans were practicing husbandry in distant parts of the globe, working with unfamiliar species.

However, we have seen that the researches conducted within the confines of the Menagerie went far beyond any such narrowly economic concerns. In particular, the question of animal "intelligence" preoccupied many of those who employed its resources. The extent and nature of this faculty was explored in a wide range of animals in various ways. But always the discourse returned to the question of how the animal mind compared to that of humans. Predictably, there was no consensus on this ideologically charged issue. Instead, a constant unresolved tension is evident between an urge to assimilate animal intelligence to that of humans and a determination to preserve a unique status for the mind of man.

The work of the Menagerie may in fact be seen, in its broadest signification, as a contribution to the creation of Man as an object of study for the emergent human sciences. These sciences were imbued with a similar utilitarian and instrumental outlook: they purported to serve the needs of the new society that emerged in the aftermath of the upheavals that followed the Revolution. The question of how to manage and govern such a society while maintaining stability and prosperity depended ultimately on how the object of that governance was conceived. The animal inhabitants of the Menagerie were among the materials that served in the creation of a new understanding of humanity. The study of animal *moeurs* and the nervous structures that underlay them drew its full significance from the bearing they were seen to have on placing human nature in starker relief.

Instead of any simple human/animal polarity, a much more nuanced picture emerged in which the boundaries between the two shift as each category served to limn the other. Flourens was among those most anxious to insist on the unique status of humankind's God-given intelligence. Yet even he could write a character sketch of one specimen that made the animal seem almost human.

The orangutan in question lacked "the impatience, the petulance of other apes; his demeanor was serious [*triste*], his gait grave, his movements measured"—characteristics that might indeed befit a scientist. This animal was one day the object of study by Flourens and an elderly acquaintance—an "*observateur fin et profound*"—who had accompanied him to the Menagerie for the first time. The animal was clearly fascinated by this gentleman's unusual appearance and the fact that he walked with difficulty by the aid of a walking stick. While the orangutan complied with all the demands the investigators made of it, Flourens noted that its "eye was always fixed on the object of its attention."[86]

As the two naturalists began to withdraw, the ape "approached his new visitor, took, with gentleness and mischief [*malice*], the stick that he held, and pretending to support himself on it, bent his back, slackening pace, he made in this fashion a circuit of the room where we were, imitating the posture and walk of my old friend. He returned the stick himself, and we left him convinced that he also knew how to observe."[87]

Notes

1. Henri F. Ellenberger, "The Mental Hospital and the Zoological Garden," 1965, accessed May 23, 2013, http://www.clas.ufl.edu/users/burt/spliceoflife/ellenberger.pdf.

2. Richard W. Burckhardt Jr., "Constructing the Zoo: Science, Society, and Animal Nature at the Paris Menagerie, 1794–1838," in *Animals in Human Histories: The Mirror of Nature and Culture*, ed. Mary J. Henniger-Voss (Rochester, NY: University of Rochester Press, 2002), 231–57.

3. Some work has been done on this shadowy group of workers in the British context. See John Sheehan, "The Role and Rewards of Asylum Attendants in Victorian England," *International History of Nursing Journal* 3, no. 4 (Summer 1998): 25–33.

4. Quoted in Ellenberger, "Mental Hospital," 65.

5. Jan Goldstein, *Console and Classify: The French Psychiatric Profession in the Nineteenth Century* (Cambridge: Cambridge University Press, 1990).

6. Nikolas Rose, "Medicine, History and the Present," in *Reassessing Foucault: Power, Medicine, and the Body*, ed. Colin Jones and Roy Porter, 59 (London: Routledge, 1994).

7. Dorinda Outram, *Georges Cuvier: Vocation, Science and Authority in Post-Revolutionary France* (Manchester, UK: Manchester University Press, 1984).

8. Burckhardt, "Constructing the Zoo," 241.

9. *Notice des animaux vivans de la Ménagerie du Muséum d'histoire naturelle* (Paris: Levrault, Schoell et Comp., 1804).

10. Ibid., 5.

11. Ibid., vi–vii.

12. Ibid., viii.

13. Frédéric Cuvier, "Essai sur la domesticité des mammifères," *Mémoires du Muséum* 13 (1825): 407.

14. Ibid., 408.

15. Ibid., 407.

16. Ibid., 408.

17. Ibid.

18. Ibid., 409.

19. Ibid.

20. Ibid., 412.

21. Ibid., 414.

22. Ibid., 415.

23. Claude Bernard, *Introduction à l'étude de la médecine expérimentale* (Paris: J.-B. Baillière, 1865).

24. Cuvier, "Essai," 454.

25. Ibid., 420–21.

26. Ibid., 422.

27. Ibid., 424.

28. Pierre Flourens, *De l'instinct et de l'intelligence des animaux*, 3rd ed. (Paris: L. Hachette, 1851), 6–7.

29. Ibid., 170.

30. Bruno Latour, *Science in Action: How to Follow Scientists and Engineers through Society* (Cambridge, MA: Harvard University Press, 1987), chap. 6.

31. Burckhardt, "Constructing the Zoo," 236–37.

32. *Notice*, 25.

33. *Galignani's New Paris Guide* (Paris: A.&W. Gagliani, 1839), 441–42.

34. Ibid., 442.

35. As Shapin has pointed out, "Historians of science have shown little inclination to study the roles of technicians or other support personnel involved in making and recording scientific knowledge. Steven Shapin, "The Invisible Technician," *American Scientist* 77 no. 6 (1989): 554.

36. On the relative veracity ascribed to the testimony of different categories of witness, see Steven Shapin, *Social History of Truth: Civility and Science in Seventeenth-Century England* (Chicago: University of Chicago Press, 1994).

37. *Notice*, 1–2.

38. Ibid., 2.

39. Ibid., 12.

40. Burckhardt, "Constructing the Zoo," 237.

41. *Notice*, 17.

42. Goldstein, *Console and Classify*, chap. 3.

43. Étienne Geoffroy Saint-Hilaire and Frédéric Cuvier, *Histoire naturelle des mammifères*, 2 vols. (Paris: A. Belin, 1833), 1:i–ii.

44. Ibid., viii–ix.

45. Ibid., ix.

46. Frédéric Cuvier, "De la sociabilité des animaux," *Mémoires du Muséum* 13 (1825): 1.

47. The locus classicus is Julien Offray de la Mettrie, *L'homme machine* (Leyden, The Netherlands: Elie Luzac, 1748).

48. Cuvier, "De la sociabilité," 7.

49. Ibid., 26.

50. Ibid.

51. Ibid., 26–27.

52. Ibid., 27.

53. Geoffroy and Cuvier, *Histoire naturelle*, 1:8.

54. Ibid.

55. Ibid., 7.

56. Ibid., 9–10.

57. Ibid., 12.

58. Ibid.

59. Ibid., 13.

60. Frédéric Cuvier, "Essai sur la domesticité des mammifères," *Mémoires du Muséum* 13 (1825): 417.

61. Geoffroy and Cuvier, *Histoire naturelle*, 1:7.

62. Similar preoccupations with defining, while also problematizing, the boundaries between human and animal and civilized and savage were evident in the contemporary fascination with the so-called Hottentot Venus. See Tracy Teslow, *Constructing Race: The Science of Bodies and Cultures in American Anthropology* (New York: Cambridge University Press, 2014), 153.

63. Geoffroy and Cuvier, *Histoire naturelle*, 5.

64. Ibid., 32.

65. Ibid.

66. Ibid., 2:38.

67. Flourens, *De l'instinct*, 32.

68. Ibid., 142–43.

69. Ibid., 38.

70. Ibid., 39.

71. Ibid., 65.

72. Ibid., 61.

73. Pierre Flourens, *Examen de la phrenologie* (Paris: Paulin, 1842).

74. Flourens, *De l'instinct*, 61.

75. J. M. S. Pearce, "Louis Pierre Gratiolet (1815–1865)," *European Neurology* 56 (2006): 264.

76. Robert M. Young, *Mind, Brain, and Adaptation in the Nineteenth Century: Cerebral Localization and Its Biological Context from Gall to Ferrier* (Oxford: Oxford University Press, 1970), 141–42.

77. François Leuret, *Du traitement moral de la folie* (Paris: J.-B. Baillière, 1840).

78. François Leuret and Pierre Gratiolet, *Anatomie comparée du système nerveux considéré dans ses rapports avec l'intelligence*, 2 vols (Paris: J.-B. Baillière, 1839, 1857), 1:517, 529–30.

79. Ibid., 1:488.

80. Ibid., 1:476.
81. Ibid., 1:484.
82. Ibid., 1:534.
83. Ibid., 1:539.
84. Ibid., 2:477.
85. Ibid.
86. Flourens, *De l'instinct,* p. 144.
87. Ibid.

Chapter Two

"Physiological Surgery"

Laboratory Science as the Epistemic Basis of Modern Surgery (and Neurosurgery)

Thomas Schlich

The first surgical operations on the nervous system originated as part of what contemporaries and later historians have called "physiological surgery."[1] The proponents of that type of surgery—among them early neurosurgeons—relied on experimental physiology as an important practical, epistemological, and rhetorical resource.[2] Experimental science shaped their particularly thorough and gentle operating style; it provided them with reasons for carrying out particular interventions; it guided them in the way they conducted these interventions in practice; it gave them a frame of reference to evaluate their own and their colleagues' work; and it helped them secure the profession's and the public's trust.

In this essay I will trace the history of physiological surgery in the late nineteenth and early twentieth centuries, discuss its characteristics, and examine how it emerged within the dynamics of rapid technical change in surgery. I will examine its emergence as a result of the interaction of specific practices and knowledge of various types and also look at its function for justifying the expansion of modern surgery in general and early neurosurgery in particular.

This essay thus explores how the context of the origin of neurosurgery was shaped by a technical approach to body function. Body function was explored and controlled by technical means, and the knowledge produced in this way was seen as being exclusively technical knowledge, hiding, in fact, the intellectual conditions and preconceptions necessary for pursuing such an approach. By the same token, surgical interventions into the body and its functions were also increasingly defined as a purely technical matter. This is, of course, still the general approach in neurosurgery and neuroscience.[3] This essay shows that this technical approach first emerged in relation to the body in general and was only applied to the brain more specifically in the context of physiological surgery. It thus points to a more general context of origin of modern neurosurgery and neuroscience. In doing this, it contributes to revealing the technical contingency of the modern approach to the brain and the interventions into this organ. The history of neurosurgery thus becomes decentered: from this perspective, neurosurgery looks not like an overarching, teleological project in its own right, but like a subtopic of larger narrative of a specific technological-surgical approach to the body in general, a narrative that emphasizes the practical, contingent contexts of the production of knowledge. It's about surgeons trying to fix their patients' problems by technical means rather than about a quest for the essence of human nature.[4]

Surgeons' interest in experimental research on body functions goes back at least to the eighteenth century. John Hunter famously tried to identify the first principles of wound healing through "anatomical experiment."[5] Later surgeons used animal experiments for trying out new interventions and techniques.[6] In 1823 Astley Cooper mentioned animal experiments as a means of investigating bone healing in humans,[7] and German surgeons at that time discussed the significance of physiologists' organ removal experiments for their field.[8]

Experimental physiology itself was in many ways surgical in character and origin.[9] The work of early physiologists, such as François Magendie and Claude Bernard, was closely related to a "tradition of testing surgical procedures on animals."[10] Much of experimental physiology continued to be based on deliberate, well-aimed surgical interventions in experimental animals,[11] performed "with boldness, technique, and localistic ways of seeing informed by surgical training."[12] Bernard repeatedly described this technical approach in his *Introduction* of 1866, where he demands "separating or altering certain parts of the living machine, so as to study them and thus to decide how they function." In order to investigate body functions, physiologists in the laboratory selectively changed the conditions under which life processes occurred and then registered the reaction with the help of physical and chemical measurement methods. In this way, Bernard explained, the researcher could exert control over life phenomena. Since the processes that can be controlled in laboratory animals are in principle also controllable in patients, the future of medicine lay in extending the technological power of experimental physiology to the field of therapy.[13] Experimental physiology as a discipline arose in the nineteenth century, at first in France and in Germany, followed by other countries such as the United States and Great Britain.[14]

Resective Surgery

However, for a long time it was not experimental physiology that was viewed to be the scientific basis of surgery but pathological anatomy. Traditionally, surgeons focused on body structures. They dealt with localized disease processes, which called for the corresponding surgical interventions in the affected sites: extirpations or amputations, for example.[15] This "localist" view of disease became dominant for medicine in general. Diseases were characterized by structural changes at a certain place in the body. Doctors used the signs they found at the body's exterior through physical examination to identify these localized lesions inside the body. The criteria that had hitherto served to describe and classify external diseases—inflammation, tumors, and so on—were now applied to internal diseases as well. Pathological anatomy was the scientific discipline that dealt with the description and classification of these structural changes.[16]

Thus, in the mid-nineteenth century, surgeons were heavily leaning on various versions of pathological anatomy as the scientific rationale of their work. Surgeons were interested in the way diseases changed body structures and how they could intervene in these structures to deal with the changes. Many of them went through a training period in pathological anatomy as part of their preparation for a surgical career, often maintaining a lifelong active interest in the approach and cultivating their skills in dissection and pathological examination.[17] In accord with the focus on structure, the most successful approach in modern surgery up to the 1880s was the removal of diseased body parts and tissues, called resective surgery. Surgeons thought they could "operate away" disease, for example, in cancer or in infectious diseases such as tuberculosis or gall bladder inflammation.[18] This anatomical rationale provided the basis of an unprecedented expansion of operative surgery.

One of the top surgeons of the late nineteenth century, Theodor Billroth, embodies this type of surgery at its zenith.[19] His example also shows how the resective strategy was not purely structurally oriented but included functional considerations as well. Categories like resective surgery thus only represent ideal types. They cannot do justice to the complexity of surgical practices at any given time.[20] As one can see from his biography, Billroth's roots lay in the anatomical approach. Billroth started his surgical career as a resident with Bernhard von Langenbeck in Berlin—one of the surgical authorities who based surgery firmly on a localistic understanding of disease and who used Rudolf Virchow's cellular pathology as the scientific foundation and guide for his surgery.[21] During that time, Billroth published extensively on pathological changes of body structures.[22] In fact, for a while he oscillated between a career in pathology or surgery. He had hoped to be offered the new Chair of Pathology in Berlin, which eventually went to Rudolf Virchow, but when he was invited to a pathological anatomy post in Greifswald in 1858, he declined because of the low salary and budget of the institute. Such a career pattern between science and medical practice was not untypical for a time when the boundaries of the individual disciplines were still fluent.[23]

For Billroth the matter was decided in 1860 when he accepted a professorship of surgery in Zurich. In the following years, he created a whole range of procedures for removing diseased organs for which he was admired by his colleagues, who came from neighboring universities to see his extensive tumor operations. He also wrote his programmatic "Fifty Lectures on General Surgical Pathology and Therapy," first published as a book in 1863, in which he argued that surgery has to be based on pathological anatomy.[24]

In 1867 Billroth was appointed head surgeon and professor at the University of Vienna. The choice reflected the intention to introduce the innovative approach of the Langenbeck School, which stood for the expansion of surgery into the body's interior. He was seen as the candidate, as the wording of the official decision of the medical faculty of March 16, 1867, goes, who had the best reputation not only in practical surgery but also in his physiological and pathological-anatomical research.[25] Billroth continued to work on a whole range of major resective operations, many of them for the surgical eradication of cancer. He extirpated parts of the thyroid, the esophagus, and the larynx. In the 1880s, he developed innovative procedures for the resection of the stomach, operations that are still called "Billroth I" and "Billroth II" after him.[26] In preparation he had performed extensive pathological research and animal experiments to convince himself that the presence of gastric acid would not prevent stomach wounds from healing so that he could reconnect the remaining portions of the gastrointestinal tract after taking out the stomach.[27]

We can see how extending the resective approach and removing the stomach forced Billroth to deal with the physiological consequences of the organ's absence and to develop strategies for reconstructing his patients' body function.[28] One technological strategy, surgical removal, was followed by another such strategy, surgical reconstruction, as a logical corollary. It was clear to him that this was only possible if he went beyond traditional pathological studies. Research on dead bodies provided little information on how removal of an organ affects the organism and how to restore the function of the organ. The functional-physiological perspective necessary for restoring body function was not new for Billroth. For his medical dissertation he had already worked on a pathophysiological topic, and under the supervision of the physiologist Ludwig Traube, had conducted twenty-eight experiments on dogs, rabbits, doves, and ducks.[29]

However, Billroth's experiments aimed less at investigating body function in the sense of physiological research. Instead, he wanted to try out surgical operations and find ways of managing their consequences and side effects.[30] Nor did Billroth single out physiology as the epistemic basis of surgery. He continued to advocate training in pathology as the necessary preparation for a surgical career,[31] and like other academic surgeons of the time, demanded to base surgical operations on a "sound anatomical and physiological foundation"[32]—the usual phrasing when academic practitioners argued for more science in surgery in a general way. The switch to privileging experimental physiology versus pathology would occur only in the generation of Billroth's students. However, as Tatjana Buklijas has argued, their reorientation was probably favored by their teacher's policy of selecting his trainees on the basis of their scientific talent and have them experiment extensively on animals before trying out procedures in the operating theater. It was therefore arguably under the influence of their training with Billroth that the generation of surgeons practicing around 1900, such as Anton von Eiselsberg and Johannes Mikulicz, worked in innovative ways in the areas of transplantation, shock, blood circulation, and asepsis.[33] In this way, Billroth can be seen as a transitional figure between resective and physiological surgery.

Billroth was not the only surgeon to move in this direction. For example, Ernst von Bergmann, von Langenbeck's successor in Berlin, also showed an interest in experimental science, even though he embodied in many ways the typical resective type of surgeon: operating fast and securely, he enjoyed extensive interventions, laying open deeply located operation sites with quick, deep cuts. Amputation of the breast, resection of the hip joint, extirpation of the kidneys or the tongue were the operations he was good at, and he performed difficult operations on blood vessels and operations for tumors in the neck region with particular aptitude.[34] At the same time, Bergmann was one of the foremost representatives of science-based surgery.[35] He followed an explicit agenda of grounding surgical practice in experimental science (which in his case meant mainly bacteriology), claiming that the rules of surgery were to be deducted directly from the scientific observation of the life processes.[36]

Radical Surgery

The extension of the resective approach came to be called "radical surgery."[37] Radical surgery had cellular pathology as its rationale. For radical surgeons, cancer, for example, was a disease produced by the abnormal proliferation of cells, and the way to cure it was by eliminating all cancerous cells from the patient's body. However, radical surgery needed more than a scientific rationale to be put into practice. In the 1870s, cancer was already seen as a surplus of cells, but surgeons were still reluctant to perform operations in the abdomen, chest, and skull for fear of suppuration, sepsis, shock, and hemorrhage.[38] Only once these complications were seen as controllable did the young generation of surgeons go ahead and open up ever more body cavities. The modern surgeon, von Bergmann's student Kurt Schimmelbusch wrote in 1892, could without worries open up the abdomen, the skull, and touch all the organs that for the older generation had been a *noli me tangere* (don't tread on me).[39]

At first the "center of the radical spirit" was in the German-speaking countries with protagonists such as Billroth and Langenbeck and their students, but the approach was taken up with particular interest in the United States, where by 1890 "most surgeons were willing to operate . . . on organs . . . that they would have refrained from violating in 1870."[40] However, especially in the American context, radical surgeons argued that their approach was, in reality, conservative. Using the tools of the new scientific surgery to cure diseases radically, in the sense of completely, they said that they needed to destroy certain parts of the body in order to preserve others. Appendectomy, with its early excision of the whole inflamed appendix, is an example. Hernia, thyroid tumors, breast cancer, and prostatic and uterine hypertrophy were dealt with in a similarly radical way.[41] Along this line of argument, radical and conservative surgery were no longer necessarily "two dramatically opposing tendencies," as William W. Keen suggested,[42] but could be reconciled by "careful diagnosis and full understanding of the underlying disease processes, together with the aid of the new laboratory methods."[43] What we see here, was not a "simple shift from conservative to bold invasive surgery." Instead, the new approach had opened up a new "range of principles and practices" for surgeons to pursue.[44] A good example of the new practices was William Halsted's surgery, with its meticulous and risk-minimizing approach and its connection to physiological surgery.[45]

As head of the surgery department of the Johns Hopkins Hospital, Halsted had established a style of performing surgery that was new for the American context. His surgery was characterized by fastidious and demanding operating techniques and the significance he placed on laboratory science. His inspiration came from what he had seen in the German-speaking countries during his two-year stay in Europe, in particular at Billroth's clinic. From the start, the newly founded Johns Hopkins Hospital and University had placed great emphasis on experimental research after the German model, and many of its doctors and scientists had been trained in German laboratories. The German-trained pathologist William Welch was put in charge of setting up the faculty. He hired Halsted to become the first head of the new surgery department because of Halsted's experience in laboratory-oriented surgery in Austria and Germany. Before Halsted took up his surgery post, he worked at the pathologist's laboratory, where his experimental surgery on dogs was as careful as surgery done on humans. In his laboratory work, Halsted studied problems of surgical interest, such as intestinal suture techniques and surgical bacteriology, but he also investigated body function, for example of the thyroid gland.[46]

For Halsted, surgical practice had to be based on experimental science. "The hospital, the operating room and the wards should be . . . laboratories of the highest order," he wrote. Surgeons should be trained as scientists,[47] but, as he stressed, "not in a dissecting room" but "in a laboratory of experimental surgery in contact with living beings."[48] This is why his French colleague and admirer René Leriche characterized him as Claude Bernard's true surgical heir.[49] Halsted's "cult of physiological surgery," as later commentators called it, also had a moral aspect to it. True proponents of physiological surgery, the idea went, did not aspire to economic gain but devoted themselves completely to the advancement of science through original and rigorous research.[50] Thus, being purely technical and scientific appeared as a sign of disengagement with commercialism and self-interest, technicality the very antithesis of unethical behavior.[51] Halsted's physiological approach became formative of American surgery as his students moved on to occupy important positions in the field and other surgeons were converted to his approach too.[52]

Halsted was radical in his surgical treatment insofar that it went to the root of his patients' problems. His technique of hernia repair stabilized the inguinal canal in a way that his patients would never have hernia problems again. His radical breast amputation aimed at the complete eradication of all cancer cells from the body.[53] Halsted first described his radical mastectomy in 1888 but kept modifying the technique in the following years. It essentially consisted in removing, in one block, the whole affected area without approaching the actual tumor with the knife, "as if it were a tissue loaded with bacteria which could be transferred to the surroundings or into the circulation."[54] This was a surgical feat that required gentle and thorough technique as well as an infrastructure of control technologies to protect the patient's life and health during the operation.

More Control and Surveillance: Shock

Encouraged through aseptic control and a pathological rationale, radical surgeons performed more extensive operations than ever before, "often with spectacular success."[55] With these new operations, however, new complications came to the fore, most significantly surgical shock. Once more the agenda of surgical research was set by the harmful consequences of previous technological developments. We can see this in the work of George W. Crile in Cleveland. Crile had adopted Halsted's radical approach and, among other things, used his radical mastectomy as the model for a new operation for neck tumors, called "radical neck dissection." Like Halsted, he removed the tumor, the lymph nodes, and all adjacent structures in one operation, hoping to cure the cancer by cutting it out in its entirety.[56] Such extensive interventions came with specific effects on the patient's organism. To be sure, the systemic impact of injury was not a new problem for surgery, but it was now a side effect of the treatment; it was caused by the surgeon. In the 1880s, most surgeons thought that the shock symptoms—pallor, sweating, fast pulse, loss of consciousness, and even death—observed in their patients were the result of a malfunction of some part of the nervous system. Crile suggested a broader concept. In his theory, the mechanisms of shock included the circulatory, the endocrine, and the muscular systems, which as he saw it, all collaborated in the body's fight to survive. So for him, shock was not part of the process of dying. It was a marshaling of the body's defenses in its struggle to survive.[57]

Most importantly, Crile brought the phenomenon of shock into the laboratory. He conducted experimental studies on series of 148 animals and proposed that a decline in blood pressure could account for all the symptoms in shock.[58] Crile performed this research in the context of the newly emerging network of physiological surgery: he had started his investigations after a visit at Theodor Kocher's Swiss hospital in 1895 and performed the first sixteen animal experiments in Victor Horsley's laboratory at University College London,[59] both surgeons being, as we will see, important pioneers of the physiological approach. In correspondence with his scientific orientation, the Cleveland surgeon demanded that only those drugs which had been shown in the laboratory to increase the arterial tension should be used for the treatment of shock. By 1910 most of his colleagues had indeed stopped the use of stimulants and were switching to intravenous fluids, transfusion, adrenalin, and other means to raise blood pressure.[60] In his human patients, Crile used the sphygmomanometer with an inflatable cuff to measure blood pressure and recorded the course of blood pressure in curves—the paradigmatic visualization technology of experimental physiology. In graph after graph he displayed the fluctuations in arterial pressure during surgery. He showed how the readings went down in patients who succumbed to shock and up after successful treatment. In this way he made shock measurable and offered a reliable means to diagnose it and monitor its treatment. No longer did surgeons rely on the weakened pulse or a sinking state of consciousness alone.[61]

Crile's work changed the way surgeons investigated shock. New ideas about shock now needed to come with an experimental backing. As Peter

English has phrased it, Crile's research was "one of the paths by which physiologists came to surgery and surgeons to physiology."[62] With blood pressure measurement, another control technology coming from physiology was added to the surgical control network. Harvey Cushing, for example, started employing the measurement of blood pressure routinely in all operations. Crile himself added an assistant to his surgical team to watch blood pressure and adjust anesthesia, intravenous fluids intake, and medication.[63] The continuous evaluation of the patient's vital functions became part of surgical routine. Before the operation, laboratory values, measurement of red and white blood cells, hemoglobin, and a variety of tests on the urine were performed. During the procedure, a minute-by-minute chart of pulse, respiration, and blood pressure kept surgeons informed about the patient's body functions. Then, "after the operation, the staff closely watches blood pressure as a means of spotting hemorrhage, and white blood cells and temperature to indicate infection, and urine flow to warn of the first signs of renal damage."[64] The ability to provide pre- and post-op care became a benchmark for distinguishing the "true surgeon" from the "mere operator." With increasing complexity of patient care, the number of journal articles about physiological (as opposed to technical) subjects and the space devoted to physiological aspects in surgery textbooks grew in the first decades of the twentieth century. Physiology became more and more part of the surgeon's job, and physiological surgery began to be seen as "applied physiology."[65]

From Structure to Function: Transplants

For the proponents of physiological surgery, experimental physiology was not only a means of finding new ways to perform successful operations. For them, experimental physiology was the epistemic basis of surgical practice. This tendency is nicely visible in the early history of organ transplantation—an intervention that embodies the switch from resective surgery to physiological surgery in a paradigmatic way and which emerged from a confluence of surgery and laboratory science between 1880 and 1920. Its history started with the Swiss surgeon Theodor Kocher in the early 1880s.[66] As it was typical for his generation, Kocher was initially above all interested in body structures and looked to pathological anatomy as the epistemic foundation of surgery. In parallel, however, he also performed experiments and sought out the assistance of physiologists, such as the director of the physiology institute of the University for Bern, Hugo Kronecker. Some of Kocher's experiments dealt with questions of a technical nature—the effect of projectiles on the body, the dynamics of head injuries, or where and how to cut skin in order to insure good healing. But some of his investigations also looked into the rationale for surgical operations, for example, his research on the pathophysiology and etiology of thyroid diseases. Kocher aimed at elucidating body functions in order to guide surgical intervention, and he eventually came to be convinced that surgical practice needed to be informed by knowledge derived from physiological experiments.[67] Thus, in a speech he gave in 1902 as president of the German Society of Surgery, Kocher reminded his colleagues that a real surgeon is above all a natural scientist.[68]

Kocher's work on the thyroid gland, which would eventually lead him to the organ replacement concept and to transplantation, is a good example of surgery's move toward a physiological perspective. Kocher's starting point was the problem of goiter, a common affliction in his Bern homeland. The abnormal enlargement of the thyroid gland was a potentially fatal condition—people could suffocate from their goiters, and for a long time surgeons could not do much about it. Because of the complicated anatomical conditions in the throat region, any attempts at removing the surplus gland tissue were followed by heavy bleeding and other complications and very often ended in the patient's death. When Billroth started operating on goiters in the years from 1860 to 1867, his death rate was at 40 percent. With increased technical sophistication, Kocher brought the mortality down to 14 percent in 1882, and to only 0.5 percent in 1906.[69] In cases of recurrent goiter, he was even able to take out the whole thyroid gland. He felt justified in doing this because the gland's function was unknown, whereas the dangers of goiters were obvious. Eventually, however, it turned out that the patients who had undergone total organ removal developed a typical set of long-term problems. Adults had swollen hands and faces and suffered from chronic fatigue. Children showed stunted development. When he became aware of this side effect, Kocher attempted to reverse the organ removal and put the gland back into the organism. For this purpose in 1882, he took thyroid tissue from goiters he had removed from other patients and implanted them into the throat region of one of his post-thyroidectomy patients. This first implantation did not have much of an effect, but it represents the first organ transplant in the modern sense of replacing an organ in order to treat a complex internal disease.[70]

The consequences of total thyroidectomy put thyroid research on the agenda of both surgery and experimental physiology. Physiologists and surgeons removed the thyroid gland from experimental animals to observe the impact of the organ's absence. In order to separate the organ-specific effect from other side effects of the operation, they took out the gland completely without touching other structures and then observed the symptoms that would follow this intervention. In a second step, some investigators implanted thyroid tissue at another place in the same animal as a cross test. If the symptoms that occurred after the organ ablation could be reversed through this transplant, the organ must have been the crucial factor, they concluded. Eliciting and then stopping the symptoms of thyroid failure by first removing and later transplanting the organ became the most important method for identifying its functions. With this procedure, the experimenters followed Bernard's program of extending the researcher's control of life phenomena to the point where they could switch the phenomena on and off at will. Along these lines, Kocher's original removal of the thyroid gland in humans came to be understood as an inadvertently performed physiological experiment, a "vivisection humaine."[71]

Numerous investigators in Germany, Austria, Switzerland, and Italy took up the topic and performed transplant experiments. Kocher reported later that "after the discovery, which rested on clinico-pathological observations, had been thus transferred to the sphere of physiology, there followed the attempts to provide by *transplantation* a substitute for the thyroid's function, which was now recognized to be a vital one. [The physiologist Moritz] Schiff had already made such attempts earlier on dogs, Sir Victor Horsley and [Anton] von Eiselsberg repeated them on animals, [the Swiss surgeon Heinrich] Bircher and I made some attempts on humans with transitory, but variable success."[72] Billroth's student von Eiselsberg investigated thyroid function in cats by transplanting the organ within the same animal.[73] Victor Horsley in England performed thyroid ablation experiments on apes to explore the role of the organ.[74] In 1885 Horsley, who was active as both a surgeon and an experimental physiologist, was able to offer the first convincing animal model of thyroid deficiency in humans.[75] Following the same logic, scientists and doctors included other organs in this research strategy, such as the parathyroid gland, pancreas, suprarenal gland, kidney, ovaries, and testicles.[76] Halsted, too, participated in transplantation research conducting experiments on the parathyroid gland.[77]

In parallel to their experimental work, surgeons started using transplants for the treatment of human patients too. Transplantation of the pancreas, for example, was used as a physiological experiment in animals to determine the organ's function but also as an attempt at treating diabetes in humans.[78] The surgeon Ernst Unger transplanted monkey kidneys onto a human patient in 1910 (the transplants never took up their function) after having carried out countless animal experiments on kidney transplants in the experimental biology department of the Pathological Institute in Berlin.[79] Often these innovative surgeons routinely performed the same operations on animals and on human patients for either research or therapy and switched effortlessly from the laboratory to the operating room and back. The boundaries between laboratory science and surgery became blurred: experiments served as justification for surgical interventions as much as the results of surgical interventions spawned new experiments.[80] Horsley switched fields several times from surgery to experimental physiology and back again.[81] He had started his thyroid experiments in 1884 in Edward Schäfer's physiological laboratory at University College London, a research university environment following the continental model. In the German-speaking world, physiology had become established both conceptually and as a discipline in the so-called second wave of foundations of new physiological institutes from the 1870s to the 1890s.[82] This well-established discipline was a potential partner for collaboration for surgeons. The surgeon Ferdinand Fuhr, for example, gained his postdoctorate habilitation degree in surgery in the 1880s with the transplantation experiments he carried out at the physiological institute of the University of Giessen.[83]

There are many more examples of the close exchange between surgery and laboratory science in the context of organ transplantation. In the first decade of the twentieth century, the French American surgeon and later Nobel Laureate Alexis Carrel performed extended series of kidney transplants in his laboratory at the Rockefeller Foundation in New York (in which he demonstrated that autotransplants can be successful, whereas allotransplants performed with the identical technique are not). In 1909 and 1910, the vascular surgeon Eugen Enderlen and the pathologist Max Borst in Würzburg also reported on substantial numbers of kidney transplants in animals.[84] Emil Knauer, a clinical gynecologist in Graz, Austria, carried out ovarian transplants in animals for purposes of physiological research. We can see how veritable local transplant cultures developed at the intersection of clinic and laboratory. Thus, Sigmund Exner's physiological laboratory in Vienna was a real hub of transdisciplinary activity: Exner sponsored animal experiments on testicle transplantation; supported Josef Halban, one of Austria's most renowned gynecologists, to establish the field of gynecological endocrinology with his transplantation experiments; and had his son Alfred work on the transplantation of blood vessels and organs.[85] Exner's laboratory was also the place where in 1902 the surgeon Emerich Ullmann performed the first kidney transplant in an animal.[86] The experimental-physiological approach provided a common basis for practitioners from different backgrounds to participate in the project of organ transplantation.[87]

The conceptual and epistemic role of experimental physiology for surgery becomes particularly clear when we look at how clinical reality had to be adjusted to comply with laboratory reality to make the organ replacement concept viable. Organ replacement was only practicable if it was associated with a disease that was defined as an organ deficiency in the laboratory.[88] In some cases existing disease entities, such as cretinism, diabetes, or renal failure, were linked to the absence of a particular organ, such as the thyroid (in childhood), kidney, and pancreas. In other cases, new disease entities were created according to the observable effects of organ removal. The model was the clinical picture caused by thyroid removal, which was called *cachexia thyreopriva*. Following this example, *cachexia parathyreopriva* became the disease that ensued after the removal of the parathyroid, *cachexia ovaripriva* followed the removal of the ovaries, *cachexia pituitaria* or *hypophyseopriva* followed the removal of the pituitary gland, and "specific cachexia" the removal of testicles. All of these diseases were to be successfully treated with organ replacement.[89]

Experimental physiology, with its control over bodily functions, became the explicit model of surgical therapy. Kocher emphasized how the total surgical extirpation of the thyroid would cause the typical syndrome "with the reliability of an experiment" and how, vice versa, treatment with thyroid preparations would eliminate the clinical manifestations of thyroid insufficiency likewise with the same degree of certainty. He had, as he said, applied this principle when he performed the first thyroid transplant in 1883.[90] Similarly, von Eiselsberg reported in 1914 that transplantations in humans had been carried out "by analogy to animal experiments."[91] The patient's disease was to be controlled as perfectly as the biological phenomena of experimental animals in the physiological laboratory.

A New Surgical Healing Strategy

The practice of organ transplantation represented a more general reorientation in surgical healing strategies. By the 1880s, the established approach of removing diseases through resective surgery had risen to hitherto unattained heights of technical perfection. Its field of application was extended to ever more body parts. However, there were also signs that this approach was reaching its limits. As early as 1873, the English surgeon John Erichsen had warned that "the knife cannot always have fresh fields for conquest; and although methods of practice may be modified and varied, and even improved to some extent, it must be within a certain limit. That this limit has nearly, if not quite, been reached will appear evident if we reflect on the great achievements of modern operative surgery."[92] He reiterated his point thirteen years later, claiming that "every artery in the human body accessible to the surgeon's scalpel has been tied. . . . Every limb has long since been amputated up to its highest point . . . every large joint has been excised."[93] Now, Erichsen argued, surgeons had to move beyond practical achievements and turn their efforts toward scientific research.

The case of the thyroid gland is a concrete example of how the extension of the resective principle had met its limits and how the unexpected consequences of this practice forced surgeons to change their concepts. This was not so easy. Even when he noticed that the logic of resection had led him to inflict damage on his patients, Kocher at first stayed within the familiar localist framework. His explanations of the aftereffects of thyroidectomy followed the familiar logic of repairing damaged body structures: He attributed them to a localized and purely mechanical influence of the organ removal on the local blood circulation and on respiration, and he initially tried to reconstruct the local anatomical conditions in the throat region in order to reverse the resection.[94] Only when he and other doctors and scientists started to interpret the organ implantation as the replacement of a systemic organ function did they switch to a new, physiologically oriented approach. The new kind of organ replacement no longer followed the localist pattern. Organ transplantation did not aim at the reconstruction of the original anatomical conditions but at replacing organ function independent of its localization.[95] It is no coincidence that this transition from local to systemic considerations began with the thyroid gland. In terms of its function, the gland is an internal organ with complex functions for the whole organism. Topographically, however, it is at the body surface. It is well visible and accessible to surgical manipulation, and because of the specific problem of goiter, an appropriate target of local intervention.[96] Here, the development followed the contingencies of human anatomy.

The two generations of surgeons that followed Billroth—Kocher, Halsted, Horsley, and others—were the ones to turn to transplantation and at the same time to the new physiological type of surgery.[97] As a reference science, descriptive pathological anatomy was replaced by experimental physiology with its epistemological strategy of investigating of the body's function through active control of the living organism.[98] Pathological anatomy no longer provided the theoretical basis for surgical innovation but took on the role of an auxiliary science.[99] Surgeons used the pathologist's service for making reliable diagnoses, for example, during the operation itself.[100] Now the anatomically oriented approach of the preceding generation seemed to be irrational. Thus, in 1892 Horsley wondered about the earlier, purely anatomically oriented research on the thyroid. To him it was obvious that an approach that tried to explain the function of an organ on the basis of its structural details was bound to fail. Horsley saw "the only true method of inquiry" in the experiment. He was puzzled about how so much had been written and argued about the thyroid without even one of the authors having tested his theses with a simple experiment.[101] Similarly, von Eiselsberg characterized the localistically guided operations of the past as "ignorant interventions," which by their unintended side effects nonetheless eventually revealed "the harmony of biological interrelationships."[102] The Billroth student embodied this generational change in surgery. He explored the transplantation of the same organ, the thyroid, that his teacher was famous for removing. Similarly, another student of Billroth's, Johannes Mikulicz, worked experimentally on various topics, among them thyroid transplantation and shock. He also went beyond the traditional localist domain by cofounding with Bernard Naunyn, a leading German internist, the interdisciplinary periodical

Mitteilungen aus den Grenzgebieten von Medizin und Chirurgie (Contributions from the Borderlands of Medicine and Surgery) (1896).[103]

Various surgical authors commented on the reorientation of their discipline at that time. Themistocles Gluck in Berlin, a student of Langenbeck's and Bergmann's, was famous for his plastic surgery techniques with tissue transplantation and endoprostheses. For him, writing in 1891, the interventional audacity of the preceding decade had made room for an interest in biological regeneration, with transplant surgery as one of its applications.[104] In 1913 Erwin Payr, an important protagonist in organ transplantation and the new head surgeon at the University of Leipzig, announced in his inauguration lecture that surgery had finally made the transition from a morphologically founded practice of removing diseased tissue to a new "physiological-biological" direction, characterized by surgeons' use of experimental science. The new surgery's ambitions went beyond healing of the patients' wounds and their mere survival to include the restoration of body function in a longer-term perspective.[105] In the United States, Robert T. Morris proclaimed that surgery had now reached its fourth, its "physiological" era, after having passed through a "heroic," an "anatomical," and a "pathological" phase. Surgeons of the physiological era tried to avoid any disturbance of the patient's physiology, so that it was possible "to operate upon a series of one hundred consecutive, unselected cases of acute infective appendicitis without having a single death, which a few years ago gave us a death rate of 20 or 30 per cent."[106] Along the same lines, René Leriche in France demanded that his colleagues focus their attention not so much on anatomical disorders but on the earlier processes of abnormal physiology that preceded them. The strategy of resection, he argued, was only interesting from a sportsmanlike point of view; viewed biologically, curing sick organs by eliminating them was brutal and counternatural. Surgeons needed to overcome their artisanal origins and their attachment to the anatomical-clinical method. Surgery should follow Claude Bernard's ideas and became an experimental discipline, using experiments not primarily for testing surgical operations and techniques but for illuminating physiological and pathological processes to guide surgical healing strategies.[107]

Physiological surgery was an international phenomenon. Its main protagonists in Britain, the United States, the German-speaking countries, and France visited each other, used each other's laboratories and operating rooms, read each other's publications, exchanged objects (for example, face masks, caps, gloves, and blood-pressure measuring instruments), letters, and students.[108] As part of the internationalization of science and medicine in general, surgical research had taken on a more collective and international character than ever before.

Surgery as Science and Technology

Physiological surgery originated in late nineteenth-century university medicine with its specific institutional context. The setting of the modern research university enabled doctors and scientists to pursue the experimental control of life processes as their research ideal. Its institutional framework gave doctors the time and material resources to follow their research interests relatively unfettered by requirements of medical service or the meddling of laypersons. It was in this context that mastering natural phenomena in an experimental setting became the leading scientific ideal and experimental physiology emerged as the model discipline for this approach, establishing itself as a methodologically, intellectually, and institutionally comprehensive discipline.[109]

Like members of many other academic disciplines, surgeons in that period looked to the experimental laboratory sciences for their standards of scientific respectability.[110] Research that did not come out of university medicine and did not meet its scientific standards was not recognized by mainstream surgery. For example, when the proponents of ovary removal in late nineteenth-century Britain and the United States defended themselves against being accused of propagating ovariotomy for commercial motives, they justified their practices through physiological laboratory research.[111] As in Halsted's case, we can again see the function of experimental science as a defense against the reproach of commercialism.

A later case is testicle transplantation. At first testicle transplants were done as part of the general approach of treating the circumscribed symptoms of organ deficiency as identified in the physiological laboratory. In the 1920s, however, some practitioners started to use testicle transplants for general invigoration, an effect that could no longer be pinpointed through experimental methods in laboratory animals. The most important protagonist of testicle transplantation of that period, Serge Voronoff, had never been a proponent of university medicine to start with. The institutions where he carried out his work were privately funded and thus did not need to compete for scientific recognition in the way their publicly funded counterparts did. Correspondingly, he performed no scientific research that was at all comparable to the prevailing standard in university medicine. Only the fact that he was independent of official scientific recognition because of his private practice allowed Voronoff to continue his transplants in the 1930s, when everybody else had abandoned organ transplantation.[112] Voronoff thus worked in a parallel space, determined completely by the commercial laws of patient demand and was shunned by the mainstream surgery.

So surgery's orientation toward experimental science helped the field to establish itself as a scientific research discipline at the universities and to compete successfully with other academic disciplines.[113] Kocher, for example, was acutely aware of the stakes in this regard. He had struggled all his life for the recognition of surgery in the face of what he saw as the dominance of internal medicine. In 1912 he protested about those "physicians who only recognize medical science's alma mater in 'internal' medicine and regard surgery as nothing but a technical 'specialty.'"[114] In 1909 Kocher became the first surgeon to be awarded the Nobel Prize "for his work on the physiology, pathology and surgery of the thyroid gland."[115] This was also a triumph for his discipline, and he used the occasion of the prize address to deliver a detailed account of the recent rise of surgical therapy in which, as he pointed out, surgery had gone beyond its traditional sphere of responsibility for treating accidental injuries and now provided the most brilliant cures for the majority of the "so-called internal diseases." Kocher gave an outline of the program of Bernard's physiology, emphasizing the importance of the surgical procedure in the experimental setting and the surgeon's expertise in that area. He ascribed the recent advances in physiological knowledge to the surgeons' newly acquired "ability to make all the organs accessible to direct observation, and to alter the conditions in which they exercise their functions." Physiologists had learned from surgeons to set up their animal experiments in a way that "the physiological activities of the organs can be brought to light without any distortion at all." It was in this way that surgery had discovered the function of the thyroid gland, Kocher pointed out.[116]

Just as the previous generation of surgeons had used germ theory for underpinning their practices, surgical leaders now referred to experimental physiology to legitimize their claims to expertise.[117] They used the same words that were used in the context of laboratory science, and they started to think of their operations in scientific terms, such as replicability. As we have seen in the context of organ transplants, surgeons frequently drew the parallel between their operations and laboratory experiments. Similarly, William Williams Keen pointed out in 1914 that a surgical operation on a human patient is literally a human vivisection.[118] One of Halsted's students compared his teacher's hernia operation to a physiological experiment, claiming that Halsted had devised a simple procedure that could be performed by different surgeons with the same reliable success.[119]

Surgeons saw their new operations, such as tonsillectomy, appendectomy, and in particular, thyroidectomy, as based on science. These innovative procedures reflected their scientific ethos and helped surgeons to project an image of themselves as bold, progressive, scientific reformers, rather than merely highly skilled technicians.[120] Even nonsurgeons thought that surgery was at the forefront of scientific medicine. When in 1899 the physician and physiologist John Burdon-Sanderson advocated a more significant role for physiology in guiding medical practice, he claimed that surgery was already closer to that ideal than medicine, stating that "one of the most striking points of difference [between surgeons and physicians] is that the influence of scientific discovery has been much greater in surgery than in medicine, so that surgeons who speak of their own as the scientific branch of the profession appear to have some justification for doing so."[121]

We can see how surgeons based their newly acquired high status on the technical power of science, which was the ability to heal, but also on its cultural power, the ability to provide plausible explanations within a particular cultural context. They used the recourse to science to attain cultural authority, much like physicians had used Latin in an earlier period.[122] Not only were they able to cure disease better than ever before, they were now also at the forefront of illuminating the laws of the body's function. However, the dichotomy of technical versus cultural power is spurious. Cultural power can be seen as encompassing the technical power of science since, in the words of historians Steve Sturdy and Roger Cooter, "Technical values must themselves be understood as a form of cultural value."[123]

With their orientation toward experimental science, surgeons were part of a more general trend. Between 1870 and World War I, laboratories and experimental disciplines were becoming central in the ideology of science in general. The rise of experimental science was an important factor in the development of university science in the late nineteenth century: the expansion of European and American universities between 1870 and 1914 resulted largely from the growth of the laboratory sciences, especially experimental chemistry, physiology, and physics. Expensive laboratories and institutes were set up for scientists, who were absolved of other duties so that they could pursue their research in these new settings. At the same time, laboratory science also became the new conceptual basis of modern medicine, shaping body-related knowledge in a specific way. Clinical fields as well as theoretical disciplines became more physiology-oriented. The laboratory-based experimental sciences were called upon to supply an epistemic and practical alternative to the traditional medical logic of individual experience and judgment. According to the scientific approach, the basic laws governing the functions of a biological organism were also the basis of good medical practice. Objective, scientifically produced knowledge from the laboratory was seen as the foundation for transforming medicine from a more or less erratic art into a science with clear and unambiguous rules. This reorientation was part of what has been called the laboratory revolution in medicine.[124] The laboratory revolution coincided chronologically with the rise of surgery, so that by the turn of the century, surgery and laboratory science were both generally regarded as the epitome of progress in scientific medicine.[125]

The cultural power of science helped to make surgery look like a purely technical and scientific activity. Partaking in the same modernity that characterized the image of other technical domains of the time, such as transport, mining, and industry, made surgery more attractive and acceptable than ever before.[126] In the words of medical historian Christopher Lawrence, "In surgery the fiction that medicine had nothing to do with politics, reached its purest expression. Surgical intervention could be represented as the inevitable, scientific solution to disease, in comparison to which the alternative solutions seemed inferior."[127]

Neurosurgery

Within the surgical domain, the surgery of the nerve system was a field that, early on, built its legitimation and identity on its epistemic and practical basis in experimental science. Not all surgical fields were picking up laboratory science and physiology as fast as neurosurgery did. For example, in orthopedic and fracture surgery, laboratory science became important only in the late 1950s.[128] Neurosurgery, by contrast, became the very embodiment of the ideals of physiological surgery.

Neurosurgery's close connection to experimental science is in part due to the origin of the field. Surgery on the central nerve system was in many instances initiated by the same surgeons who started physiological surgery, such as Kocher, Horsley, or von Bergmann. Neurosurgery displays the same gentle and disciplined way of performing surgical operations as it was cultivated in physiological surgery, and from their origins, surgeons working on the nerve system emphasized the integration of physiology and practical surgery. Ernst von Bergmann published the first modern textbook on neurosurgery only nine years after William Macewen's report on the first craniotomy for resection of a brain tumor. In his book, von Bergmann argued that the surgeon's knife had to be guided by the results of physiological experiments on the localization of brain functions. For his investigation of intracranial pressure, he collaborated with the physiologist Kronecker, who at that time worked at the Physiological Institute for the University of Berlin. (This was before the scientist had moved to Bern and collaborated with Kocher.) The continuous recording of the cerebrospinal fluid pressure in Bergmann's study was performed with Kronecker's kymograph.[129]

Von Bergmann's interest in neurosurgery was shared by his friend Theodor Kocher. Besides being an early physiological surgeon, Kocher was also one of the first protagonists in the field of neurosurgery.[130] He conducted experimental work on the topic and was the author of a book on the surgery of the brain published in 1910.[131] Kocher was in contact with other surgeons in the field, such as Fedor Krause and Antoine Chipault, as well as the British pioneers of neurosurgery, William Macewen and Victor Horsley.[132] Horsley, for his part, was both a pioneer of neurosurgical work and a prototypical physiological surgeon. Both Bergmann and Kocher perceived Horsley as an inspiring model as a physiologist and a scientific surgeon.[133] The personal network of early practitioners of neurosurgery also extended across the Atlantic. Kocher was one of the rare friends of the otherwise reclusive Halsted, who was also in touch with von Bergmann.[134]

However, for this generation of surgeons the establishment of neurosurgery as an independent discipline was inconceivable. Von Bergmann, for example, as a faculty member at the University of Berlin, decidedly opposed any neurosurgical subspecialization.[135] It was Harvey Cushing's generation that created the subspecialty in North America and elsewhere. Cushing, a trainee of Halsted's, had developed an interest in the surgery of the nervous system during his time at Johns Hopkins. In 1899 and 1900 he performed a number of successful resections of the ganglion of the trigeminal nerve for intractable pain. This was a very delicate operation, which took him "literally to the edge of brain surgery." To reach the ganglion he had to open the skull, though not the meninges. The *New York Journal American* sensationalized Cushing's operations right away and called his innovation "probably the most daring operative procedure ever attempted by a surgeon." This reaction shows how this type of surgery was perceived as taboo-breaking at the time, arousing curiosity but also anxiety. In 1900–1901 Cushing went on a trip to Europe. He first visited Horsley in London, who had pioneered a number of neurosurgical procedures, among them one of the first resections of the trigeminal ganglion. Cushing was not happy with what he saw and judged the Englishman to be "a better laboratory worker than an operator." He then visited Kocher in Bern, some of whose scientific publications he had read three or four years earlier. Because of the similarity of Kocher's style to Halsted's, Cushing felt at home in Kocher's operating room.[136] The young American stayed for six months, spending much of his time performing experiments on dogs and monkeys, investigating the topic of intracranial pressure. His experiments were supported by Kronecker, who had special expertise in the measurement of blood pressure. This physiological study was Cushing's first sustained piece of animal research and took him deeper into brain physiology.[137] Upon his return to Johns Hopkins, Halsted provided Cushing with the opportunity to develop a specialization in the surgery of the nervous system with regard to both clinical work and experimental research.[138] Cushing embraced Halsted's ethics of experimental science to such a degree that his work became, as Leriche characterized it, the fulfillment of Halsted's spirit.[139]

The first generation of American neurosurgeons around Cushing adopted his combination of modest and conscientious operative style, anti-commercialist ethics, and experimental epistemology. They used their association with the experimental laboratory and its particular kind of knowledge production as their marker for belonging to a specifically defined elite and thus availed themselves of a cultural repertoire that engendered trust in their moral reliability and respectability in order to distance themselves from commercialism and corruption.[140] As we have seen earlier, in the discourse of the United States at that time, a scientific ethos was considered an antidote to commercialism. In a speech delivered by Evarts A. Graham, professor of surgery at Washington University in St. Louis, to the Southern Medical Association in 1925, Graham observed that overemphasis on the technical side of surgery went together with unwise operating and commercialism. Instead, original contributions to scientific research, based on an understanding of pathology and physiology, represented the real measure of accomplishment in surgery.[141] Cushing himself was the paragon of the ideal type of surgeon who was fit for neurosurgery—a highly cultured, self-possessed, and discrete physician and scientist, cultivating a cautious, non-spectacular surgical style, thoroughly grounded in experimental work in the laboratory.[142] Later generations of neurosurgeons inherited the epistemic approach from physiological surgery, so that, as Delia Gavrus describes it in this volume, Wilder Penfield, for example, insisted that rational therapy and in particular surgery had to be anchored in laboratory science. Gavrus shows too that Penfield also uses the terminology of "radical" surgery to characterize the removal of scar tissue from the brain as a definite cure for particular types of epilepsy.

As a new field, neurosurgery was burdened with a particular need to defend itself against the perception that its interventions were too risky and unpredictable, especially since, as Cushing had seen after his first ganglion operations, its taboo-breaking character aroused public interest. The special anxiety about intervening into the brain in particular was also obvious from the intent public interest and ambivalence concerning spectacular and over-ambitious attempts at psychosurgery, from which the academically based group of neurosurgeons was eager to distance itself.[143] We can also see the misgivings toward brain surgery and the way Cushing's style of surgery was able to dispel them in the (ultimately unsuccessful) nominations to the Nobel Prize that were submitted for Cushing in 1931 and 1932. The nominators, a surgeon and a neurologist, emphasized that thanks to Cushing's diligent and scientifically based preparations, operations of intracranial tumors were no longer the *danse macabre* that they used to be.[144]

Neurosurgery, with its audacious, taboo-breaking new interventions, was perhaps a particularly conspicuous case of the public ambivalence toward the extension of surgery. But many general surgeons were also performing interventions into the human body in unprecedented ways, and they equally needed the profession's and the public's trust in order to continue doing that. Their link with experimental science helped them to secure this trust. Through surgeons' cultivation of experimental science, the idea of exerting control over the phenomena of life in the laboratory could be extended into the operating theater.[145] It conveyed a feeling that surgeons were indeed in control of what they were doing. Moreover, its epistemic base in experimental science helped modern surgery to project an image of being purely technical. Physiological surgery was technical in the sense that, as Theodore Porter has phrased it, there was only "little opportunity for waywardness." Technicality made a "stance of self-effacing objectivity," a "pose of disengagement," possible.[146] The idea of a solid scientific basis and technical competence was paired with the trust of surgeons as dispassionate, detached, and objective technical experts, who were free of bias and vested interest and who could offer surgery as the "inevitable, scientific solution" to the problem of disease.[147]

Notes

1. Peter English, *Shock, Physiological Surgery, and George Washington Crile: Innovation in the Progressive Era* (Westport, CT: Greenwood Press, 1980); Ulrich Tröhler, "Surgery (Modern)," in *Companion Encyclopedia of the History of Medicine*, ed. William F. Bynum and Roy Porter, (London: Routledge, 1993), 2:993–99; Peter Kernahan, "Franklin Martin and the Standardization of American Surgery, 1890–1940" (PhD diss., University of Minnesota, 2010), 28.

2. Delia Gavrus, "Men of Strong Opinions: Identity, Self-Representation and the Performance of Neurosurgery" (PhD diss., University of Toronto, 2011), 36, 52–59, 167.

3. For this see Katja Guenther, "Coda," in this volume.

4. See Delia Gavrus and Stephen T. Casper, "Introduction," in this volume.

5. Andrew Cunningham, *The Anatomist Anatomis'd: An Experimental Discipline in Enlightenment Europe* (Farnham, UK: Ashgate, 2010), 140–42, 246; Stephen Jacyna, "Medicine in Transformation," in *The Western Medical Tradition 1800–2000*, ed. W. F. Bynum and Anne Hardy, 33 (Cambridge: Cambridge University Press, 2006).

6. Sally Frampton, "'The Most Startling Innovation': Ovarian Surgery in Britain, c. 1740–1939" (PhD diss., University College London, 2013), 76–77.

7. [Astley Cooper], "Surgical Lecture, *The Lancet*, 1 (October 5, 1823): 3–4.

8. Lisa Haushofer, "Addition by Subtraction: Surgery, Experimental Physiology and the Removal of the Spleen in Nineteenth-Century Germany" (unpublished manuscript, 2013), 5–6. My thanks go to the author for making the manuscript available to me.

9. John E. Lesch, *Science and Medicine in France: The Emergence of Experimental Physiology, 1790–1844* (Cambridge, MA: Harvard University Press, 1984).

10. George Weisz, *The Medical Mandarins: The French Academy of Medicine in the Nineteenth and Early Twentieth Centuries* (Oxford: Oxford University Press, 1995), 162.

11. Lesch, *Science and Medicine*, 5–8, 12–14, 50–124, 199–218.

12. John Harley Warner, "The History of Science and the Sciences of Medicine," *Osiris* 10 (1995): 186.

13. Claude Bernard, *Introduction to the Study of Experimental Medicine*, trans. Henry Copley Greene (original French ed. 1865; New York: Dover, 1957), 66, 104; Lesch, *Science and Medicine*, 12–13, 80–100; John V. Pickstone, "Objects and Objectives:

Notes on the Material Cultures of Medicine," in *Technologies of Modern Medicine*, ed. Ghislaine Lawrence (London: Science Museum, 1994), 16.

14. Lesch, *Science and Medicine*, 1–30, 99–100, 159–77, 199–200; Timothy Lenoir, *The Strategy of Life: Teleology and Mechanics in Nineteenth-Century German Biology* (Chicago: University of Chicago Press, 1982), 103–6; William F. Bynum, *Science and the Practice of Medicine in the Nineteenth Century* (Cambridge: Cambridge University Press, 1994), 92–117.

15. Russell C. Maulitz, *Morbid Appearances: The Anatomy of Pathology in the Early Nineteenth Century* (Cambridge: Cambridge University Press, 1987), 12, 227–29.

16. Owsei Temkin, "The Role of Surgery in the Rise of Modern Medical Thought," *Bulletin of the History of Medicine* 25 (1951): 248–59; John V. Pickstone, "Ways of Knowing: Towards a Historical Sociology of Science, Technology and Medicine," *British Journal for the History of Science* 26 (1993): 435–49.

17. See, e.g., F. J. Gant, "What Has Pathological Anatomy Done for Medicine and Surgery," *The Lancet* 70 (November 7, 1857): 461–85. Cay-Rüdiger Prüll, "Pathology and Surgery in London and Berlin 1800–1930: Pathological Theory and Clinical Practice," in *Pathology in the 19th and 20th Centuries: The Relationship between Theory and Practice*, ed. Cay-Rüdiger Prüll, 81 (Sheffield, UK: EAHMH, 1998).

18. Ulrich Tröhler, "Theodor Kocher: Chirurgie und Ethik," *Gesnerus* 49 (1992): 125–26.

19. Georg Fischer, "Billroth, Theodor," in *Allgemeine Deutsche Biographie*, 1902, accessed June 15, 2014, http://www.deutsche-biographie.de/sfz4491.html.

20. Critical of this typology is found in Tatjana Buklijas, "Surgery and National Identity in Late Nineteenth-Century Vienna," *Studies in History and Philosophy of Biology and Biomedical Sciences* 38 (2007): 756–74.

21. Markwart Michler, "Langenbeck, Bernhard von," in *Neue Deutsche Biographie* (Berlin: Duncker & Humblot, 1982), 13:580–82, accessed June 15, 2014, http://www.deutsche-biographie.de/pnd11887490X.html.

22. Ernst Kern, ed., *Theodor Billroth: 1829–1894, Biographie anhand von Selbstzeugnissen* (Munich: Urban & Schwarzenberg, 1994), 36–45; Buklijas, "Surgery," 760–61; Prüll, "Pathology and Surgery," 74.

23. Kern, *Billroth*, 21, 39–42; Buklijas, "Surgery," 760–61; Prüll, "Pathology and Surgery," 74.

24. Leopold Schönbauer, "Billroth, Christian Albert Theodor," in *Neue Deutsche Biographie* (Berlin: Duncker & Humblot, 1955), 2:239–40, accessed June 15, 2014, http://www.deutsche-biographie.de/pnd118510916.html; Kern, *Billroth*, 63; Theodor Billroth, *Die allgemeine chirurgische Pathologie und Therapie in fünfzig Vorlesungen: Ein Handbuch für Studierende und Aerzte* (Berlin: Reimer, 1869).

25. Buklijas, "Surgery," 761. The decision of the Medical Faculty was quoted by Eduard Albert in his speech on occasion of Billroth's twenty-fifth-year anniversary at the University of Vienna, *Berliner Klinische Wochenschrift* 29 (1892): 1096. Fischer, "Billroth."

26. Kern, *Billroth*, 155–56. Buklijas, "Surgery," 761–62.

27. Kern, *Billroth*, 166. W. Kozuschek and C. Waleczek, "Die Entwicklung der Magenchirurgie im 19. Jahrhundert," in *Theodor Billroth: Ein Leben für die Chirurgie*, ed. W. Kozuschek, D. Lorenz, and H. Thomas, 28–51 (Basel, Switzerland: Karger, 1992).

28. Besides the gastrointestinal connections, he worked, for example, on constructing a better artificial larynx. Buklijas, "Surgery," 762–63. Kern, *Billroth*, 163.

29. Buklijas, "Surgery," 760–61. Billroth also criticized Virchow for focusing too much on localized lesions and failing to take into account changes in the organism. See ibid. and Kern, *Billroth*, 45.

30. Thus, later surgeons would give Billroth particular credit for testing new techniques on animals first. E. Payr, *Die physiologisch-biologische Richtung der modernen Chirurgie: Antrittsvorlesung gehalten am 11. Dezember 1912 in der Aula der Universität Leipzig* (Leipzig: S. Hirzel, 1913), 10.

31. Prüll, "Pathology and Surgery," 76.

32. Buklijas, "Surgery," 758.

33. Ibid., 762, 772.

34. Arend Buchholz, *Ernst von Bergmann* (Leipzig: F. C. W. Vogel, 1911), 434.

35. Ewald, "Die 55: Versammlung deutscher Naturforscher und Aerzte zu Eisenach," *Berliner Klinische Wochenschrift* 19 (1882): 609–10.

36. Ernst von Bergmann, "Die Gruppierung der Wundkrankheiten," *Berliner klinische Wochenschrift* 19 (1882): 677–79, 701–3; Ernst von Bergmann, "Ueber antiseptische Wundbehandlung," *Deutsche Medizinische Wochenschrift* 8 (1882): 559–61, 571–72. On von Bergmann's turn toward the bacteriological laboratory, see Thomas Schlich, "Asepsis and Bacteriology: A Realignment of Surgery and Laboratory Science," *Medical History* 56 (2012): 308–43.

37. Gert H. Brieger, "From Conservative to Radical Surgery in Late Nineteenth-Century America," in *Medical Theory, Surgical Practice: Studies in the History of Surgery*, ed. Christopher Lawrence (London: Routledge, 1992), 216–31.

38. English, *Shock*, 25.

39. Curt Schimmelbusch, *Anleitung zur Aseptischen Wundbehandlung* (Berlin: Hirschwald, 1892). See also English, *Shock*, 21, 30; Brieger, "Conservative to Radical Surgery," 221; Stephanie J. Snow, *Operations without Pain: The Practice and Science of Anaesthesia in Victorian Britain* (Basingstoke, UK: Palgrave Macmillan, 2006), 187; Thomas Schlich, "Farmer to Industrialist: Lister's Antisepsis and the Making of Modern Surgery in Germany," *Notes and Records of the Royal Society* 67 (2013): 245–60. For the generational change, see Carl Langenbuch, "Aus den Sectionssitzungen des VII: Internationalen medicinischen Congresses zu London," *Berliner klinische Wochenschrift* 19 (1882): 31–32.

40. English, *Shock*, 31–32, 21.

41. Brieger, "Conservative to Radical Surgery," 216–17, 221–22. English, *Shock*, 20–21. On the older tradition of conservative surgery, see Snow, *Operations*, 29.

42. W. W. Keen, "Address in Surgery," *Journal of the American Medical Association* 28 (1897): 1109.

43. Brieger, "Conservative to Radical Surgery," 222.

44. Roger Cooter, *Surgery and Society in Peace and War: Orthopaedics and the Organization of Modern Medicine, 1880–1948* (Basingstoke, UK: Macmillan, 1993), 21.

45. Brieger, "Conservative to Radical Surgery," 229.

46. W. G. MacCallum, *William Stewart Halsted, Surgeon* (Baltimore: Johns Hopkins University Press, 1930), 23–24, 58–71; Samuel James Crowe, *Halsted of Johns Hopkins: The Man and His Men* (Springfield, IL: Thomas, 1957), 15.

47. William Halsted, "The Training of the Surgeon," The Annual Address in Medicine (Yale University, New Haven, CT, June 27, 1904), published in *Johns Hopkins Bulletin* 15 (1904): 267–75, repr. in William S. Halsted, *Surgical Papers* (Baltimore: Johns Hopkins Press, 1924), 530.

48. MacCallum, *Halsted*, 161–62.

49. René Leriche, *Souvenirs de ma vie morte* (Paris: Éditions du Seuil, 1956), 184–88.

50. MacCallum, *Halsted*, 162–63.

51. Theodore M. Porter, "How Science Became Technical," *Isis* 100 (2009): 305.

52. Crowe, *Halsted*, 37–60, 123, 236; Halsted, *Training*, 522–23; MacCallum, *Halsted*, 186; B. Noland Carter, "The Fruition of Halsted's Concept of Surgical Training," *Surgery* 32 (1952): 521; Leriche, *Souvenirs*, 185–86; Allan O. Whipple, "Halsted's New York Period," *Surgery* 32 (1952): 549, 550.

53. On the kind of operations that Halsted focused on, see MacCallum, *Halsted*, 85.

54. Ibid., 91.

55. English, *Shock*, 34.

56. Ibid., 105.

57. Ibid., 177–78, 213.

58. George Washington Crile, *An Experimental Research into Surgical Shock: An Essay Awarded the Cartwright Prize for 1897* (Philadelphia: J. B. Lippincott, 1899), 7; English, *Shock*, 99, 213.

59. Ulrich Tröhler, *Der Nobelpreisträger Theodor Kocher 1841–1917: Auf dem Weg zur physiologischen Chirurgie* (Basel, Switzerland: Birkhäuser, 1984), 39. In his book, Crile thanks Victor Horsley "for many valuable suggestions, and for permitting me to perform the first sixteen animal experiments in his laboratory at the University College, London." See Crile, *Surgical Shock*, 8.

60. Ibid., 113. Subsequent investigators found that the critical factor in shock was not the diminished blood pressure as such but the reduced volume of circulating blood. Ibid., 213.

61. English, *Shock*, 99.

62. Ibid., 147.

63. Ibid., 92–105.

64. Ibid., 35–36.

65. Kernahan, "Franklin Martin," 29–31.

66. Thomas Schlich, *The Origins of Organ Transplantation: Surgery and Laboratory Science, 1880s–1930s* (Rochester, NY: University of Rochester Press, 2010), 31–58.

67. Tröhler, *Nobelpreisträger*, 17–44, 178.

68. Ibid., 180.

69. Ibid., 89.

70. Schlich, *Origins*, 31–46.

71. Ibid., 33–46; "vivisection humaine" quote from H.-Cl. Lombard, "Sur les fonctions du corps thyroïde d'après des documents récents," *Revue Médicale de la Suisse Romande* 3 (1883): 593.

72. Theodor Kocher, "Concerning Pathological Manifestations in Low-Grade Thyroid Diseases," Nobel Lecture, December 11, 1909, in *Nobel Lectures: Physiology or Medicine 1901–1921* (Amsterdam: Elsevier, 1967), 332–33.

73. Schlich, *Origins*, 46.

74. Victor Horsley, "The Brown Lectures on Pathology," *British Medical Journal* 2 (1885): 111.

75. Schlich, *Origins*, 38–41.

76. Ibid., 59–132.

77. MacCallum, *Halsted*, 145.

78. Schlich, *Origins*, 65–77.

79. Ernst Unger, "Nierentransplantationen," *Berliner klinische Wochenschrift* 47 (1910): 573; Schlich, *Origins*, 122–32.

80. Ibid., 53–132, 150–59.

81. For the British context, Horsley was somewhat of an anomaly at that time. He was one of a group of English researchers who tried to base medical practice on physiological science. These researchers had all spent time in German laboratories and wanted to establish physiology as an exact and autonomous science in the university context according to what they had seen in the German-language countries. See Stephen Paget, *Sir Victor Horsley: A Study of His Life and Work* (New York: Harcourt, Brace and Howe, 1920); Christopher Lawrence, "Incommunicable Knowledge: Science, Technology and the Clinical Art in Britain 1850–1914," *Journal of Contemporary History* 20 (1985): 503–20; Merriley E. Borell, "Origins of the Hormone Concept: Internal Secretions and Physiological Research, 1889–1905" (PhD diss., Yale University, 1976), 193–95.

82. Timothy Lenoir, "Laboratories, Medicine and Public Life in Germany 1830–1849," in *The Laboratory Revolution in Medicine*, ed. Andrew Cunningham and Perry Williams, 14–15 (Cambridge: Cambridge University Press, 1992). Richard L. Kremer, "Institutes for Physiology in Prussia, 1836–1846: Contexts, Interests and Rhetoric," in *The Laboratory Revolution in Medicine*, ed. Andrew Cunningham and Perry Williams, 72–74 (Cambridge: Cambridge University Press, 1992).

83. Fuhr characterized such a cooperation as a new phenomenon. Ferdinand Fuhr, "Die Exstirpation der Schilddrüse: Eine Experimentelle Studie," *Archiv für experimentelle Pathologie und Pharmakologie* 21 (1886): 412.

84. Schlich, *Origins*, 122–32.

85. Hans H. Simmer, "Robert Tuttle Morris (1857–1945): A Pioneer in Ovarian Transplants," *Obstetrics and Gynecology* 35 (1970): 323; Hans H. Simmer, "Innere Sekretion der Ovarien als Ursache der Menstruation: Halbans Falsifikation der Pflügerschen Hypothese," in *Festschrift für Erna Lesky zum 70: Geburtstag*, ed. Kurt Ganzinger, Manfred Skopec, and Helmut Wyklicky, 123–48 (Vienna: Brüder Hollinek, 1981); Schlich, *Origins*, 100–101, 155.

86. Emerich Ullmann, "Experimentelle Nierentransplantation: Vorläufige Mittheilung," *Wiener klinische Wochenschrift* 15 (1902): 281.

87. This happened in part in connection with endocrinology. See Borell, "Hormone Concept."

88. Thomas Schlich, "Changing Disease Identities: Cretinism, Politics and Surgery (1844–1892)," *Medical History* 38 (1994): 421–43.

89. Schlich, *Origins*, 158. See also Kocher, "Die Pathologie der Schilddrüse: Zweites Referat," in *Verhandlungen des Kongresses für Innere Medizin, Dreiundzwanzigster Kongress Gehalten zu München, vom 23–26: April 1906*, ed. E. von Leyden and Emil Pfeiffer, 81 (Wiesbaden: J. F. Bergmann, 1906).

90. Kocher, "Concerning Pathological Manifestations," 336–37, 346.

91. Anton von Eiselsberg, "Zur Frage der dauernden Einheilung verpflanzter Schilddrüsen und Nebenschilddrüsen," *Verhandlungen der Deutschen Gesellschaft für Chirurgie* 43 (1914): 656.

92. [John Eric] Erichsen, "Mr. Erichsen's Introductory Address," *The Lancet* 102 (October 4, 1873): 490.

93. John Eric Erichsen, "An Address Delivered at the Opening of the Section of Surgery," *British Medical Journal* 2 (August 14, 1886): 314–16.

94. See Tröhler, *Nobelpreisträger*, 129–33.

95. F. Marchand, *Der Process der Wundheilung mit Einschluss der Transplantation* (Stuttgart: Enke, 1901), 375.

96. The testicle is a parallel example. Cf. Schlich, *Origins*, 99–115.

97. Cf. Ulrich Tröhler, "Die Wechselwirkung von Anatomie, Physiologie und Chirurgie im Werk Kochers und einiger Zeitgenossen," in *Theodor Kocher 1841–1917*, ed. Urs Boschung (Bern, Switzerland: Huber, 1991), 65–69.

98. Tröhler, "Surgery (Modern)," 984–85.

99. Schlich, *Origins*, 165–82; see, e.g., the division of labor between the pathologist Stoerk and the surgeon Haberer in Vienna, Oskar Stoerk and Hans v. Haberer, "Ueber das anatomische Verhalten intrarenal eingepflanzten Nebennierengewebes," *Verhandlungen der Deutschen Gesellschaft für Chirurgie* 37 (1908): 693.

100. James R. Wright, "The Development of the Frozen Section Technique, the Evolution of Surgical Biopsy, and the Origins of Surgical Pathology," *Bulletin of the History of Medicine* 59 (1985): 295–326; James R. Wright, "The 1917 New York Biopsy Controversy: A Question of Surgical Incision and the Promotion of Metastases," *Bulletin of the History of Medicine* 62 (1988): 546–62; L. S. Jacyna, "The Laboratory and the Clinic: the Impact of Pathology on Surgical Diagnosis in the Glasgow Western Infirmary, 1875–1910," *Bulletin of the History of Medicine* 62 (1988): 384–406.

101. Victor Horsley, "Remarks on the Function of the Thyroid Gland: A Critical and Historical Review," *British Medical Journal* 1 (1892): 216.

102. Anton Freiherr von Eiselsberg, "Zur Behandlung der Tetania parathyreopriva," *Archiv für klinische Chirurgie* 118 (1921): 410.

103. Ulrich Tröhler, "Mikulicz-Radecki, Johannes von," in *Dictionary of Medical Biography*, ed. W. F. Bynum and Helen Bynum, vol. 4, 877–78 (Westport, CT: Greenwood Press, 2006).

104. Th. Gluck, "Referat über die durch das modern chirurgische Experiment gewonnenen positiven Resultate, betreffend die Naht und den Ersatz von Defecten höherer Gewebe, sowie über die Verwerthung resorbirbarer und lebendinger Tampons in der Chirurgie," *Archiv für klinische Chirurgie* 41 (1891): 187–239.

105. E. Payr, *Die physiologisch-biologische Richtung der modernen Chirurgie* (Leipzig: Hirzel, 1913), 9–18.

106. Robert T. Morris, *Dawn of the Fourth Era in Surgery* (Philadelphia: W. B. Saunders, 1910), 119–21.

107. Leriche, *Souvenirs*, 67–69. Roselyne Rey, "René Leriche (1879–1955): Un œuvre controversée," in *Cahier pour l'histoire de la recherché, Les sciences biologique et médicales en France, 1920–1950* (Paris: CNRS Editions, 1994), 5 (cites René Leriche, *La Chirurgie à l'ordre de la vie* [Paris: La Presse française et étrangère, Zeluck, 1945], 38).

108. MacCallum, *Halsted*, 100; Tröhler, *Nobelpreisträger*, 2, 39; Crile, *Experimental Research*, 8. On Mikulicz sending gloves, caps, and face masks to his American colleague W. W. Keen, see W. W. Keen, "Transactions of the Section on General Surgery of the College of Physicians of Philadelphia," *Annals of Surgery* 27 (1898): 209–27, 225–26. On Cushing convincing Crile to use Riva-Rocci's instrument for measuring blood pressure (which Cushing had seen in Italy), see Tröhler, *Nobelpreisträger*, 62.

109. Schlich, *Origins*, 48–150; Pickstone, "Ways of Knowing," 449–52.

110. A point that surgical authorities such as Kocher emphasized over and over again. Cf. Tröhler, "Wechselwirkung"; Bynum, *Science and the Practice*, 222.

111. Frampton, "Most Startling Innovation," 209.

112. David Hamilton, *The Monkey Gland Affair* (London: Chatto & Windus, 1986), 1–19, 62, 124–25.

113. Schlich, *Origins*, 150–53.

114. Kocher, "Pathologie der Schilddrüse," 59; cf. also Tröhler, "Wechselwirkung," 67, 151.

115. "Theodor Kocher—Facts," Nobel Media AB, accessed June 15, 2014, http://www.nobelprize.org/nobel_prizes/medicine/laureates/1909/kocher-facts.html.

116. Kocher, "Concerning Pathological Manifestations," 330, 331.

117. Kernahan, "Franklin Martin,"179–80.

118. Susan E. Lederer, *Subjected to Science: Human Experimentation in America before the Second World War* (Baltimore: Johns Hopkins University Press, 1995), xiv.

119. MacCallum, *Halsted*, 90.

120. Joel D. Howell, *Technology in the Hospital: Transforming Patient Care in the Early Twentieth Century* (Baltimore: Johns Hopkins University Press, 1995), 62.

121. J. Burdon-Sanderson, "An Address on the Relation of Science to Experience in Medicine," *British Medical Journal* 2 (1899): 1333–35, quote on 1333.

122. Warner, "History of Science," 178.

123. Steve Sturdy and Roger Cooter, "Science, Scientific Management, and the Transformation of Britain c. 1870–1950," *History of Science* 36 (1998): 449.

124. Pickstone, "Ways of Knowing," 449–52; Andrew Cunningham and Perry Williams, eds., *The Laboratory Revolution in Medicine* (Cambridge: Cambridge University Press, 1992).

125. Warner, "History of Science," 182.

126. Schlich, "Farmer to Industrialist."

127. Christopher Lawrence, "Democratic, Divine and Heroic: The History and Historiography of Surgery," in *Medical History and Surgical Practice: Studies in the History of Surgery*, ed. Christopher Lawrence (London: Routledge, 1992), 32.

128. Cooter, *Surgery and Society*, 234–37; Thomas Schlich, *Surgery, Science and Industry: A Revolution in Fracture Care, 1950s–1990s* (Basingstoke, UK: Palgrave, 2002), 86–109.

129. Gerhard Hildebrandt, Martin Nikolas Stienen, and Werner Surbeck, "Von Bergmann, Kocher, and Krönlein: A Triumvirat of Pioneers with a Common Neurosurgical Concept," *Acta Neurochirurgica* 155 (2013): 1797. For Bergmann on physiology guiding the surgeon's knife, see Ernst von Bergmann, *Die Chirurgische Behandlung von Hirnkrankheiten*, 2nd ed. (Berlin: Hirschwald, 1889), 2.

130. Tröhler, *Nobelpreisträger*, 49–54, 61; Hildebrandt, Stienen, and Surbeck, "Von Bergmann," 1796–97.

131. Gerhard Hildebrandt, Werner Surbeck, and Martin N. Stienen, "Emil Theodor Kocher: The First Swiss Neurosurgeon," *Acta Neurochirurgica* 154 (2012): 1105–15.

132. Tröhler, *Nobelpreisträger*, 58, 61.

133. Hildebrandt, Stienen, and Surbeck, "Von Bergmann," 1796.

134. Ira M. Rutkow, "William Halsted and Theodor Kocher: 'An Exquisite Friendship,'" *Annals of Surgery* 188 (1978): 630–37.

135. Hildebrandt, Stienen, and Surbeck, "Von Bergmann," 1796.

136. Michael Bliss, *Harvey Cushing: A Life in Surgery* (New York: Oxford University Press, 2005), 126–40, 126, 130, 135; Rutkow, "Halsted."

137. Bliss, *Cushing*, 142. For a good description of this work, see ibid., 142–45; Tröhler, *Nobelpreisträger*, 61; Hildebrandt, Stienen, and Surbeck, "Von Bergmann," 1790–97.

138. Bliss, *Cushing*, 146, 155–56.

139. Leriche, *Souvenirs*, 186.

140. Gavrus, "Men of Strong Opinions," 27–36.

141. Peter D. Olch, "Evarts A. Graham, the American College of Surgeons, and the American Board of Surgery," *Journal of the History of Medicine and Allied Sciences* 27 (1972): 250.

142. Gavrus, "Men of Strong Opinions," 62–72.

143. Ibid., 254–315.

144. Nobel Archive, Marcus 1931 (Swedish neurologist Henry Marcus). Nobel Archive, Bumke 1932 (German surgeon Oswald Bumke) (my thanks to Nils Hansson for making this material available to me).

145. Thomas Schlich, "Surgery, Science and Modernity: Operating Rooms and Laboratories as Spaces of Control," *History of Science* 45 (2007): 231–56.

146. Porter, "How Science Became Technical," 294, 305.

147. Lawrence, "Democratic, Divine and Heroic," 32.

Chapter Three

Configuring Epidemic Encephalitis as a National and International Neurological Concern

Kenton Kroker

Novelty and Scale

The history of epidemic encephalitis offers a profound challenge to any assumption that, in the early twentieth century, pathologies of the nervous system were somehow the exclusive province of a systematic body of specialized knowledge known as "neurology." Admittedly, the condition only began to receive wide recognition once it had been dubbed "encephalitis lethargica," a term which certainly sounds sufficiently neurological, as it describes a site (the *encephalon*, the brain), a pathological state (*-itis*, an affliction or inflammation), and a primary symptom (a profound *lethargy*). Its neurological pedigree might also be inferred from the fact that it was a neuroanatomist, Constantin von Economo (1876–1931), who, based upon his bedside and postmortem observations in a Viennese neuropsychiatric clinic, gave the condition its name in 1917. Economo's description of feverish and sleepy patients with unusual ocular palsies quickly spread. By the end of the following year, dozens of European and American medical practitioners, many of them claiming some expertise in nervous pathologies, had taken up Economo's term to describe this strange new disease. But the novelty, the epidemic character, and the protean nature of encephalitis lethargica quickly served to breach the boundaries of neurological expertise. Commentators debated whether the disease was truly new or whether it had simply been overlooked in the past. But all agreed its complex symptomatology made it extremely difficult to diagnose. In the absence of clear, standardized neurological or immunological signs (as could be found in cases of syphilis or meningitis), the only way to better understand the disease was to gather together more cases. But encephalitis lethargica's epidemiological profile was occult, at best. The causal organism was unknown, and it was unusual to find even two fresh cases in a single institution (never mind a household). Extending disease surveillance (then described as medical or epidemic "intelligence") was therefore a priority. And the only way to accomplish that was to move beyond the little world of the neurologists (to adapt a phrase from Ludwik Fleck) and enroll a wider range of other practitioners and publics.

This articulation of a system of expertise and control over a neurological condition extending well beyond the boundaries of specialized neurological knowledge must be a key point of contact for historians and social scientists with an interest in understanding how the sciences of mind and brain function in the contemporary world. It is well recognized that the current configuration of "neuro" sciences emerged as a highly interdisciplinary mix in the 1960s.[1] But given the ways in which mind/brain conditions incite structures of self-ascription, self-management, and the sociopolitical orchestration of behavior, we would do well to expand our horizons beyond discourse (no matter how interdisciplinary) and think instead of the publics who receive, react, and even redirect such expert knowledge.[2] A neurological epidemic is an excellent place to begin. By definition, epidemics are historical events: they unfold over time, among a population. By tradition, they are laden with social anxiety and conflict: they must be managed among and against other sites of social concern (commerce, warfare, sexuality). They are inevitably framed as threats to social order demanding large-scale intervention, and thus emerge as public (and publicized) objects quite differently than do nonepidemic diseases. Equally, epidemics that emphasize neuropathologies often invoke the specter of a compromised life more so than that of a horrific death: the loss or perversion of the victim's self-mastery, be it described in terms of the will, thought, or behavior, takes center stage. And in such domains, expertise can spread very far, indeed. Contemporary examples, such as autism, even invoke the central place of parental expertise in their current configurations.[3]

So a focus on the techniques, technologies, or therapies involved in establishing and understanding encephalitis lethargica as an epidemic must of necessity transcend the narrow confines of the neurological field. Aside from the usual suspects (neurologists, psychologists, psychiatrists), a host of others, including medical officers of health, educators, general practitioners, bacteriologists, politicians, parents, lawyers, and librarians all contributed to delineating encephalitis lethargica as an epidemic. And given the fact that its status as an epidemic was the central reason for its meteoric rise from the margins of neurology, it would be misleading for the historian to privilege the neurological over any other of the voices that produced such a cacophony during the 1920s.

What follows, then, is an attempt to reconstruct *epidemic* encephalitis as a novel neurological object of widespread concern. My focus here will be on the international dimensions of the epidemic, which are best described in *scalar* terms, in the sense that Nicholas King has used the word to evoke the different politics that shape the concept of emerging diseases, depending upon the geographical and political representations deployed.[4] Here, I speak of *scalar ontologies*, as the different epistemological practices, many of them shaped by broad public consumption, ultimately established different forms of epidemic encephalitis at the international level, as well as in national and local contexts. King's model also reminds us that, on every level, epidemic encephalitis was *constituted* as something very like an "emerging disease," even though its attendant framework of risks was much different than, say, those of H1N1 influenza in the early twenty-first century. In terms of establishing a new social, political, and epistemological object, what epidemic encephalitis lacked in contagiousness it more than made up for in its latent, unpredictable, and chronic natures. The relevant techniques, technologies, and therapies I describe were not a typical part of the neurological armamentarium of the day. Diagnostic technologies (reflex hammers, cinematography, blood counts, cross-immunity tests, histopathological images, to name a few) certainly did play a role in the encephalitis story. But too much attention to these devices would serve to mask the core set of technologies deployed in the quest to configure and to confront encephalitis lethargica *as an epidemic*. These core technologies were social and bibliographic in nature. So, following a recent plea to reconsider the enduring importance of "paper technologies" in the scientific medicine of the early twentieth century,[5] I will outline instead the attempts to serialize the disease through multiple forms and levels of surveillance. I also consider the reasons why emerging bureaucratic structures, such as the League of Nations' Health Organization, took up the problem of epidemic encephalitis as a *therapeutic* concern. Here, the question was less of curing (or even treating) epidemic encephalitis as it was of mitigating the damage it might cause to the large-scale interventions that were these new bureaucracies' raison d'être. Here, we find some evidence of the thesis expressed in Katja Guenther's coda to this volume; namely, that the deployment of technique can sometimes conceal as well as reveal.

The Thing-in-Itself

The most obvious question very quickly becomes the most complicated in such a scheme. For what *was* epidemic encephalitis, really? And don't we need to establish this first, before we go on reconstructing the thing's history? While this question has some limited currency in current attempts at historical epidemiology,[6] historians of medicine need to approach the question with great caution, for it assumes the answer is to be found in terms of contemporary nosology. But even contemporary biomedicine has not resolved the question as to what caused the epidemics, so historians should make no assumptions as to whether the outbreaks were due to postinfluenzal complications, latent herpesvirus, or some entirely different etiological agent. More problematically, the question assumes a homogeneity and stability in clinical and pathological description that simply didn't exist. In naming the disease, Economo did offer detailed descriptions of its pathological anatomy; but the perivascular "cuffing" and midbrain degeneration in the oculomotor nuclei and the substantia nigra he found in 1917 were often missing in cases nonetheless diagnosed as his "encephalitis lethargica."[7] Equally problematic was the fact that the novelty and chronic nature of the condition meant that such postmortems were infrequently conducted.

Attentive readers will note that I've now used at least two different names—"epidemic encephalitis" and "encephalitis lethargica"—for what is supposedly the same thing. And this brings us to the final objection to the question: asking what it *really* was requires that we name it. Yet this name was very much open to debate, because the historical actors realized that whatever name they agreed to inevitably implied something about the disease's essential nature. But the disease's essence was the very thing at stake in the debates! To take but two examples: first, a large proportion of cases did not feature the profound lethargy Economo observed in 1917. Many subsequent cases actually featured a profound *insomnia*. Second, the disease's contagious nature was never experimentally demonstrated. Rather, some investigators inferred the disease's contagious nature by drawing together results from cross-immunity studies (the rhetorical effects of which have been described by historians under the rubric of "immunological devices"), combined with a speculative taxonomy of "neurotropic viruses," itself a classificatory system that depended upon, rather than informed, the stability of the encephalitis lethargica diagnosis.[8] In contrast, epidemiological analysis revealed only that the condition appeared widespread, but infrequent, and with very few concentrated outbreaks. Attempts to pass infectious material from encephalitic patients through experimental animals never achieved the consensus necessary to claim the cause had been isolated. So the names (of which there were many) were based on whatever evidence the would-be namer had ready to hand: a lucky shot at a postmortem; a wife's report of her husband's curious "eye seizures"; a bacteriological analysis of some macerated neural matter set under pressure through an unglazed porcelain filter; a chance observation of a patient struggling to control the cup of tea as he brought it to his lips; a fatigued construction worker recalling a bout of flu years earlier; or a

Medical Officer of Health's cold comfort in telling parents that a disruptive student's appalling conduct was due to an infectious brain disease, rather than to either of the twin dysgenic horrors of insanity or mental deficiency.

During the second and third decades of the twentieth century, dozens of names were forged from these elements (and many more besides). The two most common were under continuous scrutiny by some of the most prominent medical researchers of the day, and the usage of each fluctuated over time. To choose any one of them and reconstruct its history is a linguistic convenience that does violence to the very awkward situation in which neurologists (among others) found themselves: their conventional tools proved largely incapable of stabilizing the name of the very thing they felt to be of such great value to advancing their knowledge and promoting their interests.

So they developed other tools and then adapted them to various levels of analysis in which different kinds of biomedical and neurological work could be done. One example of this has been well covered by historian Paul Foley, who describes how German, French, and American neurologists framed the encephalitis lethargica patient as offering a "window on the soul" that could provide their doctor-interlocutors with an inroad to a psychological understanding of the condition that moved beyond a psychoanalytic critique of the neurological field.[9] But this sort of investigation, which relied upon the patient's own detailed introspections, was not unique to encephalitis lethargica, as other neurological conditions generated similar motor symptoms. Nor did it speak to the condition's presumed specificity as an infectious disease. The overall approach to the object "epidemic encephalitis" was scalar. It changed, depending upon its frame of reference. In terms of its infectious nature, then, the better question is, perhaps, "How and under what circumstances did neurologists formulate epidemic encephalitis as an important problem for public health?"

The Struggle for Consensus

One of the most prominent features of the neurological approach to the problem of epidemic encephalitis was the neurologists' innovative approaches to consensus building regarding the disease. The fact that we would find methodological innovation in the face of enormous confusion should surprise no one. As Ian Hacking observed some years ago, "there is nothing demeaning about ignorance," particularly if one attends to his argument that randomization (surely one of the greatest innovations of modern science) was borne of research into telepathy, a field plagued by even greater contentiousness and confusion than that of neurology.[10]

My focus here will be on a small but prominent and highly active group of American neurologists focused in and around New York City.[11] While this group deployed a number of methods utilized by others in the United States, England, and France, it was the extent, the thoroughness, and the aim of the New Yorkers' efforts that set them apart from all others. One of their approaches was a more localized version of what we now describe as a "consensus conference," the most familiar of which might be the Intergovernmental Panel on Climate Change (IPCC), which shared the 2007 Nobel Peace Prize with Al Gore. In such a situation, a group of experts organize to examine a contentious issue, evaluate the available evidence, and attempt, as a group, to come to an agreement about basic issues and then communicate these to the larger community working in the same or related fields. The crisis here was focused perhaps less on the discordant accounts in the relevant literature but on the sheer bulk of the latter. Like the historical debates and priority disputes that surrounded the question of whether or not epidemic encephalitis was really and truly new, the bibliographic solution to the problem invoked a crisis of reading.

In 1920, New York neurologists founded just such a group, naming it the Association for Research in Nervous and Mental Disease (ARNMD). Its first conference was dedicated to the problem of epidemic encephalitis, cases of which had by then been discovered on both sides of the Atlantic. Of the thirty-five contributors, twenty-five were from New York City, and only three came from outside the US Northeast.[12] At the Association's inaugural conference in December, its president, the New York neurologist Walter Timme (1876–1951), bemoaned the way in which the turmoil that followed the end of the Great War had stifled "all educational and scientific advance" while at the same time failing entirely to slow down the rate of production of medical literature, which had by then become overwhelming. Increasing specialization, Timme contended, had severely delimited the scope of proper neurological interest. The problem of lead poisoning offered a poignant example of how neurologists had failed to take charge of a pressing public health concern, diagnosing it as "lead polyneuritis" and treating it without consideration for the "sociological and industrial conditions" of its production.[13] But the logic of specialization also provided a ready solution to the question of how neurologists could best "economize" their "time-energy unit": they needed to better coordinate their efforts so their expertise could be better "universalized." To that end, ARNMD members would collectively select a problem or disease to examine, carve it up into discrete, manageable aspects, and coordinate the subsequent work to prevent duplication of effort. The very first problem the association took upon itself to solve—namely, epidemic encephalitis—was an enigma that neurologists were far more likely to have encountered in the medical or even popular press than in their own offices. Only a collective approach could prevail.

As George Weisz has demonstrated, the meaning and progress of medical specialization was highly dependent upon the extant professional organization of general practitioners and the political system in which they worked. In the United States, specialties developed through specialist-run exam boards within the American Medical Association, where the general practitioner's interests were paramount.[14] American specialties tended to evolve less out of initiatives in medical pedagogy than from new technologically driven practices or novel public health concerns. Both scenarios required regulation to defend the public interest from dilettante practitioners performing self-declared specialized medicine, but on a part-time basis. American specialists thus tended to pursue these interests full time and were more liable to seek their identity in technology or in public health initiatives.

The story of epidemic encephalitis in America fits well into this professional pattern. In Timme's words, neurologists were "opportunistic" in their practice, and their professional organizations needed to better reflect this.[15] But specialization was supposed to be about more than professional identity and opportunism. It was supposed to advance knowledge. The enormous confusion wrought by epidemic encephalitis encouraged American neurologists to adopt a form of collective investigation, which by then had a long history in both the United States and Britain.[16] Harry Marks has argued that these sorts of studies were declining by the early twentieth century, but the example of epidemic encephalitis suggests a corrective to this view. The systematic evaluation of the enormous literature amassing around epidemic encephalitis was no less a "collective investigation" than was the evaluation of diphtheria antitoxin a quarter-century earlier. The difference in how these respective problems were framed is instructive. It reaffirms the significance of what has been dubbed the "laboratory revolution" in medicine, even as it exposes the limits of the latter by offering up clinical and bibliographic innovation in contrast.[17]

By the late 1890s, diphtheria antitoxin serotherapy was well-known and widespread. It was also highly suggestive in that it raised both practical questions about efficacy as well as theoretical questions about the nature of immunological defense.[18] Numerous clinical and experimental trials were devised to settle the questions, and its stabilization, standardization, and eventual replacement by prophylactic vaccination evolved over the next several decades. Surveying physicians' practices and observations through collective investigation was an important part of this investigative structure, but it was very much overshadowed by the bacteriological laboratory that produced both the diphtheria antitoxin and the major theoretical questions surrounding it. Epidemic encephalitis, on the other hand, did not share in this stabilized, industrialized system of laboratory-based production, as the results of virtually every laboratory analysis were disputed.[19] The disease appeared frequently, but sporadically, in diverse geographical locations, following no known logic of transmission. Yet reports of its incidence, histopathological examinations, experimental studies, and epidemiological speculations filled the biomedical literature. Therapy, which recent scholarship has shown to have provided many practical and rhetorical tools for the promotion of neurology as an independent specialty,[20] was extremely fractured in the case of epidemic encephalitis. Indeed, the ARNMD investigation insisted that scientific therapeutics for such a disease could only begin with the identification of the causal microbe, and it derided the most popular therapy of the day (the fixation abscess) as "medieval."[21]

The Matheson Commission—Bibliographic Transcendence

The stubborn refusal of epidemic encephalitis to submit to such a rational system of analysis continued to animate the collective investigation led by New York neurologists well into the 1920s. The result was the Matheson Commission (MC) report, named for its patron, William J. Matheson (1856–1930), an industrial chemist and encephalitis sufferer. The authors indicated at the outset that theirs was no mere report. They described it instead as a "survey," designed to "collect and, so far as possible, to correlate the work done on the etiology and treatment of epidemic encephalitis and to bring together the data available on its epidemiology."[22] The authors not only prepared a bibliography from all major bibliographic sources (the *Index Medicus*, the *Quarterly Cumulative Index*, and the *Catalogue of the Surgeon General's Library*); they also traveled overseas, across England and to The Hague, Brussels, and Paris to conduct personal interviews with and tour the laboratories of current and former encephalitis researchers. They then compressed a decade's worth of encephalitis research, drawn from tens of thousands of documented cases and published in thousands of scientific articles, into a single tome. The nature of the book indicates its anticipated use: it was an 850-page stitched quarto volume with thin leaves and a black flexible imitation leather cover with nothing but "Epidemic Encephalitis" and the Columbia University Press logo stamped on the front and along the spine. Half-abstract, half-bibliography, with an index for author and subject, the MC report was designed to be given away as a desk reference to help physicians negotiate what would likely be a rare encounter with a mysterious and potentially debilitating disease.

Like the ARNMD conference report, the MC's survey was an attempt to establish authority by compressing expertise into a digestible, portable format. Certainly mobile. But immutable? In contrast to the ARNMD's reliance upon prominent neurologists drawn from prestigious institutions in a geographically limited location, the MC report attempted to transcend such limitations by appealing to a strict neutrality: "In preparing the chapters on epidemiology, post-vaccinal encephalitis and etiology," the authors noted in their introduction, "it has been our aim to present an unbiased summary of the contributions of different authors. No attempt has been made to criticize the work or draw conclusions designed to express our own opinions."[23] Its authority drew from its bibliographic comprehensiveness, not the expert judgment of a select panel. And rather than reifying a laboratory event as an immutable fact, it circumscribed an object of research and practice that, for all the incoherence of the community that surrounded it, could nonetheless be projected into the future.

The strategy is revealing. The 1920s witnessed enormous changes in the structure of medical practice, particularly in the way that inscriptions came to circumscribe what counted as "scientific medicine." Physiological research and its participation in the quest for "mechanical objectivity" was perhaps the cutting edge of this movement.[24] It was accompanied by an onslaught of record keeping, particularly in American hospitals of the period.[25] The management of an ever-increasing volume of medical literature, however, has received rather less attention from historians.[26] "Cooperative bibliography," of which the MC's report was a variant, had been established as an integral part of medical knowledge since the middle of the nineteenth century.[27] In the United States, prominent medical practitioners viewed such practice as an important component of its national public health system, and as an original contribution to the growth of medical science. Unlike classical medical bibliography, in which a single medical practitioner reviewed extant literature either on a particular topic or medical system, cooperative bibliography featured a division of labor between multiple, specialized bibliographers (often women) working in libraries who would collect and classify medical literature, managed by a director who also developed or refined the attendant classificatory system. The system did not necessarily reflect any extant nosology and was instead more illustrative of trends in medical publication. Rather than being dedicated to a single disease, the scope of cooperative bibliography was, in principle, indefinite and constantly changing to reflect current medical knowledge. Its potential audience was also far more extensive, as it encompassed all medical practitioners and researchers with an interest or a perceived need to "keep up" with the latest developments in medical science. One could almost say progress was the single most important effect of such a practice.

The most prominent American example of cooperative bibliography was developed by John Shaw Billings (1838–1913), the first head of the Library of the Surgeon-General's Office. Aside from overseeing a massive expansion of the library's holdings, Billings's revision of the *Index-Catalogue of the Library of the Surgeon-General* during the late 1870s was notable for organizing the library's monographs and journal articles according to cross-referenced topics and was by far the largest such catalogue ever developed. His *Index medicus*, a private venture, aimed at indexing all the latest periodical literature on a monthly basis. "I question whether America has made any larger contribution to medicine than that made by Billings," mused William H. Welch at a 1914 meeting held in Billings's honor. "That in my judgment is our greatest contribution to medicine."[28] A year later, Fielding Garrison's address to the medical faculty of Syracuse University described bibliography as "an enlarged system of bookkeeping" with effects as indispensable for the progress of medicine as for business. Indeed, Garrison continued, "we are disagreeably reminded of this fact in connection with the present European war, for on this simple idea is based the whole Prussian system of 'efficiency'; the idea that, in war or business, every slightest detail is important, the duties of the milkman, baker, printer, or mechanic, as well as those of the soldier and strategist."[29]

So at least some leading practitioners deemed collective bibliography every bit as important for progress in medical knowledge, practice, and pedagogy as were systematized patient records or replicable, mechanical inscriptions of physiological events generated in the laboratory. Many prominent neurologists evidently agreed, particularly when it came to making sense of epidemic encephalitis as something more than a clinical curiosity. An enormous bulk of publications had appeared on the topic in the decade preceding the MC bibliography's publication in 1929: almost 4,700 journal articles, reports, monographs and books, themselves based upon nearly 53,000 officially reported cases worldwide, were recorded therein. The infrequency of the disease and its widespread nature meant that, unlike other infectious diseases, epidemic encephalitis only rarely offered an opportunity to study multiple cases at once. Organizing the extant medical literature around a single topic appeared to make this possible, at least on paper. The systematic application of consensus meetings and bibliographic surveillance held out the promise for neurologists that they could make the disease more than a fascinating but rare clinical oddity.

Epidemic Encephalitis and the Emergence of International Health

Epidemic encephalitis's status qua epidemic was at the core of how this disease emerged at the international level. Neurology, however, appears to have enjoyed less influence here, as the major issues involved epidemiological concerns of both tracing (if not delimiting) the disease's progress across borders and preventing it from interfering with one of the oldest and most symbolically laden of all public health initiatives—smallpox vaccination.

Pandemic influenza presented an enormous challenge to an emerging international sanitary order in the early twentieth century. As the extent of pandemic influenza's destructive potential was unveiled during the autumn of 1918, existing public health measures in every nation rapidly proved themselves to be insufficient, illusory, misguided, and ultimately futile. Neurological knowledge was brought along for the ride, as epidemic encephalitis was initially conceptualized by several prominent observers as an after-effect of particularly virulent waves of pandemic flu. The rapid devastation of this pandemic fundamentally transformed the emphasis of modern epidemic control, as national and international systems alike shifted from their mandate of infectious disease eradication to one that instead focused on a more "ecological" vision of managing the equilibrium of morbidity rates within a given population.[30] This is not to say that the ideal of disease eradication disappeared entirely during the 1920s: vaccination against smallpox, for example, continued to hold up this lofty goal.[31] But pandemic influenza had an unquestionable effect on how public health authorities approached the conceptualization and control of other long-standing diseases. A number of outspoken epidemiologists began to criticize their field's reliance upon the laboratory, and some proposed reviving the neo-Hippocratic notion of "epidemic constitutions" to challenge the dominance of concepts of bacteriological specificity.[32] Although such commentators initially invoked the sudden appearance of epidemic encephalitis in the historical register as proof of their theories, by the end of the 1920s, most researchers had rejected any strong correlation between flu and epidemic encephalitis. Modern-day biomedical revisionists, by contrast, have encouraged the consideration of a causal relationship between the two, typically suggesting that improved surveillance would likely have revealed the same.[33] But this idealized picture subverts the actual order of events: epidemic encephalitis was less the victim of a lack of proper epidemiological surveillance than it was the creation of novel attempts to expand such surveillance at an international level.

Internationalizing Epidemic Encephalitis

The process of converting a conventional exercise in medical bibliography (listing all extant publications on the topic under consideration) to treating a list of references as a potential index of morbidity began with a series of British public health reports on epidemic encephalitis dating back to 1922. Its primary author, Allan C. Parsons (c. 1872–1947), a medical officer with the newly created Ministry of Health, attempted to provide "some idea of the widespread experience of encephalitis lethargica" by calculating the "comparative literary output in the various countries concerned."[34] To this effect, he listed, in alphabetical order, the national origin of all medical publications on the disease and the total number of items published from each country. From this latter number, Parsons then derived the total number of cases referred to in each country's publications. So, for example, France's 59 publications to that date made reference to some 529 cases, while Italy's

42 publications referred to 186 cases. In contrast, Egypt and Cuba each produced one publication mentioning only one case each. It was almost certain that within at least some nation's publications, multiple references were made to the same discrete case. (The French literature, for example, tended to include a higher number of authors reading nearly identical reports to different professional societies, which were then counted as two discrete publications.) But the report was silent as to this possibility, just as it ignored whether or not there was duplication of cases among publications from different nations (as might well have been the case for those authors who published in multiple countries).

Parsons's faith in his ability to sketch out national morbidity figures on the basis of counting case references was surely informed by the lack of any reasonable alternative. International comparisons were certainly of interest, particularly in the case of a new but rare infectious disease. But unless countries published this data, the ready-made seriality derived from counting cases in what was supposedly a complete collection of the relevant literature made a great deal of sense. It effectively relied upon a transnational and professional sense of curiosity and an incitement to publish among medical researchers that was part and parcel of what it meant for medicine to be "scientific" during the 1920s. And it was as good a comparative strategy as could be had when most countries either had not made encephalitis lethargica a notifiable disease, or had they done so, were hardly able to enforce such notification. The extent of Britain's somewhat exceptional status in this regard shone through in Parsons's report, where the first appendix, rife with detailed clinical notes culled from several clinicians, was followed by five tables of data on cases involving pregnancy, case-to-case infection, lumbar puncture and postmortem findings, and various sequelae among more than six hundred cases, each of which featured a discrete "notification number," thereby avoiding duplication of cases and enabling their cross-referencing.[35] This empirical bent of the report's seemingly comprehensive surveillance was reinforced by the fact that the report actually made very few references to the appendices at all.[36] The data, it seems, were expected to speak to the reader directly.

The League of Nations' Health Organization (LNHO) continued the British ministry's technique of using national publication data to help frame the international incidence of epidemic encephalitis. Like the LNHO's technical committee, which helped design indices to standardize biological products (especially sera and vaccines), the epidemiological wing of the LNHO attempted to evaluate public health performance across national boundaries, thereby "internationalizing" health.[37] In the absence of standards regarding diagnosis and notification, crafting an international epidemiology for a new and obscure infectious disease through literary surveillance must have made a good deal of sense.[38] The prominence of George S. Buchanan

(1869–1936) within the LNHO clearly also helped shape this approach to internationalizing epidemic encephalitis. Buchanan was a career medical bureaucrat whose penchant for administrative clarity and efficiency helped translate the complexities of contemporary medical science for Britain's growing health bureaucracy.[39] Starting as a medical inspector for the Local Government Board in 1895, Buchanan rose to the international stage in 1914, when he became the British delegate to the Office internationale d'hygiène publique (OIHP). When plans for a League of Nations committee on international health began to take shape in mid-1919, Buchanan (now senior medical officer in charge of the Medical Intelligence Service in the Ministry of Health) encouraged his counterparts to adapt OIHP to the task.[40] This proposal ultimately failed, and the diplomatically oriented OIHP frequently conflicted with the LNHO's more activist agenda. The latter evolved out of the League's Epidemics Commission, a temporary organization devised to help prevent the spread of epidemic typhus from the Soviet-Polish border following the end of the Great War. Buchanan, however, felt this level of intervention should be the exception for the new Health Organization, not the rule. Nor, he argued, would any nation agree to "a superman for international health" permanently directing a massive new research enterprise from Geneva.[41] His more modest proposal was of an organization primarily dedicated to the efficient management of epidemic intelligence; in particular, a permanent committee dedicated to the coordination, standardization, compilation, and redistribution of epidemiological and public health data from around the world. The benefits of such an organization at the international level were twofold: its pointed and repeated requests for information would encourage nations to adopt a single and rational system of notification (he singled out France as a particularly problematic case), and its efficiencies would "produce a minimum of interference and annoyance in international traffic and commerce."[42]

When the International Health Board of the Rockefeller Foundation (RF) agreed to financially support the League's Provisional Health Committee in 1922, the offer came with one condition: the committee had to clearly outline its mandate. Committee members quickly linked up the RF's own interest in epidemiological intelligence with Buchanan's template for the same. But the very question of what, in fact, constituted an epidemic quickly arose. In the fourth session of committee meetings that took place in Geneva in mid-August 1922, the French champion of public health reform, Léon Bernard (1872–1934), expressed skepticism at using RF money for studying any but the most obvious contagions, insisting that "it was not possible to extend the meaning of the word 'epidemic' to include other than infectious diseases."[43] Buchanan disagreed, and proposed instead that the money from the RF be used to gather information on any disease, regardless of its status as a contagion. Given that the fact (but not the nature) of encephalitis's contagiousness was agreed upon by most, gathering international data on its incidence must have seemed a good compromise between these two positions. More importantly, the international circulation of case studies might help overcome the disease's novelty and its low morbidity rate, both of which made it extremely difficult to diagnose. Following Buchanan's constructivist argument that international disease surveillance would pressure individual nations to improve their own national systems of epidemic intelligence, the League's repeated requests for statistics on encephalitis lethargica would then increase the number of cases reported, with the hopeful end of solving the riddle of its contagiousness.

Buchanan appeared to have Parsons's work on epidemic encephalitis in mind, for he quickly put forward Parsons as someone particularly well qualified to undertake such an international survey should the newly christened LNHO choose to focus on encephalitis lethargica as a topic of investigation.[44] The inquiry began in earnest in 1923 with a letter from the LNHO circulated to health officials around the world. Noting that "the available information regarding this infectious disease has hitherto been limited, in point of fact, to monographs on well-defined epidemics," the letter indicated the LNHO's desire to formulate knowledge of the disease "from a general standpoint," and to that effect, requested both updated statistics regarding the number of cases since the beginning of the year as well as a weekly telegram (paid for by the League's Health Section) indicating the "number of fresh cases" or the absence of the same.[45]

The intelligence gathering was short-lived, as the LNHO's Director, Ludwik Rajchman (1881–1965), informed correspondents on February 8, 1924, that the organization could no longer cover the cost of telegraphs. By then, dossiers had been created for each nation that had responded. Dossiers are missing for many nations that received the LNHO letter, including Soviet Russia, Portugal, Yugoslavia, and Germany (whose lack of participation was explicitly noted in some instances). Other nations sent data on a regular or semiregular basis, but their responses could be heavily qualified. The correspondent from Czechoslovakia, for example, sent several telegrams but noted that many of the cases described therein were "without symptoms that could be otherwise attributed to influenza."[46] The LNHO delegate from the Netherlands, Dr. N. M. Josephus Jitta (1858–1940), complained that notification of the disease was not obligatory in his country, so the numbers he offered were not reliable.[47] The implication here was that the disease was likely underreported. But the United States, which reported larger numbers of cases than most other corresponding nations, appeared to be suffering from the opposite situation. The US dossier contains a copy of a press release from the US Public Health Service quoting Surgeon-General Hugh Smith Cumming to the effect that, as epidemic encephalitis was reportable in very few states, most data reported were based on newspaper stories. Worse, the disease was easily confused with many other diseases and so "its prevalence is therefore likely to be unduly magnified."[48]

Cumming's suggestion that some state public health agencies were compiling morbidity statistics through newspaper reports offers a somewhat populist counterpoint to Parsons's bureaucratic confidence in taking published articles as an index of encephalitis's worldwide prevalence. Given its complex symptomatology, the continued absence of diagnostic standards for the disease, differing nosological traditions, and the uneven global distribution of legislation to notify and its subsequent enforcement, it is clear that any quantitative assessment of epidemic encephalitis's worldwide prevalence was speculative at best. The League's own published incidence rates were spotty and never provided a global count of cases. Indeed, when the League's publications did offer such a measure, it cited the MC's 1929 total of "more than 50,000" recorded cases between 1919 and 1927 rather than referring to any of its own publications.[49] This completed the circular pattern of citation, as the MC report itself had relied heavily on the LNHO measures to compile the very same data.

My point here is not so much to put what limited statistics we do have regarding epidemic encephalitis into question (although historical epidemiologists might be well-advised to do so in their retrospective analyses). Encephalitis researchers during the 1920s were keenly aware that they were operating in a domain of extraordinary uncertainty, bordered on one side by fears of exaggerating the extent of the epidemic and thereby revealing their ignorance, and on the other by concerns that an underestimation of the extent of this occult disease might wreak havoc on emerging national and international public health institutions. What made this situation novel was the fact that despite the severe lack of identifiable and accessible "clinical material," there was no lack of published data. The long-term trajectory of encephalitis encouraged the latter to emerge as a surrogate for the former. But while one aspect of the international interest in the disease was clearly epidemiological and projective, another was developing that was far more engaged in protecting extant public health achievements.

A Latent Threat to International Health

Epidemic encephalitis did pose an immediate threat to international public health, but concerns were less with extant victims than with the innumerable future victims who might harbor latent and otherwise harmless viruses that could be accidentally activated in the process of the most celebrated of all public health initiatives: vaccination.

The modern history of vaccination has been an integral feature of what is now known by convention as "biomedical citizenship." For more than two centuries, the extension of and resistance to compulsory smallpox vaccination have been important stages on which various strategies of biopower have unfolded. Historical accounts of this dynamic quite naturally organize themselves at the level of the nation-state.[50] At the international level, however, historical analysis has been effectively dominated by the World Health Organization's attempts to eradicate smallpox. The main biomedical figures themselves established the central narrative, with 1958 marking the formal beginning of eradication as a stated goal, followed by the WHO's 1967 Intensified Smallpox Eradication Programme, and culminating in the global eradication of the disease a decade later.[51] Historians have narrated a similar trajectory, elaborating upon national, geographical, political, or technological details.[52] But smallpox vaccination was in fact an object of international health in the pre-WHO days. It is true that smallpox's endemic status in virtually all nations (as well as the increasing prominence of its less virulent forms) put the disease outside the interwar international health movement's dedication to containing the spread of infectious disease.[53] But its potential linkage with encephalitis through adverse vaccination reactions made smallpox a distinctive object of international health nonetheless. In keeping with the epidemiological tenor of the times, it was less the eradication of smallpox than surveillance and standardization of vaccine that emerged as the stated goals of the technical commission of the LNHO. Despite the fact that so little was known about epidemic encephalitis, the LNHO and its counterparts in the British Ministry of Health were publicly at pains to distinguish the neurological complications that occasionally accompanied vaccination from the epidemics of encephalitis that had no geography, yet seemed to lurk everywhere.

British Origins

Death had long been recognized as a risk of smallpox vaccination, but it was not until the early 1920s that this phenomenon took on a distinctly neurological character. In December 1922, Hubert M. Turnbull (1875–1955), the long-standing director of the Institute of Pathology at the London Hospital, and James McIntosh (1882–1948), director of the Bland-Sutton Institute of Pathology at Middlesex Hospital, conducted postmortem exams of four patient who died within two weeks of being vaccinated. They discovered the brains and spinal cords of the victims showed an infiltration of cells around the blood vessels, as well as a general "softening" around vessels in the white matter of the brain, which they described in terms of "demyelination."[54] The authors were careful to describe this encephalo-myelitis as finding "its closest affinity in poliomyelitis and encephalitis lethargica," but that it was distinct from the latter less in "detail" than in the lesions' "distribution and sites of maximal incidence."[55]

Any link between postvaccinal and epidemic encephalitis opened up considerable problems for vaccinationists. While smallpox had been on the rise in Britain for several years, its virulence had noticeably decreased. The Vaccination Act of 1907 had allowed for conscientious objection, meaning that parents could refuse to vaccinate their children, provided they signed a declaration affirming that they believed vaccination would do harm to their child. From the perspective of Britain's extensive public health system, it was bad enough to have to acknowledge difficult and potentially fatal complications of a vaccination for what was (rightly or wrongly) perceived as an increasingly mild and rare disease. But the notion that smallpox vaccination could somehow unleash a latent, undetectable virus in the body that might then generate the horrific effects of epidemic encephalitis was even worse. In such a scheme, the specter of the "healthy carrier," by then a well-established principle in epidemiological reasoning and a touchstone of the new public health, loomed large. But it was also seriously disfigured. In contrast to cases of typhoid carriers (for example), whose status could be detected by bacteriological analysis, the hypothetical carrier of the encephalitis virus was entirely invisible *until* a preventative vaccination was deployed, at which time encephalitis lethargica (or a postvaccinal variant) might appear.

In their 1926 paper, Turnbull and McIntosh noted that they had alerted the ministry regarding their investigation in 1922. But they only completed their pathological and experimental work in January 1924. By that time, their informal network of clinicians, pathologists, and Medical Officers of Health (MOH) had gathered together an additional three cases. In the interim, the ministry had struck a commission led by Sir Frederick W. Andrewes (1859–1932), a well-known pathologist and professor at London University. This commission issued two internal reports over the next two years, and it took Turnbull and McIntosh's still-unpublished work as its starting point. The reasons for why this latter work remained unpublished until 1926 are uncertain, but it seems likely that ministry officials explicitly requested it not be published until they could orchestrate a complete study of the question.[56] This meant finding more fatal cases of postvaccinal encephalitis that could be used to generate a reliable histopathological profile of the condition, which could then help distinguish its clinical picture from those of epidemic encephalitis and polio.

The Andrewes Commission reported internally to the ministry, which by February 1926 determined that the problem was serious enough to strike a Committee on Vaccination in conjunction with the Medical Research Council. The significance of the inquiry was clearly indicated by the choice of chair, for it was none other than Humphry Rolleston (1862–1944), Regius Professor of Physic at Cambridge, president of the Royal College of Physicians, and physician-in-ordinary to King George V. Rolleston is perhaps better-known for chairing a 1924 committee investigating the problem of opiate addiction and the use of opiates by British doctors,[57] but the two committees shared a common purview of reinscribing older therapeutic or preventative agents within a new, expansive, centralized system of public health surveillance, enforcement, and research.[58] The committee's terms of reference focused on evaluating means of standardizing the production and use of vaccine lymph and evaluating the risks posed by its use as well as the means that might be used to mitigate such risk.[59] Finding additional cases without raising alarm was crucial. As notification of complications following vaccination did not fall under the same category as notification of infectious disease, one of the vaccination committee's first actions was to enroll as many medical practitioners as possible in its surveillance efforts. In April 1926, the committee, having announced its mandate two months earlier, published its request that medics report all incidents of "disease of the central nervous system with an acute onset" in which "vaccination has preceded the onset of the symptoms within a period of four weeks."[60]

The eighty-seven cases ultimately reported upon did little to mitigate the ignorance regarding the etiology of encephalitis in either its postvaccinal or epidemic guises. In fact, the Rolleston Committee's 1928 report did not appear to advance from the majority opinion expressed in its 1924 predecessor. Both reports outlined the three main hypotheses; namely, that postvaccinal encephalitis was due solely to vaccinia virus, that the appearance of encephalitis was entirely unrelated to the fact of vaccination, or a pathological interaction between vaccinia and a preexisting (or subsequent) neurotropic virus or viruses triggered an encephalitis. But because the epidemiological, clinical, experimental, and histopathological evidence regarding all kinds of encephalitis was still so vague, none of these explanations could be definitively ruled out. In the end, the 1928 report concluded that "present evidence" (which was distinguished from recognized fact) indicated "vaccinia cannot be held solely responsible for the nervous sequelae," and that "in the present state of uncertainty" regarding encephalitis lethargica, vaccinia's interactions with its causal agent or with that of poliomyelitis should be taken as a working hypothesis upon which to conduct further research.[61]

By the time the final Rolleston Committee report was released in early 1931, things had gotten so confusing that editorial commentators in the *British Medical Journal* offered a sociological explanation to help set things straight. The editorial noted its "regret that a committee concerned with 'observations on the epidemiology and the clinical and pathological character of post-vaccinal nervous disease' should include no neurologist" and concluded that the different positions adopted on the question were really little more than a reflection of disciplinary orientation. Those who argued vaccinia alone was the cause tended to champion epidemiological analysis and experimental evidence. They noted that postvaccinal encephalitis was characterized by a relatively stable "incubation period," that vaccinia could be demonstrated to cause encephalitis in experimental animals, and that vaccinia could be recovered throughout the human brain following vaccination. Those who favored the virus "activation" theory, on the other hand, stuck closely to the pathological evidence, noting that the histopathology of experimentally produced encephalitis in animals looked very little like human postvaccinal encephalitis and quite a bit more like the rare encephalitic complications following various viral diseases, including measles and influenza. The editorial conclusion effectively relegated the past decade's efforts to understand neurotropic viruses through histopathological methods to the dustbin of history: "We may justly wonder whether we are not here dealing with phenomena which are beyond the scope of our present neuro-pathological concepts, and involve more complex events than the simple invasion of the nervous system by an infecting organism."[62]

Vaccine Standards Migrate to Diagnosis

The LNHO's Commission on Smallpox and Vaccination, on the other hand, adopted a flexible theoretical perspective from the outset. This is perhaps not surprising, given that, unlike the British Ministry of Health, the LNHO was not directly or even indirectly responsible for the health of its "citizens." The object of its interventions was the nation-state. The LNHO was a forum for creating an entirely new perspective on health as an object of international collaboration and research. Like the League itself, the LNHO lacked most forms of coercive power and operated instead through introducing and sustaining novel systems of surveillance, coordination, standardization, and publication. It was not in the business of scientific discovery (as was the MRC, for example), focusing instead on international technoscientific alignment, instigated and evaluated in large part through the novel format of international metastudies.[63] It tended to view vaccination as much more than a preventative measure: it was also a tool for gaining a toehold for the new public health where none had previously existed (among refugees from the Greco-Turkish conflict in 1919, for example, or in Shanghai in 1930).[64]

The theoretical perspective in question was the idea that the novel neurological epidemics that appeared in the early twentieth century were in fact the result of viral variability. Constantin Levaditi (1874–1953) led a research group at the Institut Pasteur who spent the better part of the 1920s developing a theoretical and experimental framework for explaining how *les ectodermoses neurotropes* (the neurotropic ectodermosis group of viruses) could account for the changing fortunes of the viruses of herpes, vaccinia, poliomyelitis, rabies, and epidemic encephalitis inside and outside the bacteriological laboratory.[65] Levaditi emphasized the common embryonic origins of dermal and neural cells to explain why this group of neurotropic viruses could vary in their virulence: sometimes they would have great affinity for cells in the dermis and evoke the skin reactions that characterized, for example, herpes labilis; other times, they would be strongly neurotropic and produce neurological symptoms characteristic of epidemic encephalitis. Experimentally, Levaditi relied upon his demonstration that corneal scarification with herpes virus in a rabbit could generate an encephalitis, while neural material taken from an encephalitic patient could generate dermal reactions in the same animal. There also appeared to be a number of complex cross-immunity reactions in each.

While the ability to generate an experimental encephalitis using herpes virus was relatively uncontroversial, many prominent bacteriologists—in particular, Simon Flexner, director of the Rockefeller Institute for Medical Research in New York—doubted whether Levaditi's group had in fact isolated the virus of encephalitis at all. But Levaditi's taxonomy had many supporters on the continent. So when cases of postvaccinal encephalitis began to appear in the Netherlands in conjunction with an outbreak of epidemic encephalitis in 1923, a number of investigators took Levaditi's schema as a starting point for a general investigation. Given the relatively small number of cases, their widespread incidence, and the significance of smallpox vaccination for most nations' public health systems, the problem seemed ready-made for an LNHO investigation involving international cooperation.

Following multiple reports of postvaccinal encephalitis in the Netherlands, Jitta began in April 1925 to push for the LNHO to create a committee to investigate the possibility that repeated passage of vaccina was increasing their virulence and increasing their affinity for neural (as opposed to dermal) tissue. The committee was led by the Portuguese delegate, Professor Ricardo Jorge (1858–1939), and its composition was ultimately approved in late October, with a formal conference to be held January 4–9, 1926, at The Hague.[66] The LNHO's director, Ludwik Rajchman, advised Jorge from the very beginning to do everything he could to keep the commission's interest in evaluating the relationship between epidemic and postvaccinal encephalitis out of the public eye. Standardization of the vaccine was one thing; the mere thought that the vaccine might be somehow responsible for the horrors of epidemic encephalitis, quite another.[67] Jorge, a neurologist by training, was himself highly skeptical of there being any connection between the two. The timing of the postvaccinal and lethargic encephalitis outbreaks in Holland, he argued, was irrelevant, given that the sixty-two documented cases in Britain showed little linkage to any other local outbreaks. Moreover, Jorge agreed with his many British counterparts that the histopathology of the two conditions appeared to be completely different. This position, of course, assumed a stable pathology for epidemic encephalitis, something yet to be proven in the eyes of many investigators.

Jorge seemed to have little interest or respect for Levaditi's work, and he greatly feared the latter's suggestion that in the case of postvaccinal encephalitis, the rare but devastating effects of vaccination might result from activation of a latent and otherwise harmless virus, in the same way that the epidemics of encephalitis since 1917 might have been caused by the activation of a latent herpes virus. But such theories proved impossible to ignore. Not only had Levaditi's work on epidemic encephalitis gained international attention, his process of producing decent quantities of standardized vaccinia by serial passage through rabbit brains (also known as neurovaccine) was widely viewed as a serious alternative to lymph production in cows. The internationalist composition of the League's committee also made it difficult to marginalize Levaditi, for there needed to be at least one French representative for every German on any committee, and both a German (Heinrich Alexander Gins) and a German-speaking Swiss (Robert Doerr) had already made their way onto a list of expert delegates by the time Jorge got around to making formal invitations.

Jitta had initially framed the problem of postvaccinal encephalitis in Levaditi's terms, but Jorge was optimistic that the more sober and tentative conclusions put forward by his British counterparts would win the day. Jorge was diplomatic in his correspondence with Levaditi, but he was not above personal attacks when discussing the Parisian with Rajchman. Casting doubt on both the validity of his ideas and the utility of his neurovaccine, Jorge cautioned against giving too much prominence to Levaditi's theories in LNHO discussions. The problem of encephalitis, Jorge complained, had fueled the "fertile imagination" of this "great experimenter," who, he ultimately concluded, was little more than a "novelist of the laboratory, whose judgment was entirely unreliable."[68] Jorge's opinion appeared somewhat tempered after he toured Levaditi's laboratory in mid-July. He found the latter "amiable" but continued to express concern over how he had framed the problem of postvaccinal encephalitis to the French newspapers.[69]

Mediating Encephalitis at The Hague

The January 1926 conference at The Hague did little to resolve any of these tensions. Levaditi relentlessly promoted his neurovaccine as a way of achieving a higher degree of both purity and control over vaccinia. He implied that his system of vaccine production was superior to the more conventional approach utilizing calf lymph, because the former avoided the risks of increasing vaccinia's virulence and perhaps triggering an encephalitis in those harboring a latent virus. He also threw Turnbull and McIntosh's histopathological work into question by delimiting the similarities between conventional vaccine and neurovaccine. Where Turnbull and McIntosh had demonstrated that conventional vaccine could produce an encephalitis in an experimental monkey, Levaditi claimed he had been entirely unable to produce similar effects with his new neurovaccine.

For his part, Buchanan unsurprisingly stuck close to the epidemiological trail, where British accomplishments were perhaps the least vulnerable to criticism on an international stage. He noted that while the Dutch outbreak did indeed feature a similar seasonal incidence between postvaccinal and lethargic encephalitis, no such correlation could be detected in the series of British cases. This fact, combined with the arguments of Turnbull and McIntosh regarding the more "generalized" nature of the postvaccinal lesions, led him to conclude that postvaccinal encephalitis was entirely distinct from the epidemics of encephalitis lethargica so well-documented in Britain. The German delegate, Gins, proposed a precautionary strategy, advocating a suspension of all smallpox vaccination during outbreaks of epidemic encephalitis. The Swiss delegate, Georg Sobernheim, rejected this as entirely impractical, as such a move would almost certainly provide fuel for the antivaccination movement. In an appendix to the LNHC's report on the conference's six meetings, the Czech delegate, Franz Lucksch, cast the entire project of separating the two diseases into doubt by arguing that epidemic encephalitis was in all likelihood multiple diseases, one of which was postvaccinal encephalitis.

In his internal report to the LNHO, Jorge concluded that he sensed among the conference delegates "an obvious tendency in favour of identifying it [postvaccinal encephalitis] with *encephalitis lethargica*, without going so far as to state it outright."[70] In public, Levaditi's critics insured that however unclear explanations of postvaccinal encephalitis might be, the notion that it was either analogous to or an integral part of epidemic encephalitis was definitively rejected.[71] In its place was the claim, based on the disseminated pathological picture, that encephalitis was an accidental and fairly rare feature of the viral landscape in general, and could be found in a number of viral infections, including measles, herpes, and influenza. Vaccinia (as the virus used to vaccinate against smallpox) was thus implicated as the most significant cause of postvaccinal encephalitis. But the latter, now that it had been definitively detached from epidemic encephalitis, was now subject to calculation and control as a risk associated with vaccination. Recommendations released by the commission the following month emphasized the need for further epidemiological data documenting the frequency of such major postvaccinal complications, as well as the need to work toward the international standardization of vaccina's production, potency, and deployment.[72]

Success on these fronts was limited. Subsequent meetings of the commission in 1927 and 1928 reported details of experimental and epidemiological reports from various nations, with little resolution. The 1927

Berlin meeting, for example, established four different methods (from four different national traditions) of establishing vaccinia virulence and then proceeded to endorse them all.[73] National public health media dutifully reported the differing incidence rates of postvaccinal encephalitis, from a low of one case per seven hundred thousand vaccinations in Germany to a high of one per four thousand in the Netherlands.[74] But with no international standards of vaccine potency or application in effect, it was impossible to draw any firm conclusions from a comparison of these rates. What *was* certain was that epidemic encephalitis had been effectively eliminated from the constellation of factors that could potentially explain postvaccinal encephalitis. In the face of a wide-ranging, open-ended inquiry into the interactions between a novel neurological disease and a well-established technique of preventative medicine, national systems of public health surveillance and control had successfully reasserted themselves.

Conclusions

What can these national and international configurations of a mysterious epidemic disease tell us about interwar neurology? The most powerful way of framing the question, I would argue, is to consider the concerted and diverse attempts investigators undertook to make epidemic encephalitis visible. On the one hand, such efforts would hardly seem necessary: the gross motor disturbances of parkinsonian gait, tremors, oculogyric crises or ataxic limbs were nothing if not spectacular disturbances of the victims' nervous systems. But acute cases were often fleeting, and chronic instances of the disease rare (or, at least, rarely diagnosed as such). Neurologists struggled to grasp the incidence of the infection in the general population and failed to successfully formulate an accurate natural history of the disease over the long term. The latency of the condition, both as an acute infection that could easily be confused with influenza and as a chronic neurological condition whose diverse outcomes seemed reducible to no systematic neurological assay, was the primary object of interest for those neurologists who took the "epidemic" aspect of encephalitis lethargica seriously. The logic of the ARNMD suggested that this latency was as much within the published literature as it was among the population at large. The ARNMD's solution to making epidemic encephalitis visible was thus to devise a way to systematically sort through all the available literature on the topic, while at the same time combining it into a form that could gain universal assent and be widely circulated. The group's bibliographic surveillance project, which culminated in the Matheson Commission's 1929 publication on epidemic encephalitis, represents a novel technique to transcend the boundaries of neurological knowledge and practice. Under the rubric of a little-known neurological condition, it both compiled masses of published literature that went far beyond conventional neurological publications and simultaneously attempted to disseminate this knowledge to an audience with little neurological expertise, in the clear hope they would more readily identify the condition and thereby help illuminate the extent of its latency.

At the international level, on the other hand, neurological knowledge appears to have played a much less ambitious role. Despite the active involvement of several neurologists, the LNHO's concern with epidemic encephalitis was not piqued until it appeared to threaten vaccination—a cornerstone of an emerging international health. Like the ARNMD, the LNHO was designed to coordinate and disseminate expertise across extant boundaries (enacted by medical specialization in the former case and geopolitics in the latter). Its central epistemological tools were consensus conferences and large-scale data collection. But the LNHO, like some other technical committees of the League, ultimately proved more successful than the League's efforts at peacekeeping and protecting minority populations precisely because of its limited purview.[75] Its focus and leverage came from the creation and standardization of public health tools; research and discovery, on the other hand, were not part of its mandate. In such a configuration, epidemic encephalitis proved less a curiosity in and of itself than an amorphous condition that could potentially undermine the League's mandate to extend, in a tangible way, preventative measures to preserve health. At first blush, this seems counterintuitive: identifying the smallpox vaccine as the central cause leading to postvaccinal encephalitis would seem to threaten the status of vaccination more than picking out a mysterious new infection as the culprit. But even though its precise mode of action was not understood, vaccinia was still artifice. As such, it was subject to modification by all the measures and controls then familiar to League technical committees. Epidemic encephalitis, on the other hand, was a natural force still largely resistant to human understanding. Uncovering its latency in this instance quite literally meant unleashing a terrible disease through vaccination. Where the Association for Research in Nervous and Mental Disease could use epidemic encephalitis's naturalized status as a means to extend the reach and salience of neurological knowledge, the LNHO's Smallpox and Vaccination Commission made every effort to move around and past it.

Notes

Research for this chapter was funded by a Standard Research Grant (410–2009–1803) from the Social Science & Humanities Research Council of Canada. Much of the data was collected while I was an Invited Researcher at the Centre de recherche médecine, sciences, santé et société (Cermes3), CNRS UMR 8169, Inserm U750 in 2009–10. Feedback from Jean-Paul Gaudillère and Ilana Löwy proved particularly valuable. I was able to develop considerable insight into the "globalized" structure of epidemics in my graduate STS seminar on that topic at York University in the fall of 2014—my thanks for the enthusiastic participation of students in that course. Thanks are also due to Francesc Rodríguez for his quantitative analysis of the MC bibliography, which helped shape my arguments. Finally, I want to thank Delia Gavrus and Stephen Casper for their critical engagement with and continual support of my work (through all manner of trial and tribulation).

1. Nikolas Rose and Joelle Abi-Rached, *Neuro: The New Brain Sciences and the Management of the Mind* (Princeton, NJ: Princeton University Press, 2013), 25–52.

2. Joseph Dumit, *Picturing Personhood: Brain Scans and Biomedical Identity* (Princeton, NJ: Princeton University Press, 2004); Mathew Thomson, *Psychological Subjects: Identity, Culture, and Health in Twentieth-Century Britain* (New York: Oxford University Press, 2006); Erika Dyck, *Psychedelic Psychiatry: LSD from Clinic to Campus* (Baltimore: Johns Hopkins University Press, 2008).

3. Gil Eyal et al., *The Autism Matrix: The Social Origins of the Autism Epidemic* (Cambridge: Polity, 2010).

4. Nicholas B. King, "The Scale Politics of Emerging Disease," *Osiris* 19 (2004): 62–76.

5. Volker Hess and J. Andrew Mendelsohn, "Case and Series: Medical Knowledge and Paper Technology, 1600–1900," *History of Science* 48 (2010): 287–314.

6. Sherman McCall, James M. Henry, Ann H. Reid et al., "Influenza RNA Not Detected in Archival Brain Tissues from Acute Encephalitis Lethargica Cases or in Postencephalitic Parkinson Cases," *Journal of Neuropathology and Experimental Neurology* 60 (2001): 696–704; J. A. Vilensky and S. Gilman, "Encephalitis Lethargica: Could This Disease Be Recognised if the Epidemic Recurred?," *Nature Clinical Practice Neurology* 6 (2006): 360–67; P. P. Mortimer, "Historical Review: Was Encephalitis Lethargica a Post-Influenzal or Some Other Phenomenon? Time to Re-examine the Problem," *Epidemiology and Infection* 137 (2009): 449–55.

7. Kenton Kroker, "Epidemic Encephalitis and American Neurology, 1919–1940," *Bulletin of the History of Medicine* 78 (2004): 108–47.

8. Michael Bresalier, "Neutralizing Flu: 'Immunological Devices' and the Making of a Virus Disease," in *Crafting Immunity: Working Histories of Clinical Immunology*, ed. K. Kroker, J. Keelan, and P. M. H. Mazumdar, 107–44 (Aldershot, UK: Ashgate, 2008); Kenton Kroker, "Creatures of Reason? Picturing Viruses at the Pasteur Institute during the 1920s," in *Crafting Immunity: Working Histories of Clinical Immunology*, ed. K. Kroker, J. Keelan, and P. M. H. Mazumdar, 145–64 (Aldershot, UK: Ashgate, 2008). See also Michael Bresalier, "Uses of a Pandemic: Forging the Identities of Influenza and Virus Research in Interwar Britain," *Social History of Medicine* 25 (2008): 400–24.

9. Paul Foley, "The Encephalitis Lethargica Patient as a Window on the Soul," in *The Neurological Patient in History*, ed. L. Stephen Jacyna and Stephen T. Casper, 184–211 (Rochester NY: University of Rochester Press, 2012).

10. Ian Hacking, "Telepathy: Origins of Randomization in Experimental Design," *Isis* 79 (1988): 427–51.

11. Kroker, "Epidemic Encephalitis."

12. Four were from Philadelphia, two were from Baltimore, and one was from Boston. The rest included William Boyd (professor of Pathology and Histology at the University of Manitoba); George Hassin (professor of Neurology at the University of Illinois, Chicago); and William Thalhimer (director of Laboratories at Columbia Hospital in Milwaukee). See "List of Contributors" in Association for Research in Nervous and Mental Disease (hereafter ARNMD), *Acute Epidemic Encephalitis (Lethargic Encephalitis): An Investigation by the Association for Research in Nervous and Mental Diseases* (New York: Paul B Hoeber, 1921), ix–xi.

13. ARNMD, *Acute Epidemic Encephalitis*, xvii.

14. George Weisz, *Divide and Conquer: A Comparative History of Medical Specialization* (Oxford: Oxford University Press, 2006), 127–46.

15. ARNMD, *Acute Epidemic Encephalitis*, xix.

16. Harry M. Marks, "'Until the Sun of Science . . . the True Apollo of Medicine Has Risen': Collective Investigation in Britain and America, 1880–1910," *Medical History* 50 (2006): 147–66.

17. Andrew Cunningham and Perry Williams, eds., *The Laboratory Revolution in Medicine* (Cambridge: Cambridge University Press, 1992). A cogent critique can be found in Michael Worboys, "Was There a Bacteriological Revolution in Late Nineteenth-Century Medicine?," *Studies in History and Philosophy of Biological and Biomedical Sciences* 38 (2007): 20–42.

18. Kenton Kroker, "Immunity and Its Other: The Anaphylactic Selves of Charles Richet," *Studies in History and Philosophy of Biological and Biomedical Sciences* 30 (1999): 273–96; Christopher Gradmann, "Locating Therapeutic Vaccines in Nineteenth-Century History," *Science in Context* 21 (2008): 145–60; Pauline Mazumdar, "Antitoxin and *Anatoxine*: The League of Nations and the Institut Pasteur, 1920–1939," in *Crafting Immunity: Working Histories of Clinical Immunology*, ed. K. Kroker, J. Keelan, and P. M. H. Mazumdar, 177–97 (Aldershot, UK: Ashgate, 2008).

19. Kroker, "Creatures of Reason?," 145–64.

20. Delia Gavrus, "Men of Dreams and Men of Action: Neurologists, Neurosurgeons, and the Performance of Professional Identity, 1920–1950," *Bulletin of the History of Medicine* 85 (2011): 57–92; Katja Guenther, "Exercises in Therapy— Neurological Gymnastics between *Kurort* and Hospital Medicine, 1880–1945," *Bulletin of the History of Medicine* 88 (2014): 102–31.

21. ARNMD, *Epidemic Encephalitis*, 157.

22. Matheson Commission, *Epidemic Encephalitis: Etiology, Epidemiology, Treatment: Report of a Survey by the Matheson Commission* (New York: Columbia University Press, 1929). Hereafter MC.

23. Ibid., xiii.

24. François Dagognet, *Etienne-Jules Marey: A Passion for the Trace*, trans. Robert Galeta with Jeanine Herman (New York: Zone, 1992); Marta Braun, *Picturing Time: The Work of Étienne-Jules Marey (1830–1904)* (Chicago: University of Chicago Press, 1992); Lorraine Daston and Peter Galison, *Objectivity* (New York: Zone, 2007).

25. Joel D. Howell, *Technology in the Hospital: Transforming Patient Care in the Early Twentieth Century* (Baltimore: Johns Hopkins University Press, 1995); Marc Berg and Paul Harterink, "Embodying the Patient: Records and Bodies in Early 20th-Century US Medical Practice," *Body & Society* 10 (2004): 13–41.

26. For a notable exception, see Alex Csiszar, "Seriality and the Search for Order: Scientific Print and Its Problems during the Late Nineteenth Century," *History of Science* 48 (2010): 399–434.

27. Estelle Broadman, *The Development of Medical Bibliography*, Medical Library Association Publication No. 1 (Baltimore: Waverly Press, 1954).

28. Welch quoted in Lucretia W. McClure, "A Student of History: Perspectives on the Contributions of Estelle Brodman," *Journal of the Medical Library Association* 96 (2008): 255–61.

29. Fielding Garrison, "The Uses of Medical Bibliography and Medical History in the Medical Curriculum," *Journal of the American Medical Association* 66 (1916): 319–24.

30. J. Andrew Mendelsohn, "From Eradication to Equilibrium: How Epidemics Became Complex after World War I," in *Greater than the Parts: Holism in Biomedicine, 1920–1950*, ed. Christopher Lawrence and George Weisz (New York: Oxford University Press, 1998).

31. Martin David Dubin, "The League of Nations Health Organization," in *International Organizations and Health Movements, 1918–39*, ed. Paul Weindling (Cambridge: Cambridge University Press, 1995): 56–80, 73.

32. Francis Graham Crookshank, *Epidemiological Essays* (London: K. Paul, Trench, & Trubner, 1930); Olga Amsterdamska, "Demarcating Epidemiology," *Science, Technology, & Human Values* 30 (2005): 17–51.

33. R. T. Ravenholt and W. H. Foege, "Influenza, Encephalitis Lethargica, Parkinsonism," *The Lancet* 2 (1982): 860–64; Vilensky and Gilman, "Encephalitis Lethargica"; C. P. Manriz, "Influenza Caused Epidemic Encephalitis: The Circumstantial Evidence and a Challenge to the Nay-Sayers," *Medical Hypotheses* 28 (1989): 139–42; P. P. Mortimer, "Historical Review: Was Encephalitis Lethargica a Post-Influenzal or Some Other Phenomenon? Time to Re-Examine the Problem," *Epidemiology and Infection* 137 (2009): 449–55.

34. Alan C. Parsons, A. Salusbury Macnalty, and J. R. Perdrau, *Reports on Public Health and Medical Subjects No. 11: Report on Epidemic Encephalitis* (London: Ministry of Health, 1922), 330.

35. Ibid., 171–255.

36. A notable exception can be found in the preface (written by George Newman, the ministry's chief medical officer), which noted that the appendix showed very small numbers of case-to-case case contagion, thereby supporting the notion that it was spread by undetected healthy carriers; the nervous sequelae listed in another appendix demonstrated a lack of complications from other infections (ibid., viii).

37. Lion Murard, "La santé publique et ses instruments de mesure: Des barèmes évaluatifs américans aux indices numériques de la Société des Nations, 1915–1955," in *Body Counts: Medical Quantification in Historical and Sociological Perspective*, ed. G. Jorland, A. Opinel and G. Weisz, 266–308 (Montreal: McGill-Queen's University Press, 2005); Mazumdar, "Antitoxin and *Anatoxine*"; Iris Borowy, *Coming to Terms with International Health: The League of Nations Health Organization, 1921–1946* (Frankfurt am Main: Peter Lang, 2009).

38. The MC deployed a similar approach, including with its 1929 report a table (XI) of the international incidence of the disease, in which the origins of each

nation's figures were described as coming from literary ("L R") or official ("O R") reports.

39. Major Greenwood, "Sir George S. Buchanan, C.B., M.D., F.R.C.P.," *British Medical Journal* 2, no. 3958 (October 17, 1936): 788–9.

40. Borowy, *Coming to Terms with International Health*, 41–48, 84–85. Buchanan became president of the OIHP in 1932 and typically advanced its interests over those of the LNHO.

41. George S. Buchanan, "An Address on International Organization and Public Health," *British Medical Journal* (March 5, 1921): 335.

42. Ibid., 332.

43. See "Second meeting, 15 August 1922, 10 a.m.," in League of Nations Health Committee, *Minutes of the Fourth Session, Held at Geneva, 14–21 August 1922*, 12 (hereafter LNHC Minutes). Held at the United Nations Office at Geneva Library, League of Nations Archive (LNA), ref. C.555.M.337.1922.III.

44. See "Third meeting, 16 August 1922, 10 a.m.," LNHC Minutes, 13–14.

45. See t/s circular letter, dated March 23, 1923, in League of Nations (LN), Correspondence, "Enquiry Respecting Encephalitis Lethargica 1923," LNA, R.869, Doc. no. 27370.

46. LN, "Enquiry Respecting Encephalitis Lethargica 1923," LNA, R.869, Doc. no. 27386.

47. Ibid., Doc. no 273782.

48. Ibid., Doc. no 27888. Cumming's observation was also reported in the *New York Times*, "'Flu' the Precursor of Sleeping Sickness, March 18, 1923, 4.

49. "Epidemic and Other Forms of Encephalitis," *Weekly Epidemiological Record* 14 (December 14, 1939): 543.

50. For examples, see James Colgrove, *State of Immunity: The Politics of Vaccination in Twentieth-Century America* (Berkeley: University of California Press, 2006), and Jennifer Keelan, "Risk, Efficacy, and Viral Attenuation in Debates over Smallpox Vaccination in Montreal, 1870–1877," in *Crafting Immunity: Working Histories of Clinical Immunology*, ed. K. Kroker, J. Keelan, and P. M. H. Mazumdar, 29–54 (Aldershot, UK: Ashgate, 2008).

51. Frank Fenner, D. A. Henderson, and I. Arita et al., *Smallpox and Its Eradication* (Geneva: World Health Organization 1988); William H. Foege, *House on Fire: The Fight to Eradicate Smallpox* (Berkeley: University of California Press, 2011).

52. Examples include Sanjoy Bhattacharya, *Expunging Variola: The Control and Eradication of Smallpox in India, 1947–1977* (London: Sangam, 2006); Christopher Rutty, "Canadian Vaccine Research, Production and International Regulation: Connaught Laboratories and Smallpox Vaccines, 1962–1980," in *Crafting Immunity: Working Histories of Clinical Immunology*, ed. K. Kroker, J. Keelan, and P. M. H. Mazumdar, 273–800 (Aldershot, UK: Ashgate, 2008).

53. Bernardino Fantini, "Les organisations sanitaires internationales face à l'émergence de maladies infectieuses nouvelles," *History and Philosophy of the Life Sciences* 15 (1993): 436.

54. H. M. Turnbull and J. McIntosh, "Encephalo-Myelitis Following Vaccination," *British Journal of Experimental Pathology* 7 (1926): 181–222.

55. Ibid., 219–20.

56. Turnbull's entry in *Munk's Roll* states that "early publication was prohibited at the time by the Ministry of Health." See the Royal College of Physicians, "Lives of the Fellows," accessed May 29, 2014, http://munksroll.rcplondon.ac.uk.

57. Virginia Berridge, *Opium and the People: Opiate Use and Drug Control Policy in Nineteenth and Early Twentieth Century England* (London: Free Association Books, 1999).

58. Christopher Gradmann and Johnathan Simon, eds., *Evaluating and Standardizing Therapeutic Agents, 1890–1950* (Basingstoke: Palgrave Macmillan, 2010).

59. "Variola Research," *British Medical Journal* 1, no. 3398 (February 13, 1926): 293–94.

60. Committee on Vaccination (Ministry of Health), "Request to Medical Practitioners," *British Medical Journal* 1, no. 3408 (April 24, 1926): 748.

61. As quoted in MC, *Epidemic Encephalitis*, 132–33.

62. "Vaccination and Encephalitis," *British Medical Journal* 1, no. 3654 (January 17, 1931): 104–5. Such qualifications regarding the limitations of neurological knowledge might well have been fueled by the recent debacle over the (quickly discredited) discovery of a vaccine for multiple sclerosis, which similarly turned on the question of the accuracy of neurological diagnosis. See Stephen T. Casper, "Trust, Protocol, Gender, and Power in Interwar British Biomedical Research: Kathleen Chevassut and the 'Germ' of Multiple Sclerosis," *Journal of the History of Medicine and Allied Sciences* 66 (2011): 180–215.

63. Borowy, *Coming to Terms with International Health*, 285–86.

64. Ibid., 309–10.

65. Kroker, "Creatures of Reason?," 145–64.

66. Details on the committee can be found in the League's annual report for 1926, and in LN, "Correspondence Concerning Complications Resulting in Certain Cases from Anti-smallpox Vaccination," LNA, R.960 (1925), Classement no. 12B, Doc. no. 43681. A summary of the conference was published as "Small-Pox, Alastrim, and Vaccinia," *British Medical Journal* 1, no. 3398 (February 13, 1926): 299–300.

67. Letter from Ludwick Rajchman to Ricardo Jorge, June 12, 1925, LNA, R.960 (1925), Classement no. 12B, doc. no. 43681.

68. Letters from Ricardo Jorge to Ludwick Rachjman, July 3 and 11, 1925. It should be noted that Jorge's letter does not identify Levaditi by name, indicating only that "in Paris, I will be seeing M. . . ." But the reference to neurovaccine and subsequent discussion makes it clear that Levaditi is the subject of Jorge's commentary.

69. Letter from Ricardo Jorge to Ludwick Rachjman, July 2, 1925.

70. LNA, R.961V (1926), classement no. 126, doc. no. 50779. April 1926.

71. For examples, see Simon Flexner "Postvaccinal Encephalitis," *Transactions of the Association of American Physicians* 44 (1929): 181. See also the draft versions of this paper held in the Flexner Papers of the American Philosophical Association, Philadelphia, B:F365 "Encephalitis, Postvaccinal." See also Ricardo Jorge, "Post-Vaccinal Encephalitis: Its Association with Vaccination and with Post-Infectious and Acute Disseminated Encephalitis," *The Lancet* 219, no. 5656 (January 23, 1932): 215–19.

72. LN, "Press Communiqué on the Hague Conference, January, 1926," LNA, doc. no. 49079.

73. LN, "Post-vaccinal Encephalitis: Report of Sub-committee on Its Session of January 1927," LNA, doc no. 57089.

74. Charles Armstrong, "Postvaccinal Encephalitis," *Public Health Reports* 44 (1929): 2041–44.

75. Susan Pedersen, "Back to the League of Nations," *American Historical Review* 112 (2007): 1091–1117.

Chapter Four

Circuits, Algae, and Whipped Cream

The Biophysics of Nerve, ca. 1930

MAX STADLER

> There will be nothing that the average man sees, hears or buys that will
> not be controlled, regulated or affected in some important respect by
> an electronic tube!
>
> —O. H. Caldwell, 1930

The intimate entanglements of electrical technologies and nervous phenomena belong to the better charted territories in the history of the
neurosciences. The metaphors of the telegraph, switchboard, battery, or
computing machinery make for familiar reading, as do narratives of laboratories in the midst of urban electrification or of scientists chasing impon-
derable fluids, nervous "messages," and "codes": from Leyden jars to Cold
War electronics, historians of science have explored at great lengths the
careers of animal electricity. Their actors, too, typically were quick to point
to the signal importance of such entanglements. "The history of electrophysiology has been decided by the history of electric recording instruments," as the great Edgar Adrian ventured in his *Mechanism of Nervous
Action* (1932), his fellow British countrymen still recovering from the
Faraday Centenary the year before (generally a cause for the celebration
of electric progress, of course).[1]

The very "gadgets" of physiology thus may have fostered the "kind of electrical double-talk concerning nerve" in which everyone indulged. Thus pondered Columbia neurophysiologist Harry Grundfest some twenty years later
at the First Macy Conference on the "Nerve Impulse" in 1950—just having

lived through yet another (this time electronic) upheaval in the annals of electrophysiology.[2] Nuances apart, historians have mostly found themselves in agreements with such verdicts.[3] And a very similar picture of entanglement will be belabored in the present essay, which deals with the production of electrophysiological knowledge in the proverbial "radio-age" of the 1920s and 1930s. But in doing so, I aim to add a historiographical twist to the story of nervous activity. This essay is less interested, that is, in showing how electrical things shaped, or did not shape, the sciences of the nervous system; nor is it to demonstrate that instruments or metaphors are important—historians of science already know that. Rather, it aims to show how these electrical things, their uses, and the knowledge effects they had may prompt us to reconsider the nature of those very sciences. Thus, below circuits and nerves *will* be featured—along with such items as algae and whipped cream.

The point, if you will, is to defamiliarize us from a neuroscientific past that always already has revolved, however unsophisticatedly, around a coherent object: the mind/brain. The interwar pursuit of bioelectricity, as we shall see, is one such site of apparent incoherence; or, put positively, a site where quite different, more "fractured" kinds of lineage become palpable. The period, to be sure, also saw the origins of electroencephalography, or the infamous "war" of the "soups and sparks," but such episodes do not exhaust the sheer breadth of items that meant puzzles to electrically minded scientists.[4] Attending to the material cultures of electricity that got enrolled in the process helps to see this, as this chapter argues. For these weren't "instruments" so much as aggregations of electrical elements—themselves rhizomatic, omnipresent, and indeed, ready to hand; in turn, they spawned experimental techniques of rearranging, reassembling, and retooling that could be put to multiple uses. The elucidation of the nerve impulse was one of them.

As the (then newly launched) journal *Electronics* advised in 1931, "The best radio designer is the one who draws on and skilfully assembles the existing experiences of the best makes of components and parts."[5] It would have been an apt description for the radio-age physiologist, too; and in many ways, then, this essay is concerned with the inverse problem pursued in this volume by Frank Stahnisch on "materials"; not with the scientific things that migrate, but with the technical things, the components and parts, that were, in a sense, already there.

Prelude: 1939

To enter the interwar sciences of organic circuitry, let us take the story a bit back first. The year 1939, as specialists will know, was important in terms of the nervous impulse. That summer, at the Plymouth Marine Biological

Station in England, young Alan Hodgkin and his (younger still) collaborator Andrew Huxley pulled off the delicate feat of measuring the nervous action potential *across* the surface of a *single* nerve fiber, "intracellularly."[6] Both descendants of the famed Cambridge school of physiology, they promptly unearthed a somewhat puzzling phenomenon that hitherto had escaped physiological investigators. For various (mostly technical) reasons, physiologists traditionally had tended to busy themselves with *extra*cellular measurements; that is, to measurements *along* the surface of a nerve. The phenomenon in question—a "reversal" or "overshoot," as Hodgkin and Huxley labeled it, of the cellular potential during activity—was indeed something unheard of in the annals of electrobiology. Or rather, it was defying the received wisdom (which had it that a cell's electric potential should vanish, not reverse its polarity).

Across the ocean that summer at Woods Hole, Massachusetts, and not coincidentally deploying a very similar setup—Hodgkin had just recently returned from there—the biophysicists Kenneth Cole and his colleague Howard Curtis broke new ground as well.[7] For their part, Cole and Curtis managed to detect, by similarly "direct" means, a change of resistance of the nerve membrane during activity. Or to be precise, they detected a change of the nerve's "impedance"—crudely, its *alternating* current resistance. This too was no negligible achievement, for little was known about the physical properties of this elusive structure except "indirectly" and by means of speculation; and even less was known about its dynamic behavior. The accompanying record is an iconic one (see fig. 4.1): a photograph of the surface of a cathode ray tube screen, the tube itself connected, via a multistage amplifier, to a microelectrode; the electrode, in turn, carefully inserted into the interior of a squid giant axon.

The subsequent, considerable career of the squid giant axon as an experimental object need not concern us here; neither will Hodgkin and Huxley's rise to fame in the early 1950s or, for that matter, what contemporaries were quick to identify as one of the "brightest chapters of neurophysiology and even biology of all time"—their seminal, computational model of the nervous impulse.[8] It is a seemingly technical detail that interests me here: the change in "impedance" pictured above. Or more precisely, it is the world of biophysical practice it emerged from: an electrobiological world that was stranger, I shall argue, than the received plotline—from Galvani to *Aplysia*—would seem to suggest.[9] While, with hindsight, the records obtained by Cole—much like Hodgkin and Huxley's—do form a central role in the postwar story of protoneuroscientific consolidation, they also point to a past which fits that teleology less neatly. Indeed, as a closer look at the genealogies of the above "change in impedance" will reveal, nervous activity—let alone the activity of brains and minds—was typically not at stake as radioage scientists worked out the details of "animal" electricity. Rather, at stake

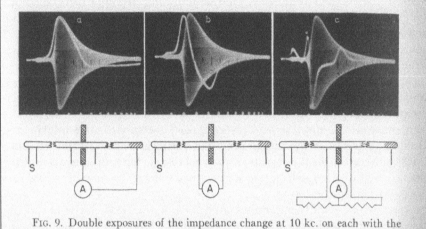

FIG. 9. Double exposures of the impedance change at 10 kc. on each with the action potential in each picture from the circuit shown below it. (a) is V, the monophasic potential, (b) is V_1, the first derivative or axial current, and (c) is V_{11} the second derivative or membrane current. The time marks at the bottom are 1 millisecond apart.

Figure 4.1. "Impedance" change in the squid giant axon. © 1939, K. S. Cole and H. J. Curtis, "Electric Impedance of the Squid Giant Axon during Activity," *Journal of General Physiology* 22, no. 5 (1939): 655, doi:10.1085/jgp.22.5.649.

were nerves, muscles, hearts, legs, arms, torsos, breast tumors, algae, even microbes and suspensions of "whipped cream"—a range of epistemic objects that come across as fairly disparate in retrospect; they do have the virtue of making it possible to conjure up a different, less brain-centered image of the neuroscientific past.

In other words, the production of bioelectric knowledge in the interwar period was a considerably more eclectic affair than what the emphasis on places such as Cambridge, eminent figures such as E. D. Adrian, or the more obvious applications—the EEG and the vacuum tube amplifier—tends to imply (important as they were).[10] By the same token, while it was a technique largely alien to "classical" nerve-and-muscle physiology, to zero in on the impedance of nerve was a far from unsystematic (or unobvious) manoeuvre vis-à-vis the study of so-called *excitable* tissue, broadly conceived (as interwar physiologists were inclined to conceive it). Much of this essay will be concerned, therefore, with the diverse range of sites, actors, and excitable "materials" that did serve the advance of bioelectrical knowledge at the time; and much of it will be concerned, consequently, with the technological infrastructure connecting those various dots: the practical culture—and conceptual universe—of the radio (or "wireless"). The incursions of the radio arts into the realms of bioelectricity—or what at first sight might seem to be at best a tangent to the True Story of neuroscience—in fact was a significant, epistemological turning point. In the study of nervous phenomena, it implicated a turn toward an epistemology of "measurement" and (so-called) "models," displacing physiologists' earlier predilection for curves, graphs, and ultimate "laws."[11] From this perspective, the 1939 episode recounted above was less of a beginning but a symptom: a case of well-honed, biophysical techniques implanted into seemingly purer realms of physiological science (we shall return to the episode in conclusion).

In what follows, I approach this gradual shift in techniques and technologies from several angles: as a matter of cultural, and conceptual appropriations—the adoption and creative (re)uses of the "wireless" arts in the biological laboratory; as a matter of practical knowledge (including therapeutic applications of electricity); and, finally, as a matter of transmogrifying biophysical objects, from algae to nerve.

The Laws of Excitation

The significance of "wireless" in this story will turn out to largely revolve around the domestication of alternating currents (AC) at the time. The reason is, by and large, simple. Traditionally, studying nerve (or muscle) scientifically meant deriving *laws*—the laws of excitation. It also meant *stimulating* the nerves (so that their activity could then be recorded). This, in turn, implied—by virtue of their excitatory powers—the use of *direct* (or galvanic) current (DC).

Historians of the physiological sciences, quite understandably, have been enthralled by the production of "inscriptions" in this type of experimentation (or so-called graphic methods), neglecting somewhat the great efforts that had always been devoted to, as it were, the reverse operation: the production of *interventions*.[12] By the 1930s, an immense variety of devices had become available to this very end, littering trade journals, scientific articles, and the catalogues of scientific instrument makers: all were means to enumerate currents, from "classic" electro-mechanical devices such as ballistic rheotoms or pendulums to rotating commutators; so-called chronaximeters; "make and break" circuits; arbitrary wave forms etched onto gramophone records; and increasingly so, fully electrical outfits. Neon lights, for example—widely used for advertising—were most suitable for the purposes of "rhythmic" stimulation: faster, more accurate, and more reliable than anything that could be achieved by electromechanical means.[13]

A whole story remains to be written here regarding these devices of synthesis, but for present purposes it will do to point out only one, central bifurcation. Whereas direct currents were, evidently, eminently suited to excite, alternating currents, curiously enough, had no such excitatory effects when applied to organic tissues (even though they were perfectly suited to electrocute microbes, rodents, and even elephants, as readers familiar with the late nineteenth-century "war of the currents" will recall).[14] Alternating, high frequency currents were less easily handled, too. As late as 1908, for example, the physical chemist Walther Nernst—always keen to weigh in on electrophysiological matters—declared in his "Theory of the Electrical Stimulus" that, all things told, it remained virtually impossible to generate alternating currents "pure" enough to even begin to ground the tremendous amount of speculation surrounding their putative organic action.[15]

But along came the "modern comforts of broadcasting" (as Adrian put it);[16] most notably, of course, along came the vacuum tube. Indeed, the many "triumphs" of the vacuum tube—exemplar of "modern universal instrumentality," as the electric boosters had it—prominently included the "production" of alternating currents—"of any desired frequency."[17] And once reined in, alternating currents swiftly accrued an increasing range of biomedical uses, too: therapeutic, diagnostic, surgical, and so on. It could, after all, be done and at the very least, there was an "intense modernism" about it (as the growing numbers of medical proponents enthused).[18]

This amounted, one might complain (as some did), to little more than the indiscriminate deployment of an immature technology. But indiscriminate or not, before long these uses did make salient a range of different electrophysiological effects and properties—different, that is, from the typical electrophysiological roster. As we shall see shortly, this prominently included the electrical properties—impedance, capacitance, and so forth— of organic materials. It was a subtle but significant departure because, as the Harvard physiologists Hallowell Davis and Alexander Forbes noted in 1936, physiologists were seemingly obsessed with something else entirely; namely, with the properties of stimulation currents and corresponding tissue responses—and hence with said "laws" of excitation.[19] Taking stock, Davis and Forbes then made a point in putting together almost thirty such laws, derived in recent years, as they explained, in the futile hope that the ongoing proliferation of experimental observations might be "covered ultimately by a single law and formula."[20]

Reflecting the daily routines of much physiological practice—stimulating and recording—these formulae and their diagrammatic representations, so-called strength-duration curves, indeed had become ubiquitous, omnipresent in journals, textbooks, and laboratory manuals. But for all the progress in precision and exactitude, the "true picture" of bioelectrical activity, it seemed, was as distant as ever.[21] The popular concepts of the day, traveling under names such as "excitation-time," "temps utile," "chronological coefficient of excitation," "time factor," "Nutzzeit," "Kennzeit," and—most infamously—the "chronaxie"—did not help it;[22] this confusing abundance of inscriptions all were variations on the same empiricist theme: the urge to establish such more or less "arbitrary" but quantitative relationships between the electrical stimulus properties on the one hand (such as its duration), and the responses of irritable tissues on the other (say, the interval between stimulus onset and impulsive reaction).

Or we should say beliefs that these laws and curves were "arbitrary," crudely empirical, merely "phenomenological" and lacking "immediate physical sense" constituted a lament that was being voiced with increasing frequency by physiologists from across the electrified world. Their practical usefulness being widely acknowledged, nothing in this veritable, DC-driven natural history of curves was at all "direct" or, for that matter, intellectually defensible: so went the gist of these complaints, which picked up steam toward the late 1920s.[23] In the words of one Cambridge physiologist, William Rushton, it was difficult to find a "physical justification" for such formal maneuvers, much less to "find a physical meaning to it."[24] Mere "fitting" of curves ventured the young Bernard Katz;[25] a "Kunstprodukt" [artifice] without "physiological correlate," decried another German physiologist.[26] Worse, deviations from the ideal, law-derived curves became suspiciously manifest especially for the "smallest times"—by 1930 these were in the range of a millionth of a second, and they were manifest as well in cases of "prolonged" stimulation, when so-called accommodation effects noticeably set in.[27]

In brief, the progress of electrical precision did not straightforwardly translate into progress when it came to making sense of the "quantitative fixation" of tissue excitation.[28] Even physiologists' best guess in the direction of "physical sense"—Julius Bernstein's so-called membrane theory—was increasingly eyed was suspicion. It had degenerated into a "means of lulling the mind," as the "axonologist" Herbert Gasser complained in 1933.[29] Not too much, of course, should be made of such crisis talk, but as an indicator of tendencies, it is instructive. For there was, significantly, a great deal of movement at the fringes of the "classic" nerve-and-muscle physiology—though this generally still failed to impress those operating at its center. Hans Schaefer's utterly comprehensive, two-volume tome *Elektrophysiologie,* finally completed in 1940, was symptomatic in this regard. The work was, according to Schaefer, confined to the more "theoretical" aspects of the subject (still including some six thousand references), but was unable to consider the "purely clinical-pathological" studies, topics of a mostly electrochemical and electrophoretic nature, the "physiology of short-waves" and of "high-voltage currents," and "all those things where the electrical [was] only technics [*Technik*]."[30]

Enter Biotechnics

Only "technics"—there was, no doubt, a lot of truth in Schaefer's exclusion principle (and by no means was Schaefer a stranger to the more technical dimensions of his subject matter). But the accumulated effect of such disciplinary stratification and streamlining, which would only intensify over the years to come, was to obscure the extent to which the "theoretical aspects," of course, had never been so neatly separate from the purely practical ones. In this regard, the 1920s and 1930s were distinguished not least by the emergence of a heterogeneous population of actors—Cole and Curtis among them—who would have felt rather comfortable with precisely the latter, technical aspects of all things bioelectrical. It was also a preoccupation usually involving simpler, and less delicate, objects than nerve (or even muscle). And for reasons explored below, these actors thus had little time for excitation laws or general solutions. Indeed measurements such as those pursued by Cole and Curtis demanded a different kind of theory: one based on models rather than laws.

To enter these terrains, consider the biophysical trajectory of Hugo Fricke (1892–1972).[31] His forays into the electrical properties of biological things will turn out to have profoundly shaped and prepared the biophysical vision of the nervous impulse, with which this essay opened. But such genealogies are all too easily obscured, as was already indicated. Operating in a world removed from the centers of the purer kinds of physiological science, Fricke's oeuvre was steeped in tumor cells, bacteria, blood corpuscles, and similarly simple objects. But neither was Fricke disconnected from the biomedical world at large; or rather, as we shall see, he did not remain so always. In 1928 Fricke became the first director of the Walter B. James Laboratory for Biophysics at Cold Spring Harbor on Long Island. For now, however, more revealing is Fricke's background: he had spent the previous decade or so as the resident biophysicist at George W. Crile's Cleveland Clinic Foundation, making a reputation for himself in the area of high-frequency measurements.

Crile, for his part, was a figure as notorious as he was distinguished.[32] "Dr. Crile Suggests That Our Bodies Are Electric Batteries" went a typical headline. Crile's daring biophysical theories predictably failed to enlist much sympathy among the more clear-headed students of living processes (more likely, such students sneered at "Crile's rather loose and uncritical methods of work").[33] Even so, Crile was an accomplished surgeon. And, propelled by a bizarre, electric vision of life as "bipolar," Crile fashioned himself into the role of true biophysical pioneer and enabler.[34] The Cleveland Clinic thus provided, for several (and much renowned) investigators, a first contact with, if not a more permanent home in the borderlands of physics and biomedicine. From here, Otto Glasser, remembered mostly as a biographer of Roentgen, was pushing the case for *Medical Physics* (1944) and *The Science of Radiology* (1933); he had joined Crile's enterprise in 1922 (after quitting his previous job with the German *BASF* concern). Meanwhile, Fricke—trained in engineering and physics in Denmark—had already been enrolled in Crile's sprawling program the previous year. And soon after, Kenneth Cole, then still a graduate student in physics at Cornell, made it on the temporary staff list as well.[35] Fricke, installed as the director of the clinic's biophysical laboratories, developed his work chiefly along two lines (as he later commended himself to the Cold Spring Harbor Laboratories): "the biological effect of radiation and the electric polarization and conductivity of biological cells."[36]

Both of these were subjects considered to be of immense significance by Crile, who had had his biophysical epiphany at least twice. First, in 1887, when Crile witnessed the death through "shock" of a fellow student whose legs had been crushed by a streetcar: "the dramatic picture of failing bodily energies and death."[37] And again, when Crile had to cope with the "intensive application of man to war" at the Western front (Crile being surgical director of the American Ambulance): millions of similar cases of "shock—a violent restless exit," as he reminisced, and phenomena leading him to reason "that man and other animals are physico-chemical mechanisms."[38] Back in Cleveland, Crile promptly initiated a series of biophysical investigations into the electrical conductivity of animal tissues, co-opting the special expertise of one Helen Hosmer, formerly of the General Electric Laboratories. The organism, Crile then inferred, was "operated by electricity"; in particular, as Crile determined, in a state of shock it was marked by a diminished conductivity especially of the brain and an increased conductivity of the liver.[39]

The framework had thus been set. As Crile hit the news with spectacular bioelectric discoveries (as happened every so often),[40] Fricke quietly embarked on figuring out the details. Most notably, toward the mid-1920s Fricke had begun to look into high-frequency measurements of blood, bacteria, and various animal tissues. Finally, here was a "precision method" that had, as Fricke explained, certain "practical implications" as well.[41] Their basic principle was simple enough, and in fact, long established. It left few traces because the goal was silence—the *absence* even of sound: equipped with, say, a telephone receiver (or similar "display"), when measuring with a so-called bridge-circuit (or "null" method) one was required to balance an unknown circuit component (or "arm") against a parallel, *known* one: silence meant balance—or, in electrical terms, "equivalence" (more on which below).[42]

What was new was the sheer range of frequencies at Fricke's disposal. As significant, a "most convenient and uncomplicated material for study" was found in tumors, something readily available at the clinic.[43] By 1926, in a paper on "The Electric Capacity of Tumors of the Breast," Fricke set out how a suspension of such malignant tissue, when injected with such high-frequency currents, "behaves as though it were a pure resistance in parallel with a pure capacity."[44] The diagnostic potential apart—certain types of malignant tumors, it turned out, featured an abnormally high capacitance— Fricke was already teasing out some of the theoretical implications as well.

As attentive readers of Crile's *Bipolar Theory of Life* (also appearing in 1926) would have known, in investigations such as this, "Dr. Fricke ha[d] found that the film which surrounds ... [biological] cells is in the order of 4/10,000,000 of a centimeter thick." Such "films of infinite thinness," according to Crile, were "peculiarly adapted to the storage and adaptive discharge of electric energy."[45] But Crile's *Bipolar Theory* need not distract us here; for present purposes, what was significant about Fricke's tumor experiments is that here was the germ of a *physical* model of the cell. Fricke, the practical biophysicist, had little time for, or interest in, establishing phenomenological correlations between stimulus and response. Nor, as the next section shows, did his biophysical peers. What mattered most to them were the physical characteristics and properties that now were exposed by rapidly undulating currents.

Medical Physics as a "Model" Science

The timing at any rate was opportune: Fricke's high-frequency forays into the electrical nature of biological membranes occurred at a time when the more business-minded men enthused that thanks to short-wave radio, these "once useless very short waves [were] becom[ing] most valuable."[46] The vacuum tube, and wireless technology generally, then turned from the experimental stage into commercial products. By 1923, 4.5 million tubes were produced annually in the United States, a figure reaching 69 million in 1929, with prices for tubes and materials plummeting. "Kaleidoscopic changes," the trade journals recorded, were underway in the electrical industry.[47] As wave-lengths diminished ever more rapidly, there emerged a true zoo of diodes, triodes, tetrodes, pentodes, thyratrons, magnetrons, rectifiers, and oscillators.

Fricke, too, was impressed. "Earlier investigations were handicapped by the experimental difficulties of producing alternating currents over a wide range of frequencies," he noted. "This difficulty was overcome by the introduction of the audion oscillator, which initiated a period of considerable progress."[48] And as Fricke knew well enough—because it had been done before (albeit with limited success) and because it was being done in many venues elsewhere—"an interesting application" of such very short waves consisted in the calculation of membrane *thickness* (on which these capacities depended). More generally, variations in tissue resistance, when subjected to alternating currents of varying frequency, allowed the physiologist to make inferences concerning the physical properties of the (preferably simple) biological objects so investigated; these included, as seen, their capacitance but also their *impedance*.

Such inferences, it is important to see, followed a somewhat different logic than the pursuit of "laws" by means of bioelectrical *stimulation*. By design, they gravitated toward the kind of physical "sense" that physiologists so sorely missed—or toward, to use the term that would grow in significance in subsequent years, *models*. Nor would they adequately be captured by filing them as a case of neuroscientific metaphor; by this time, the word *equivalence* was in the process of accruing a very definite and exacting meaning in many an electrotechnical field, most notably in telephone engineering and elec-tro-acoustics.[49] Indeed the very idea that organic materials were, somehow, electrically "equivalent" to this or that circuit was something that was being built into the practices of (bio)electrical *measurement* itself; it thus came nat-urally to anyone hailing from the technical peripheries of academic physiol-ogy (or what Schäfer above termed its "Randgebiete" [borderlands]).

From this perspective, a hodgepodge venture in medical physics such as Crile's Cleveland Clinic Foundation was fairly typical of the eclectic, make-shift technical culture that was interwar biophysical science.[50] What it lacked in prestige (or, as some might say, scientific mindedness), it frequently made up for in explorative (ab)use of electrical devices. In this, Crile's enterprise was not so much unlike the Institut für die Physikalischen Grundlagen der Medizin in Frankfurt, the Institut für physikalische Therapie in Vienna, or the Johnson Foundation for Medical Physics in Philadelphia (the latter funded by Eldridge R. Johnson of the Victor Talking Machine Company and headed by engineer-turned-nerve-physiologist Detlev Bronk). And one might add to this list many other venues, small and large, where a growing number of readily available, electrical things—from telephone-condensers, switches, and vacuum tubes to neon lamps, amplifiers, and cathode ray tubes—gradually transformed, often subtly, the face of biomedical science.[51]

What went under the name of "medical physics" was a most adventur-ous assortment of electrical instruments and gadgetry in particular.[52] It stretched from quartz lamps for home use to (increasingly) off-the-shelf devices for purposes as diverse as electrocardiography, X-rays, myotherapy, light therapy, or ultrashort wave therapy. Courtesy of firms eager to cash in on the modernity and cleanliness of such physical interventions—Radionta, Siemens, the British Hanovia Quartz Lamp Co., GEC, Icalite, Ulvira, Cox-Cavendish Electrical, and many more—there was no shortage of "new and highly technical" forms of treatment and diagnosis (so much so, in fact, as to prompt the British Medical Association to install a Register of Biophysical Assistants to regain some control over the matter);[53] even better, for those skilled enough, "handy, lucid, and comfortable" apparatus oftentimes was easily DIYed by making exclusive use of components, as one physiologist advised, "as [were] being used in radio technics and [were] available every-where, at relatively low cost and in excellent finish."[54]

Once unleashed and democratized, the proliferation of physical agents at the time—ranging from ions, UV rays, currents of high and ultra-high frequencies to the more controversial items such as radiogens and mitogenetic rays[55]—duly prompted curiosity regarding their physiological actions (if any). Of particular interest here, of course, are those investigations pertaining to the effects of the new, and newly precise, abundance of currents during the 1920s, which, as it was quickly appreciated, were most easily generated by the vacuum tube. A correlate to the ubiquity of the latter, biomedical scientists now increasingly trained their attention onto the various effects that high-frequency currents were found to provoke, or seemed to provoke, after all.

The new ultra-high frequencies especially fueled the biomedical imagination. Still in the early 1920s, as nerve-and-muscle physiologists turned to harnessing their fickle and failure-prone amplifiers for the purposes of analysis,[56] others discovered the tube's powers of synthesis. For example, Joseph Schereschewsky of the Office of Cancer Investigations of the US Public Health Service at Harvard University, was among the first to investigate the therapeutic action of such electrical waves with small animals and "inanimate models"; similar advances were due to the physician Erwin Schliephake in Germany who, in collaboration with the physicist Abraham Esau, took to the thermal "depth-effects" of such short waves, induced by means of a special "vacuum tube sender."[57] More spectacularly, figures such as the exiled Russian engineer Georges Lakhovsky would reveal the new applications of such short wave-length oscillations. Lakhovsky, "the well-known French scientist" (according to *Radio News*) by 1925 had created a *Radio Cellulo-Oscillator*, a device producing currents up to 150 million cycles-per-second. Reportedly, it had a morbid action on plant cells, tumors, and microbes; it also provided the technological substrate for Lakhovsky's many assaults on "orthodox medicine" such as, notably, *The Secret of Life* (1925) and *The Cellular Oscillation* (1931).[58]

More widespread deployment, however, found the less drastic effects of high-frequency currents. Fricke's investigations into the electrical nature of membranes are a case in point; more typically however, these effects concerned the production of heat, or what was known as diathermy. The means were the same, only the objective differed: analysis here, the useful distribution of currents in the body there. As the British textbook *Diathermy: Its Production and Uses* (1928) explained, "To generate a perceptible and measurable amount of heat in the tissues, a current . . . deprived of its power to stimulate the excitable tissues and to cause chemical (electrolytic) change [must be used]. This can be done by making it alternate at an exceedingly high rate. . . . It may be regarded as not less than 500,000 per second."[59] These peculiar thermal effects had first been noted by Tesla as early as 1891, an observation followed up in a more systematic fashion by the French physiologist Arsonval. Beginning in the early 1890s, Arsonval investigated the "sensation de chaleur désagréable" so produced, killing many a rabbit along the way through "overheating."[60] It wasn't until several years later that the medical chemist Richard von Zeynek first realized the therapeutic potential of such "Durchwärmung" (or thermo-penetration), while pursuing research in Nernst's laboratories in Göttingen. (Indeed, it was the puzzling, nonexcitatory effects of alternating currents that then had prompted Nernst to develop the aforementioned "exact, mathematico-physical theory of the phenomena of excitation" in 1908).[61] Almost simultaneously, the Berlin clinician Franz Nagelschmidt—later claiming priority—also introduced high frequencies into electrotherapeutic practice, calling it diathermy.[62]

After a slow start, which was hampered, as one leading diathermist opined, by the still mediocre "technic"—and the considerable reservations regarding the utilization of such currents—diathermy "undoubtedly occupied the prime position among the electro-physical therapies" by the late 1920s.[63] As proponents saw it, in Germany and elsewhere, high-frequency currents now provided a therapeutic means almost as "natural" as it was "rational"; there was, consequently, "scarcely a region of the body to which it ha[d] not been applied."[64] Meanwhile, as the technique was diffusing, the currents involved reached staggering proportions, or cycles-per-second. The year 1930, for instance, marked the advent of ultra-short wave therapy, when Willis Whitney, director of the General Electric research laboratories at Schenectady, New York, happened on "radio fever": "Men working in the field of a short wave radio transmitter," he found, "were having fever."[65] (Whitney promptly recruited Helen Hosmer, Fricke's former Cleveland colleague who, equipped with "powerful radio equipment," recreated the phenomenon with ease, being able to increase the temperature of both salt solutions and tadpoles by several degrees).

As a correlate to such electric business, the soon immense literature on diathermy and kindred short-wave applications was replete with attempts at elucidating the nature of AC currents, their putative physiological action, or the reality and presence of so-called specific effects (over and above the production of heat, that is); this naturally was a set of concerns typically accompanied by laments concerning the deficient physical and technical understanding of (most) medical practitioners. And it is here that our stories—the story of models-of-nerve and the story of applied biophysics—begin to intersect. For the generation of such physico-physiological knowledge was prompted in no small measure by the imperatives of high-frequency biomedical practice.

Textbooks on the subject thus routinely explained the nature of electricity and its biological effects.[66] But rather than puzzling over electricity's excitatory powers, practical biophysicists deployed a different register than academic physiologists, zeroing in on the spatial and temporal distribution of currents and on the physical properties of tissues such as dielectric constant, resistance, and "polarization capacity." Much like Fricke, who instinctively had turned to simple blood corpuscles and suspension of tumor cells, diathermy enthusiasts gravitated toward protein solutions, gelatine, or meat when investigating the "difficult subject of [bio-] electrical reactions."[67] They thus turned to the use of such simple, physical models when pondering the influence of, say, electrode shape and size on current distribution. Very nearly impossible to fathom in the abstract, high-frequency currents were most easily coaxed, for instance, into leaving their visible traces—or rather, three-dimensional zones (of coagulation) (see fig. 4.2).

In brief, the scientific cultures of bioelectricity that were taking shape around high-frequency currents differed in significant respects from the DC world of stimulus-response curves and "graphic methods." Where the latter stressed the correlations between their electric interventions and the phenomena induced, the former naturally was drawn to the physical properties of organic things; where the latter worried that the specificities of the electrical setups they employed were hopelessly entangled with—or deformed—the phenomena they induced, the former entangled things, as we shall see,

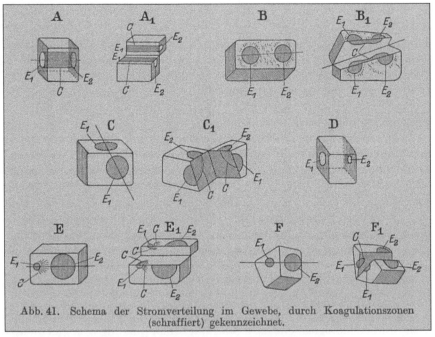

Abb. 41. Schema der Stromverteilung im Gewebe, durch Koagulationszonen (schraffiert) gekennzeichnet.

Figure 4.2. "Coagulated meat." Nagelschmidt, Lehrbuch der Diathermie für Ärzte und Studierende, Berlin, 1921, Springer-Verlag; Abbildung 41, p. 60.

on purpose: at its core resided the production of material "equivalence"—between gelatine and cells, cells and algae, algae and circuits.

To be sure, as theoretical entities, or for the purposes of calibration, quantities such as (tissue) resistance had long been of concern to physiologists. But ultimately, these projects—predicated on the regime of stimulation/response/inscription—had been geared toward other ends and constructs, many of them soon to be derided, as we have already heard, as merely phenomenological, treacherous "laws" and "formulae." In contrast, the techniques of high-frequency stimulation made salient quantities that, or so one said, had real "physical sense."

Circuits

The pursuit of circuit "equivalence" was not nearly exhausted by substituting patients for gelatine, of course. It didn't take long until such empiricist maneuvers were supplemented by a range of more theoretical considerations. As one medical scientist, this one based at the Rockefeller Institute for Medical Research, complained in 1927, hitherto, the spatio-temporal qualities of "heating effects" mainly had been studied "in vitro," preferably through "the coagulation of egg albumin or the cooking of meat and potatoes."[68] By implication, what was known about the physiological action of high-frequency currents was known mostly, and merely qualitatively, by "analogy" with what could be observed when electro-cooking various model-substances. Fortunately, the more abstractly minded biophysicists had already begun to intervene in the matter, turning such modeling-qua-substitution into a more formal affair.

For instance, Jesse McClendon. professor of physiologic chemistry at the University of Minnesota Medical School, already was pushing a more rigorous approach to such current distributions: "The extensive use of high frequency currents for heating the deeper tissues of the human body," as McClendon submitted in 1932, "has made it desirable to obtain more information on the path of the current between the electrodes and the distribution of heat in the tissues."[69] On McClendon's mind, in this regard it was the "localization of heating [that was] important." And therefore, it was essential to know the "seat of the . . . resistance." Like Fricke (who, we will remember, was after conductivity), McClendon thus availed himself to "bridge" circuits (see fig. 4.3)—"most extensively used by physical chemists, industrial chemists, and workers in biological sciences," as an assistant of McClendon's had explained in a 1928 review of the subject (characteristically, this focused especially on the beet root).[70]

Having extensively studied the electrical properties of sea urchin eggs, muscular tissue, and blood suspensions himself, McClendon was confident that, now, a "true reproduction of the circuit within the cell" could be

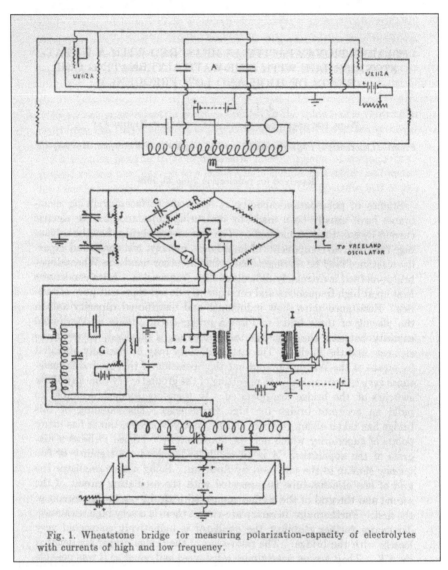

Fig. 1. Wheatstone bridge for measuring polarization-capacity of electrolytes with currents of high and low frequency.

Figure 4.3. Wheatstone bridge circuit (note the parallel "arms" in the center). J. F. McClendon, "Polarization-Capacity as Measured with a Wheatstone Bridge with Sine-Wave Alternating Currents of High and Low Frequency," *American Journal of Physiology* 91, no. 1 (1929): 80.

obtained.[71] Indeed, thanks to the art of frequency control, already a much more complex picture of the conditions in such electro-organic circuits had emerged. Unsurprisingly perhaps, much of this practice-induced theorizing revolved around the frequency dependency of a cell's (certain) electrical properties. Most notably, by the late 1920s there had been revealed the presence of a "capacitance" effect in addition to the tissue resistance; it made itself suspiciously manifest at the far, high-frequency end of the spectrum. And while its causes largely remained elusive, the clear implication was that none of the simplistic, "customary methods of obtaining balance" in a bridge circuit could result in a "true reproduction" of the unknown "circuit" that was the cell. At the very least, the more complex picture would involve, according to what quickly turned into the consensus view, a resistance (the cell interior) in series with a "leaky" condenser (the cell membrane).

Once established, such equivalent-circuit representations could be turned to manifold uses: gauging current distributions and devising means to control and improve them; diagnosing malignant tissue; or, based on measured, empirical values of conductivity, estimating the thickness—the real, physical dimensions, of cellular membranes (a good candidate for the "source of resistance" puzzling not only McClendon).[72] "Equivalence," in other words, was a theoretical concept anchored and honed in practice. Much like the "physical sense" these practical bio-electricians were fabricating, it sprang forth from the worlds they moved in (see fig. 4.4).

Cream, Algae, Nerve

Seen in this light, the turn from "laws" to models was the cumulative effect of a complex assortment of techniques, predicated on a multilayered, material logic of substitution: simple objects replacing complex ones; unknown, organic circuit elements being "balanced" by known, inorganic ones; and a set of diagrammatic and formal tools that themselves were drawn from the investigation of *technical* things: circuits. If my emphasis thus far has been on Fricke, it is because there is a direct line leading from Crile's biophysico-clinical venture to the nervous impulse as it was taking shape in 1939. For both Kenneth Cole and Howard Curtis (and, indirectly, Alan Hodgkin) were deeply familiar with the science of Hugo Fricke; this concluding section will resume their story.

Fricke's own initiation into biophysical research, as we have seen, took place in a world of blood suspensions, breast tumors, pathological conductivity changes, and X-ray dosimetry. Before long, however, Fricke found himself transplanted into the center of academic, "quantitative" biology: Cold Spring Harbor, the renowned home of the eponymous Symposia on Quantitative Biology. The first such gathering, staged in 1933 (five years

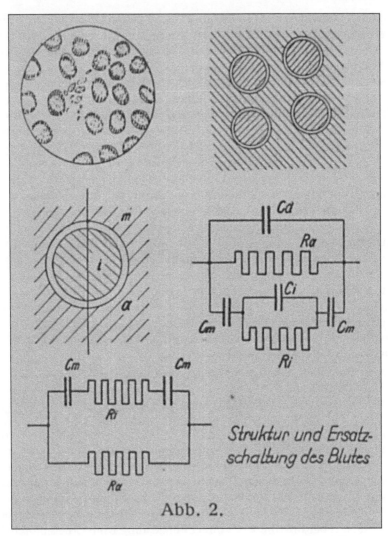

Figure 4.4. "Equivalent circuit of blood," 1937. B. Rajewsky and H. Lampert, eds. *Erforschung und Praxis der Wärmebehandlung in der Medizin einschliesslich Diathermie und Kurzwellentherapie* (Dresden: Steinkopff, 1937), Abbildung 2, p. 85.

after Fricke's arrival in Long Island), not coincidentally dealt with surface phenomena in a symposium of that name. Participants included the
likes of Herbert Gasser, Winthrop Osterhout, Eric Ponder, and Leonor
Michaelis, as well as Kenneth Cole—biophysicists, for the most, of present
or future acclaim. The "presence of such a group . . . each summer," as the
published *Proceedings* announced, would hopefully "aid the Laboratory in
its . . . aims of fostering a closer relationship between the basic sciences
and biology."[73]

The publications now issuing from Fricke's circle clearly reflected their
newly biological environs: "The study of the electric resistance of living
cells," as one of Fricke's new students mused in 1931, "has been used chiefly
in . . . special investigations on subjects such as the resistance of malignant
tumors; but such problems of general physiology as growth or death, in relation to variation of frequency, remain almost untouched."[74] Among those
who began to touch them now was Howard Curtis, an electronics-savvy Yale
physics graduate who had recently been recruited by Fricke.[75] Meanwhile,
too, Kenneth Cole had undergone a similar trajectory, gradually moving into more recognizably physiological territories as he had meandered
from an apprenticeship with Fricke at Crile's Cleveland Clinic, via the High
Tension Electrical Laboratory at Harvard, on to an assistant professorship in
physiology at Columbia University.

Unsurprisingly, then, Cole and Curtis's forays into the sciences of the
nervous system would bear the mark of their sometime teacher. Fricke, for
his part, retained a preference for the simple, red corpuscle even in Long
Island—albeit, as indicated, with a new emphasis. Once he had settled in,
Fricke began to move beyond the merely *static* properties of membranes. It
was the result of a complex set of factors: progress in high-frequency technique; the interaction with biological students who came to the picturesque
location for summer school or more permanently to be "acquainted at first
hand," as Fricke said, with the "findings" of biophysics; and not least, the
Long Island site—a strategically located nature spot, "easily accessible to
biologists residing in, or visiting, New York, and to those in passage to and
from Europe."[76] And as if inspired by his new, and less morbid, surroundings, Fricke increasingly trained his attention on the *dynamic* aspects of the
cellular life.

With Curtis's aid, the two of them soon were able to observe *variations*
in the frequency-dependent, electrical characteristics of the cell as they
induced membrane "desintegrations" through swelling in water (osmotic
lysis), by way of freezing and thawing, and with various chemicals. "The fact
that a change of the frequency dependence takes place," as they reported
in 1935, "show[ed] that the injury cannot be due merely to a rupture in the
membrane, but must be due to changes in the properties (increased perme-
ability) of the membrane as a whole."[77]

The potential significance of these new horizons was clear enough—one observed physiological *changes*. But making intelligible such behavior was, as ever, difficult. Worse, certain "characteristics" of the natural surfaces were easily "obscured . . . by reason of their lack of homogeneity."[78] Fricke, always the practical biophysicist, therefore turned to even simpler, fabricated systems. His surviving notebooks show him grappling with various "model substances." On December 17, 1934, for instance, Fricke prepared a "heavy suspension of whipping cream in H20." January brought "Lion brand evaporated milk-homogenized" and solutions of "1% of 'Cooper's' gelatin." Or again, suspensions of (relatively simple) yeast cells, he found, also exhibited sudden, drastic, and reversible drops in resistance and capacitance at high frequencies.[79] These sudden changes, they reasoned, were thus unlikely due to "minute disintegration[s]" of the lipoid layer surrounding these cells. Rather, being reversible, such behavior indicated processes that were *functional* in nature. Meanwhile, Fricke struggled with the detailed interpretation of these observations, jotting down calculations next to circuit diagrams and wondering about "condition[s] of equivalence."[80]

But to no avail. While Fricke was able to generate increasingly better guesses at the physical dimensions of these—possibly bimolecular—cellular membranes, no clear "conception as to the origin of the dielectric properties of cell membranes" was in evidence, as Fricke confessed in 1937; and neither was a conception of their *changes*.[81] Increasingly consumed with problems of radiation biology, it was not for Fricke to carry this particular case forward; rather, it was Kenneth Cole, who by then had teamed up with Curtis, to whom was due the protracted migration of high-frequency measurements into the realms of the nervous.

Cole's biophysical career path was fairly prototypical otherwise. "Accumulating batteries, magnets, and other worn out parts" during his youth already,[82] Cole had been soaking up the wireless arts all his life: at the General Electric Research Laboratory in Schenectady (where he had spent two years after high school); as a physics graduate at Cornell; in the course of a NRC fellowship with Emory Chaffee at Harvard—an authority on vacuum tubes and someone who regularly weighed in on biophysical matters (for instance, on the sterilization of fruit juices, "ultra-violet" therapeutic lamps, iono-atmospheric hygiene, or "diathermy from the view point of physics"); and most fatefully, perhaps, at Crile's biophysical clinic, where Cole went for a summer job in 1925 after responding to a note hung up in the Cornell physics department: "Wanted, at the Cleveland Clinic, two biophysicists."

Unsurprisingly, Cole's first forays into biophysical matters very much (or merely) centered on the "technics" of bioelectric, high-frequency measurement (indeed, it was a Bell labs engineer—K. S. Johnson, at the time a visiting professor at Harvard—who had introduced the young Cole to the more esoteric dimensions of circuit equivalence). And much like anyone else in

this essay, this naturally attracted him toward simple model systems: suspensions of calf blood, cat diaphragms, skin, potato slices, sea urchin eggs,
or muscle.[83] What is more, by the early 1930s, Cole had already turned to
charting out a bigger picture. In all these cases, the "frequency characteristics of tissues," as Cole informed his biophysical peers at the symposium
on surface phenomena at Cold Spring Harbor in 1933, could be traced to a
single, "variable impedance element"; its "seat," Cole confidently declared,
"is probably the cell membrane."[84]

Paralleling Fricke's own move into the more "active" (or *living*) systems,
Cole—by now at Columbia—had begun to venture into more complex
terrains as well. In collaboration with a Columbia anatomist, for instance,
Cole then turned toward the high-frequency analysis of embryo rat heart
muscle cultures—a rather more active thing than potato slices (little could
be made, however, of the heaps of confusing data the muscle cultures
produced); with Emil Bozler, a German zoologist visiting the Johnson
Foundation for Medical Physics in Philadelphia, Cole took on impedance
changes during muscular activity and rigor (these proved similarly elusive); and not least, Cole then won the attention of Warren Weaver, who
encouraged him to submit a "program of research on the electrical con-
stants of the membrane and cytoplasm of the normal and abnormal cell"
to the Rockefeller Foundation.[85]

But Cole did not yet worry much about nervous impulses, let alone the
"messages" so broadcast. The erratic behavior of the above, complex objects
already and all-too-easily sabotaged the aim of investigating the functional
changes these objects quite evidently underwent; the organic, bioelectrical
action of living things made the analytic task of the bioelectric engineer very
difficult indeed (it was [electrically] the "passive" effects that one "always
hope[d] to maintain during the measurement," as Cole noted).[86] Ideally,
experimental objects should be both, simple *and* living, but not too active:
a single cell. The "most direct attack," as Cole had noted in 1933 at the
Surface Phenomena gathering, would be to relinquish such complex materials altogether and to measure the impedance "between the interior and
exterior of a single cell . . . such that the most of the current traverses the
cell membrane."[87]

꙳   ꙳   ꙳

Our story has thus come full circle—or has come so almost: although the
ideal experimental design seemed clear enough now, regarding the study
of nerve (or, indeed, of any living cell), the prospects were still daunting.
At the time, only a few electric investigators had felt their way toward single
cells. The required minuscule microelectrodes were by and large a technology of the future. Biologists still routinely worked on isolated organs, whole

tissues, entire bundles of nerve fibers, or suspensions. The "single cells" that came into question at all, because they were large enough, weren't even real cells but unicellular algae, tulip spores, and marine eggs. They also were very fragile objects, and measuring them in the way Cole proposed meant "impaling" them—a highly precarious affair. In brief, a great many factors were in place that would have served to render the nerve impulse a far from obvious object of investigation to electrically minded investigators such as Cole: it was too complex; too delicate and "alive"; and thus too unsuited for measuring/modeling.

If, just about six years later, the *New York Times* reported that "Drs. Cole and Curtis" had uncovered "a sort of Rosetta stone for deciphering the closely guarded secrets close to the very borderland of mind and matter,"[88] it was the sudden appearance of two new experimental objects, which principally altered the position, smoothing the transition from the study of tumors, eggs, potatoes, and whipped cream to those very borderlands of mind and matter. One was the giant squid axon—a nerve axon visible to the plain eye, which the young Oxford zoologist John Z. Young rediscovered in 1936 (the same year that Young was touring the East Coast on a Rockefeller stipend).[89] The other was the simplest kind of cell imaginable: *Nitella.* Unearthed on the tropical beaches of Bermuda, here was an uncomplicated, living object—a giant algae—which, as W. J. V. Osterhout, Jaques Loeb's successor at the Rockefeller Institute, had noted in about 1927, exhibited an impulse-like phenomenon when injured: A "wave of some sort," as Osterhout said, "which we may for convenience call a death wave."[90] This death wave, as he perceptively surmised as well, clearly "resembl[ed] action currents of nerve and muscle." It only traveled much more slowly.

And it was this quasi-nerve, which provided the intermediary between complexity and simplicity, between the real thing—the nerve impulse—and the electric passivity of skimmed milk and sea urchins. Indeed, if the possibilities the squid giant axon offered in terms of membrane analysis were plainly obvious, adapting existing techniques was not. But the remedy would have come very naturally to circuit-savvy investigators such as Drs. Cole and Curtis: substitute, simplify, replace the elements in the circuit—such were the powers of circuit equivalence. "The experimental procedure and the technique of analysis," as Cole and Curtis happily conceded, were "fundamentally the same as those used in Nitella during activity."[91]

And we may conclude, then, that a great many disparate things went into the electrical fabrication of the nerve impulse: *Nitella* but also coagulated meat, sea urchins and lowly plants, high-frequency currents, diagrams, circuitry, the scenes of medical physics, the electronic arts, as well as radio-cultural forms of instrument use. Historiographically speaking, by the mid-twentieth century, the genesis and legibility of the nerve impulse thus not only depended on particular interpretational techniques, but these techniques themselves were embedded in experimental and material cultures that largely would remain invisible were one to adopt the narrow perspectives from academic nerve physiology or that of inscription devices.[92] But neither should this story of the nervous impulse be construed as a story of physicists (or engineers) colonizing biology.[93] The point that I've tried to convey is that interwar bio/medical physics was a more complex, homegrown and heterogeneous subject matter than that. Rather than being imposed from the outside, circuitry-based modeling practices, for one, reflected the variety of medico-physical practices that surged in the interwar period, notably those having to do with high-frequency currents. And more generally, as I have suggested, they reflected the permeation of interwar life-worlds with electrical technologies.[94] It was, after all, a time when "every child dabbled in resonance, filter circuits and distortions" (as one German physiologist put it).[95]

Regarding technique and technology, the turn from "laws" to "models" in neurophysiology is best conceived, accordingly, not in terms of this or that instrument's transformative role—an object and its impact. The arts of "wireless" weren't anything like that; they were a system, a culture of oftentimes DIY-esque bricolage, a set of *Kulturtechniken* (such as reading a circuit diagram). But nothing that could have exerted a single, unidirectional, let alone deterministic influence—the rhetoric of actors notwithstanding.[96] By implication, and curiously enough, "nerve" (let alone brains) may not always be the best guide to the history of the nervous system: regarding the interwar "impulse," circuits, nerve, and whipped cream went together.

Notes

Epigraph. O. H. Caldwell, "The Electron Tube . . . A Universal Tool in Industry," *Electronics* 1 (April 1930): 10–11.

1. Edgar D. Adrian, *The Mechanism of Nervous Action: Electrical Studies of the Neurone* (Philadelphia: Pennsylvania University Press, 1932), 2.

2. Harry Grundfest, "Potentialities and Limitations of Electrophysiology," in *Nerve Impulse: Transactions of the First Conference*, ed. David Nachmansohn, 18–19 (New York: Josiah Macy Jr. Foundation, 1950).

3. See, for example, Timothy Lenoir, "Models and Instruments in the Development of Electrophysiology, 1845–1912," *Historical Studies in the Physical Sciences* 17, no. 1 (1986): 1–54; Robert G. Frank, "Instruments, Nerve Action, and the All-or-None Principle," *Osiris* 9 (1994): 208–35; Laura Otis, "The Metaphoric Circuit: Organic and Technological Communication in the Nineteenth Century," *Journal of the History of Ideas* 63, no. 1 (2002): 105–28; Sven Dierig, "Engines for Experiment: Laboratory Revolution and Industrial Labor in the Nineteenth-Century City," *Osiris* 18 (2003): 116–34; Cornelius Borck, "Electrifying the Brain in the 1920s: Electrical Technology as a Mediator in Brain Research," in *Electric Bodies: Episodes in the History*

of Medical Electricity, ed. Paola Bertucci and Giuliano Pancaldi, 239–64 (Bologna: CIS, 2001); Robert L. Schoenfeld, *Exploring the Nervous System: With Electronic Tools, an Institutional Base, a Network of Scientists* (Boca Raton, FL: Universal Publishers, 2006); Henning Schmidgen, *The Helmholtz-Curves: Tracing Lost Time* (New York: Fordham University Press, 2014).

4. On the EEG, see Cornelius Borck, *Hirnströme: Eine Kulturgeschichte der Elektroenzephalographie* (Göttingen: Wallstein, 2005). On said "war," see Elliot S. Valenstein, *The War of the Soups and the Sparks: The Discovery of Neurotransmitters and the Dispute over How Nerves Communicate* (New York: Columbia University Press, 2005).

5. O. H. Caldwell, "Engineers, Components, Parts," *Electronics* 2 (November 1931): 173.

6. See Alan Hodgkin and Andrew F. Huxley, "Action Potentials Recorded from Inside a Nerve Fibre," *Nature* 144 (1939): 710–11. More broadly, see Alan Hodgkin, *Chance and Design: Reminiscences of Science in Peace and War* (Cambridge: Cambridge University Press, 1992); Max Stadler, "Assembling Life: Models, the Cell, and the Reformations of Biological Science, 1920–1960" (PhD diss., Imperial College London, 2009), chap. 4.

7. Kenneth Cole and Howard Curtis, "Electric Impedance of the Squid Giant Axon during Activity," *Journal of General Physiology* 22 (1939): 649–70; Kenneth Cole and Alan Hodgkin, "Membrane and Protoplasm Resistance in the Squid Giant Axon," *Journal of General Physiology* 22 (1939): 671–87. See also Kenneth Cole, *Membranes, Ions, and Impulses: A Chapter of Classical Biophysics* (Berkeley: University of California Press, 1968).

8. Chandler McC. Brooks, "Current Developments in Thought and the Past Evolution of Ideas Concerning Integrative Function," in *The History and Philosophy of Knowledge of the Brain and Its Functions*, ed. F. N. L. Poynter, 248 (Oxford: Blackwell, 1957).

9. For a recent example of this kind of narrative, see Eric Kandel, *In Search of Memory: The Emergence of a New Science of Mind* (New York: W. W. Norton, 2006).

10. For instance, John Bradley and Tilly Tansey, "The Coming of the Electronic Age to the Cambridge Physiological Laboratory: E. D. Adrian's Valve Amplifier in 1921," *Notes and Records of the Royal Society* 50, no. 2 (1996): 217–28; David Millet, "Wiring the Brain: From the Excitable Cortex to the EEG, 1870–1940" (PhD diss., University of Chicago, 2001); Borck, *Hirnströme*.

11. Regarding the historiography, the production of "curves" (or "inscriptions") has been of signal importance, of course. See, for instance, Frederic L. Holmes and Kathryn Olesko, "The Images of Precision: Helmholtz and the Graphical Method in Physiology," in *The Values of Precision*, ed. M. Norton Wise, 198–221 (Princeton, NJ: Princeton University Press, 1995); Soraya de Chadarevian, "Graphical Method and Discipline: Self-Recording Instruments in Nineteenth-Century Physiology," *Studies in History and Philosophy of Science* 24, no. 2 (1993): 267–91; Philipp Felsch, *Laborlandschaften: Physiologen über der Baumgrenze, 1800–1900* (Göttingen: Wallstein, 2007); and Schmidgen, *Helmholtz-Curves*.

12. Ibid., all citations. More broadly, of course, the appeal of the graphic method owed to the increasing significance that was attached to all things visual. See, e.g., Bruno Latour, "Visualisation and Cognition: Thinking with Eyes and Hands," in *Knowledge and Society: Studies in the Sociology of Culture*, ed. Henrika Kuklick, 1–40 (Greenwich, CT: Jai Press, 1988).

13. See, e.g., Gustav Oppenheim, "Die Schallplatte im Dienste der Elektro-Medizin," *Klinische Wochenschrift* 11, no. 14 (1932): 595–97; Francis O. Schmitt and Otto H. Schmitt, "A Universal Precision Stimulator," *Science* 76, no. 1971 (1932): 328–30; Archibald V. Hill, "Repetitive Stimulation by Commutator and Condenser," *Journal of Physiology* 82, no. 4 (1934): 423–31; cited in Ferdinand Scheminzky, "Über einige Anwendungen der Elektronenröhren in Widerstandsschaltung und der Glimmlampen für die Physiologie," *Pflüger's Archiv* 213, no. 1 (1926): 126–27.

14. Any biography of Edison or Tesla will feature the story of this AC/DC "war." See, for example, W. Bernard Carlson, *Tesla: Inventor of the Electrical Age* (Princeton, NJ: Princeton University Press, 2013).

15. Walter Nernst, "Zur Theorie des Elektrischen Reizes," *Pflügers Archiv* 122, nos. 7–9 (1908): 275–314.

16. Edgar D. Adrian, *The Basis of Sensation: The Action of the Sense Organs* (London: Hafner, 1928), 39.

17. William H. Eccles, "The New Acoustics," *Proceedings of the Physical Society* 41 (1929): 232–33.

18. Burton Baker Grover, *High Frequency Practice for Practitioners and Students* (Kansas City, KS: The Electron Press, 1925), 3.

19. Halloway Davis and Alexander Forbes, "Chronaxie," *Physiological Reviews* 16 (1936): 407–41.

20. Ibid., 410.

21. Cited in Hans Rosenberg, "Untersuchungen über Nervenaktionsströme," *Pflüger's Archiv* 223, no. 1 (1930): 120–21.

22. On the concept of "chronaxie," see Joy Harvey, "l'autre côté du miroir (The Other Side of the Mirror): French Neurophysiology and English Interpretations," in *les sciences biologiques et médicales en France 1920–1950*, ed. Claude Debru, Jean Gayon, and Jean-Francois Picard, 71–81 (Paris: CNRS Editions, 1994).

23. For instance, Max Cremer, "Erregungsgesetze des Nerven," in *Handbuch der Normalen und Pathologischen Physiologie*, ed. Albrecht Bethe, vol. 9 (Berlin: Springer, 1929); Hans Schaefer, "Neuere Untersuchungen über den Nervenaktionsstrom," *Ergebnisse der Physiologie* 36, no. 1 (1934): 151–248; Walter Eichler, "Über die Abhängigkeit der Chronaxie des Nerven vom äusseren Widerstande," *Zeitschrift für Biologie* 91 (1931): 475.

24. W. A. H. Rushton, "A Physical Analysis of the Relation between Threshold and Interpolar Length in the Electric Excitation of Medullated Nerve," *Journal of Physiology* 82, no. 3 (1934): 483.

25. Bernard Katz, *Electric Excitation of Nerve: A Review* (London: Oxford University Press, 1939), 66.

26. Johann D. Achelis, "Kritische Bemerkungen zur Chronaxiebestimmung am Menschen," *Zeitschrift für Neurologie* 130, nos. 5–6 (1933): 233.

27. Cremer, "Erregungsgesetze," 255–56.

28. Friedrich Lewy, "Bericht: Die Chronaxie," *Deutsche Zeitschrift für Nervenheilkunde* 129, nos. 5–6 (1933): 186–87.

29. Herbert Gasser, "Axon Action Potentials in Nerve," in *Cold Spring Harbor Symposia in Quantitative Biology*, vol. 1 (Cold Spring Harbor, NY: CSH Cold Spring Harbor Laboratory Press, 1933), 143.

30. Hans Schaefer, *Elektrophysiologie. I. Band: Allgemeine Elektrophysiologie* (Vienna: Franz Deuticke, 1940), iv.

31. E. J. Hart, "Hugo Fricke, 1892–1972," *Radiation Research* 52, no. 3 (1972): 642–46.

32. On Crile, see *George Crile: An Autobiography*, ed. Grace Crile (Philadelphia: J. B. Lippincott, 1947).

33. Winthrop Osterhout to E. S. Harris, June 13, 1928, folders "Dr Hugo Fricke" (folder 3), Special Collections, Cold Spring Harbor Laboratory, NY.

34. George Crile, *A Bipolar Theory of Living Processes* (New York: Macmillan, 1926).

35. Unless noted otherwise, biographical information on Cole is based on Kenneth Cole, oral interview transcript, National Institutes of Health oral history collection, National Library of Medicine, Bethesda, MD.

36. Hugo Fricke to Harris, July 31, 1928, folders "Dr Hugo Fricke" (folder 3), Special Collections/Cold Spring Harbor Laboratory, NY.

37. Crile, *Bipolar Theory of Life*, 3.

38. George Crile, *A Mechanistic View of War and Peace* (New York: Macmillan., 1915), vii; Crile, *George Crile*, 328, 369–70.

39. Crile, *Bipolar Theory of Life*, 7.

40. For example, "'Suns' in Man's Body Pictured by Crile," *New York Times*, November 26, 1932.

41. Hugo Fricke to Harris, July 31, 1928, folders "Dr Hugo Fricke" (folder 3), Special Collections, Cold Spring Harbor Laboratory, NY.

42. More broadly on the notion of electrical equivalence, see Emily Thompson, *The Soundscape of Modernity: Architectural Acoustics and the Culture of Listening in America, 1900–1933* (Cambridge, MA: MIT Press, 2002); Roland Wittje, "The Electrical Imagination: Sound Analogies, Equivalent Circuits, and the Rise of Electroacoustics, 1863–1939," *Osiris* 28, no. 1 (2013): 40–63.

43. Hugo Fricke and Sterne Morse, "The Electric Capacity of Tumors of the Breast," *Journal of Cancer Research* 16 (1926): 340.

44. Ibid.

45. Crile, *Bipolar Theory of Life*, 15.

46. "The Expanding Short-Wave Spectrum," *Electronics* 3, no. 3 (September 1931), 91.

47. "Raw Materials, Costs—in Tube Manufacture," *Electronics* 1, no. 8 (November 1930), 366.

48. Hugo Fricke, "The Electric Impedance of Suspensions of Biological Cells," in *Cold Spring Harbor Symposia in Quantitative Biology*, vol. 1 (Cold Spring Harbor, NY: CSH Cold Spring Harbor Laboratory Press, 1933), 117.

49. See Stadler, "Assembling Life"; Thompson, *Soundscape of Modernity;* Wittje, "Electrical Imagination."

50. Pnina Abir-Am, "The Biotheoretical Gathering, Trans-Disciplinary Authority and the Incipient Legitimation of Molecular Biology in the 1930s: New Perspective on the Historical Sociology of Science," *History of Science* 25 (1987): 1–70; Lilly E. Kay, *The Molecular Vision of Life* (Oxford: Oxford University Press, 1993); Nicolas Rasmussen, "The Mid-Century Biophysics Bubble: Hiroshima and the Biological Revolution in America, Revisited," *History of Science* 35, no. 109 (1997): 245–93; Soraya

de Chadarevian, *Designs for Life: Molecular Biology after World War II* (Cambridge: Cambridge University Press, 2002).

51. For a more detailed account, see Stadler, "Assembling Life."

52. See C. Thomas de la Peña, *The Body Electric: How Strange Machines Built the Modern American* (New York: New York University Press, 2003); Cornelius Borck, "Electricity as a Medium of Psychic Life: Electrotechnological Adventures into Psychodiagnosis in Weimar Germany," *Science in Context* 14, no. 1 (2001): 565–90.

53. See "A Review of the Medical Curriculum" (1930), ROUGHTON Papers, box 34.60u, American Philosophical Society, Philadelphia, and "Register of Biophysical Assistants," *The Lancet* 215, no. 5570 (May 31, 1930): 1195–96.

54. Wolfgang Holzer, "Modelltheorie über die Stromdichte im Körper von Lebewesen bei Galvanischer Durchströmung in Flüssigkeit," *Pflüger's Archiv* 232, no. 1 (1933): 195–96.

55. For instance, John B. Bateman, "Mitogenetic Radiation," *Biological Reviews and Biological Proceedings of the Cambridge Philosophical Society* 10, no. 1 (1935): 42–71.

56. Frank, "Instruments, Nerve Action"; Bradley and Tansey, "Coming of the Electronic Age."

57. Erwin Schliephake, "Die biologische Wärmewirkung im elektrischen Hochfrequenzfeld," *Verhandlungen der Deutschen Gesellschaft für innere Medizin* 4 (1928): 307–10.

58. Georges Lakhovsky, "Curing Cancer with Ultra Radio Frequencies," *Radio News Magazine* (February 1925), 1282–83; Georges Lakhovsky, *The Secret of Life*, trans. Mark Clement, 2nd ed. (London: Heinemann, 1939).

59. Elkin P. Cumberbatch, *Diathermy; Its Production and Uses in Medicine and Surgery*, 2nd ed. (St. Louis: C. V. Mosby, 1928), 3–4.

60. Josef Kowarschik, *Die Diathermie* (Vienna: Springer, 1913), 3.

61. Nernst, "Zur Theorie des Elektrischen Reizes," 275–76, 313.

62. Franz Nagelschmidt, *Lehrbuch der Diathermie für Ärzte und Studierende* (Berlin: Springer, 1921).

63. Josef Kowarschik, *Die Diathermie*, 7th ed. (Vienna: Springer, 1930), iii; Hans Henseler and Erich Fritsch, *Einführung in die Diathermie vom medizinischen und technischen standpunkt* (Berlin: Radionta-Verlag, 1929), 5.

64. Elkin P. Cumberbatch, "Uses of Diathermy in Medicine and Surgery," *The Lancet*, February 7, 1931, 281.

65. J. Stafford, "Radio Waves Cause Fever in Patients to Cure Dreaded Paresis," *The Science News-Letter* 18, no. 484 (1930): 36; C. M. Carpenter and A. B. Page, "The Production of Fever in Man by Short Radio Waves," *Science* 71, no. 1844 (1930): 450–52.

66. See, for instance, Kowarschik, *Die Diathermie*; Nagelschmidt, *Lehrbuch*; Cumberbatch, *Diathermy*; Erwin Schliephake, *Ondes electriques courtes en biologie* (Paris: Gauthier-Villars, 1938); Wolfgang. Holzer and Eugen Weissenberg, *Foundations of Short-Wave Therapy: Physics-Technics-Indications* (London: Hutchinson, 1935); Boris Rajewsky and Heinrich Lampert, eds., *Erforschung und Praxis der Wärmebehandlung in der Medizin einschliesslich Diathermie und Kurzwellentherapie* (Dresden: Steinkopff, 1937).

67. "Reviews and Notices of Books," *The Lancet* 215, no. 5551 (1930): 140.

68. Carl A. L. Binger and Ronald V. Christie, "An Experimental Study of Diathermy," *Journal of Experimental Medicine* 46, no. 4 (1927): 571–72.

69. Allan Hemingway and Jesse F. McClendon, "The High Frequency Resistance of Human Tissue," *American Journal of Physiology* 102 (1932): 56.

70. Roe Remington, "The High Frequency Wheatstone Bridge as a Tool in Cytological Studies; with Some Observations on the Resistance and Capacity of the Cells of the Beet Root," *Protoplasma* 5, no. 1 (1928): 353–54; Jesse F. McClendon, "Polarization-Capacity as Measured with a Wheatstone Bridge with Sine-Wave Alternating Currents of High and Low Frequency," *American Journal of Physiology* 91, no. 1 (1929): 83–93.

71. Remington, "High Frequency Wheatstone Bridge," 356–58.

72. A more exhaustive account than I can provide here would include figures such as B. S. Gossling of the GEC Research Laboratories, Wembley, a short-wave therapy expert and someone naturally straddling the "essential differences of outlook between electro-engineering and therapy." It would also have included the likes of Boris Rajewsky, the Russian émigré biophysicist who, as director of the Kaiser-Wilhelms-Institute for Biophysics, put some considerable effort into clearing up the physical foundations of high-frequency interventions. Or again, it would have included figures such as Wolfgang Holzer, a graduate of the High Voltage Institute at the University of Berlin, and also the author of *Foundations of Short-Wave Therapy: Physics-Technics-Indications* (1935), which he had co-written with the medical superintendent of the short wave section at the Vienna University Clinic for Nervous and Mental Diseases. Much like everyone else in the short-wave business, Holzer was primarily after the electrical principles involved in "the action of ultra-high frequency currents on biological materials."

73. *Cold Spring Harbor Symposia in Quantitative Biology* (Cold Spring Harbor, NY, 1933), v.

74. Basile Luyet, "Variation of the Electric Resistance of Plant Tissues for Alternating Currents of Different Frequencies during Death," *Journal of General Physiology* 15, no. 3 (1932): 283.

75. On Curtis, see Raymond E. Zirkle, "Howard James Curtis, 1906–1972," *International Journal of Radiation Biology* 23, no. 6 (1972): 530–32.

76. Hugo Fricke, memorandum "General in Biophysics," August 23, 1930, folders "Dr Hugo Fricke" (folder 3), Special Collections, Cold Spring Harbor Laboratory, NY.

77. Hugo Fricke and Howard Curtis, "The Electric Impedance of Hemolyzed Suspensions of Mammalian Erythrocytes," *Journal of General Physiology* 18 (1935): 836.

78. Hugo Fricke and Howard Curtis, "Electric Impedance of Suspensions of Yeast Cells," *Nature* 134, no. 3377 (1934): 102.

79. See Notebook V, folder "Fricke Notebook, Book V, Nov 28 '34-Dec 18 '35," box 2, Special Collections, Cold Spring Harbor Laboratory, NY.

80. Ibid.

81. Hugo Fricke to Winthrop Osterhout, February 18, 1937, folder "Hugo Fricke," box 2, Osterhout Papers, American Philosophical Society Library, Philadelphia.

82. Biographical information, as indicated, is based on Cole, oral interview transcript, National Institutes of Health oral history collection, National Library of Medicine.

83. Cole began to "duplicate" Fricke's high-frequency bridge while at Harvard.

84. Kenneth Cole, "Electric Conductance of Biological Systems," in *Cold Spring Harbor Symposia in Quantitative Biology*, vol. 1, 107–16 (New York: CSH Cold Spring Harbor Laboratory Press, 1933).

85. Kenneth Cole to Rockefeller Foundation, September 23, 1935, Rockefeller Archives RG.1.1, series 200, box 133, folder 1650; and see, for instance, Emil Bozler and Kenneth Cole, "The Electric Impedance and Phase Angle of Muscle in Rigor," *Journal of Cellular and Comparative Physiology* 6, no. 2 (1935): 229–41. Further details can be found in Stadler, "Assembling Life."

86. Cole, "Electric Conductance of Biological Systems," 114–15.

87. Ibid., 111.

88. "New Clues Found to Life Process," *New York Times*, February 27, 1938, 35.

89. See R. S. Bear, F. O. Schmitt, and J. Z. Young, "The Sheath Components of the Giant Nerve Fibres of the Squid," *Proceedings of the Royal Society of London*, series B, 123, no. 833 (1937): 496–504.

90. W. J. V. Osterhout and E. S. Harris, "The Death Wave in Nitella," *Journal of General Physiology* 12 (1928): 186.

91. Cole and Curtis, "Electric Impedance of the Squid Giant Axon," 650.

92. Owing to post–World War II developments (notably cybernetics), the word *circuits*, as is well-known, increasingly would come to signify codes, messages, and so on; this, however, tends to obscure the wider, richer histories of circuitry, which typically had little to do with cybernetics. On the former, see, for instance, Lilly E. Kay, "From Logical Neurons to Poetic Embodiments of Mind: Warren S. McCulloch's Project in Neuroscience," *Science in Context* 14, no. 4 (2001): 591–614; and Tara Abraham, "From Theory to Data: Representing Neurons in the 1940s," *Biology and Philosophy* 18, no. 3 (June 2003): 415–26.

93. On this topos, see Abir-Am, "The Biotheoretical Gathering"; and Pnina Abir-Am, "The Discourse of Physical Power and Biological Knowledge in the 1930s: A Reappraisal of the Rockefeller Foundation's 'Policy' in Molecular Biology," *Social Studies of Science* 12, no. 3 (1982): 341–82.

94. On this point, also see Jeff Hughes, "Plasticine and Valves: Industry, Instrumentation and the Emergence of Nuclear Physics," in *The Invisible Industrialist: Manufactures and the Production of Scientific Knowledge*, ed. Jean-Paul Gaudillière and Illana Löwy, 58–101 (London: Macmillan, 1998); Kristen Haring, *Ham Radio's Technical Culture* (Cambridge, MA: MIT Press, 2006); Wittje, "Electrical Imagination."

95. Otto Ranke, "Philipp Broemser," *Ergebnisse der Physiologie* 44, no. 1 (1941): 1–2.

96. Unsurprisingly, therefore, "technological determinism" has been troubling historians of electrophysiology. See Frank, "Instruments, Nerve Action"; Cornelius Borck, "Between Local Cultures and National Styles: Units of Analysis in the History of Electroencephalography," *Comptes Rendus Biologies* 329, nos. 5–6 (2006): 450–59.

Chapter Five

Epilepsy and the Laboratory Technician

Technique in Histology and Fiction

Delia Gavrus

That's a popular misconception about science, Nett. But, Science, on
the contrary, is very humanly warm and frail. It makes very human mis-
takes and has to change its views often so that, like the rest of humanity,
it can go blundering steadily forward.

—Edward Dockrill, mid-1930s

In the interwar period, Gerry Armstrong, a technician working at a prestigious Canadian hospital, spoke passionately against the invisibility of laboratory workers. Dependent on the patronage and research funds of elite
doctors and scientists, the technicians who mastered staining techniques
received no formal acknowledgment for their scientific endeavors. "I'm paid
to produce results," Armstrong reflected bitterly. "Whoever pays me has
the social and economic right to take what they are paying for."[1] This invisible labor formed the "stepping stones for somebody else's rise to fame,"
Armstrong lamented, while technicians were too worried to demand public recognition for fear of losing their jobs and "falling into the gutter."[2]
Mustering all the courage and frustration he felt, Armstrong did confront
his superiors on several occasions, receiving either blank incomprehension
or hollow placations.

Gerry Armstrong did not actually exist. He was a character conjured up
by Edward Dockrill, a real-life laboratory technician who wrote a manuscript
titled "The Means Are Nothing," a complex, nearly four-hundred-page novel
that never saw the light of print. Set mostly in the fictional bilingual town of

Tasville—a lightly disguised Montreal—the novel is a bildungsroman that slowly unspools the young hero's life as he arrives to North America from England with the explicit goal of proving his worth. Armstrong is dazzled at first by the hospital and its chief, Dr. Meadowes, and he throws himself passionately into his work in the pathology laboratory. Soon, however, disillusion sets in. After many nights of exhausting labor to perfect histological techniques, he watches helplessly as one of the senior doctors appropriates one of his own breakthroughs, publishing it to great acclaim and giving Armstrong no credit, despite having promised to share the laurels of scientific discovery. The story's climax stages an explosive encounter between Armstrong and Meadowes, the technician accusing the chief and his acolytes of "becom[ing] famous with work you never did, paid for by money you never owned."[3]

Like his fictional alter ego, Dockrill embodies what the historian Steven Shapin has called the "invisible technician,"[4] and what the historians N. C. Russell, E. M. Tansey, and P. V. Lear have described as "the forgotten members of the scientific club," whose absent histories obscure the role of teamwork in the production of science.[5] Recent historical scholarship has worked to unveil the invisible presences—whether they be technicians,[6] "human computers,"[7] women,[8] or industrialists[9]—that made the laboratory the complex scientific and social space that it was and still is. Like the work of many of his colleagues in the interwar period, Edward Dockrill's labor has been largely obscured, and his voice has remained silent despite his bold attempts to remedy the situation. Dockrill did submit his novel to a publishing house in Montreal, but realizing the thinly fictionalized identity of the protagonists, the publisher rejected it. In what Dockrill would have recognized as an ironic turn of events given the themes of his novel, the manuscript was returned not to Dockrill himself, but to the famous real-life Meadowes, Dr. Wilder Penfield.[10] It is yet another irony that, if the novel has survived to this day, it was precisely by the grace of this celebrated neurosurgeon. Although stung by what he considered to be a betrayal of loyalty, Penfield nevertheless recognized that the manuscript "surely . . . deserves a place in [the Montreal Neurological Institute] Archives,"[11] and he deposited it there, along with his own papers.

I have pieced together these two stories—that of the fictional Armstrong and the nonfictional Dockrill—from archival records and published autobiographies, from newspaper and journal articles, government records and transatlantic passenger lists. But can these stories tell us something about the mind and brain sciences of the 1920s and 1930s? At first glance, these tales appear to be at best minor episodes, diverting marginalia in a scientific field with a much more weighty history. This marginality works on two fronts. Dockrill himself, as a laboratory technician, was viewed at the time as a marginal player in the economy of the lab, an economy driven by famous scientists with research agendas and the ability to supply the requisite funds. In addition, the histological work itself, performed at Penfield's direction, was driven by a theory about the etiology of idiopathic epilepsy and by a desire to validate a directly related therapeutic intervention that ultimately failed. This failure might appear to consign Dockrill's work to historical marginality: while Dockrill's histological preparations correctly showed the existence of intracerebral vascular nerves (an existence that had been debated at the time), the application of this knowledge to therapy did not succeed, as Penfield had hoped. But the view that this double marginality—Dockrill's social marginality and the technical marginality of the work itself—makes this episode unworthy of historical exploration is problematic on two counts.

First, as cultural and social historians have repeatedly argued, it is important to pay attention to groups who have been historically marginalized—like laboratory technicians—and to ask how meaning is made from the margins.[12] These workers' identities, the manner in which they understood their professional life and made sense of their work, should matter historically. Dockrill's work in the laboratory can tell us a great deal about the complexity of the technician's work and the level of skill and tacit knowledge implicit in such work, illuminating at the same time the social economy of the laboratory and the collective nature of scientific work in the past.

Second, these stories appear marginal only in retrospect; they shed light on fascinating and central events that shaped the brain sciences in the interwar period. As I will argue, Dockrill's work functioned as both evidence and justification for a new and promising therapeutic approach that Penfield was attempting to devise for idiopathic epilepsy, an approach that relied on two surgical procedures—a cervicothoracic sympathetic ganglionectomy and a periarterial sympathectomy of internal carotid and vertebral arteries. While the approach ultimately failed and has subsequently been forgotten, in the 1920s and 1930s it certainly occupied center stage on Penfield's professional agenda. An analysis of this case study throws into sharp relief the relationship between early twentieth-century neurohistological techniques; new epistemological commitments to an ideal of bench science in medicine; and the urgent, if unfulfilled, hope of devising radical and rational therapies for a serious neurological condition. Thus, by focusing on what appeared at the time and on what appears now to be marginal (the technicians' work, a forgotten failed therapy, and the epistemic scaffolding built to support it), it becomes clear that the marginal itself is a concept that needs to be historicized.

This study, while in essence a microhistory, nevertheless highlights broader and central themes in the history of science. In particular, I draw attention to the crucial role that techniques—histological ones in the laboratory, narrative ones in the writer's room-of-his-own—play in the constitution of scientific knowledge, medical therapy, and professional identity. In so doing, this chapter moves back and forth between the actual and the fictional, putting the two in conversation and reading one against the other. In a similar fashion, scholars such as Anne Stiles have explored the rich historical ties between literature and neurology and have shown how a careful analysis of fiction can uncover surprising reactions to neurological theories du jour, such as for instance pervasive anxieties about cerebral localization in the Victorian period.[13] Fiction allowed Dockrill to explore his own professional identity in the neuropathological laboratory and to express frustrations about the invisibility of technicians. It led him to imagine a world in which, unlike in real life, the histological techniques that he perfected led to a spectacular clinical payoff.

❧   ❧   ❧

Thomas Edward Dockrill was born in 1900 in the vicinity of Manchester, England,[14] and in his youth he traveled the seas as a cabin boy, eventually disembarking in New York City and obtaining a job as an orderly on the public wards of Presbyterian Hospital. In 1923 he aimed higher, applying for a job in the hospital's pathology laboratory, where a young surgeon had secured a small room to study the brain's healing process after injury. The surgeon was Wilder Penfield, a newly hired Johns Hopkins MD who was well versed in laboratory practices, which he had studied not only at Hopkins, where such rapprochement between medicine and bench science was highly encouraged, but also at Oxford in the laboratory of Charles Sherrington, the Nobel Prize–winning physiologist.[15]

Penfield had completed a surgical internship in Boston and a fellowship at London's premier hospital for neurological diseases, and he now stood poised to choose between these two medical specialties, neurology and neurosurgery.[16] The scales eventually tipped in favor of the latter, but at the Presbyterian in the early 1920s, Penfield was eager to do more than apply his rather incipient neurosurgical skills to generally desperate cases; he wanted to continue his cytological research of the nervous system because he believed that reductive scientific work held the key for rational medical therapy. After all, such practices had worked so well for bacteriology, why not for diseases of the brain?[17]

As the historian Jean-Gaël Barbara has argued, Rudolph Virchow's work on cellular pathology and his formulation of cell theory in the middle of the previous century provided "an epistemological engine to search for new pathogenies of diseases," including those of the nervous system.[18] An encounter with the Presbyterian's pathologist, William Clark, had led Penfield to ask questions about the pathological changes that developed after brain injuries, with a view toward a potential understanding of the mechanisms responsible for epilepsy. His focus was soon directed away from the nervous tissue itself. Penfield had noted that the cells involved in the formation of these scars were not the neurons themselves, which died as a result of the injury and, as far as he could tell, did not regenerate. Rather, the scars were formed mostly by non-nervous (interstitial) support- ive cells, which mounted a powerful response to injury. In the early 1920s, the classification of these cells was still a matter of debate. Virchow had coined the term "neuroglia" to describe what he considered to be a con- nective tissue in which neurons were embedded, and over the following decades various other anatomists and pathologists described these cells and their structures in more detail. Camillo Golgi, who devised the first silver-staining methods, observed the connections between these cells and the brain's vascular system and thought that their function was to provide metabolic support.[19]

The term *neuroglia* initially referred to a particular type of these interstitial cells and was often used interchangeably with the term *astrocytes*. Two types of astrocytes were recognized early on: protoplasmic and fibrous, depending on their location in gray or white matter respectively. The Spanish anato- mist Santiago Ramón y Cajal, refining Golgi's techniques, observed and described the astrocytes in great detail, noting their many cytoplasmic pro- cesses and their position around neurons. He speculated that their purpose was to insulate neurons to maintain the function of the neuronal circuit.[20] He also observed another type of interstitial cell, which he called "the third element," but he was only able to stain its nucleus.

In his small room in the pathology laboratory, Penfield set out to visual- ize these interstitial cells with help from his new technician. It became clear very soon after hiring him, however, that Dockrill's claim of having trained as a technician in a laboratory at Queen Square, London was—at best—an imaginative stretch; but instead of firing him, Penfield set out to teach the young man, and to teach himself at the same time, Cajal's staining methods.

Generally speaking, the classic histological techniques developed over the course of the nineteenth century involved three major steps.[21] First, the tis- sue was fixed with the help of agents such as mineral acids and salts. Second, it was further hardened, preserved, and dehydrated with other fluids such as alcohol. Third and last, in order to prepare the tissue to be sliced very thinly, it was embedded in paraffin or celloidin with the intermediary help of clear- ing reagents (usually a type of oil that could mix with the melted paraffin). Once a thin section of the tissue was obtained by means of a microtome, it was placed on a microscope slide, and the entire process was reversed: the paraffin was melted with a clearing agent, which was then removed by alcohol, which in turn was washed away with water. The tissue was now ready to be stained with a dye that brought into focus the constituent parts, and eventually it was topped up with a drop of acid-free Canada balsam solution upon which a cover glass was placed.[22]

In the case of the central nervous system, the silver-staining methods of Golgi were particularly useful. In the last decades of the nineteenth century, Cajal improved Golgi's silver stain by tweaking concentrations, temperatures, exposure to light of the silver salts, and other such variables.[23] It was a delicate, time-consuming, and labor-intensive process that invited constant refinement. Penfield had found that traditional methods of staining involving paraffin and classic dyes, which were popular in Britain and which he had learned at Oxford, had failed to clearly reveal the neuroglia. At Sherrington's suggestion, Penfield had also had some success with Cajal's method for staining neurons, which apart from the particular silver and gold salts, involved the use of frozen sections instead of paraffin.[24]

Penfield now attempted to use the same technique for interstitial cells. Armed with Cajal's original papers, which he found at the New York Academy of Medicine, and with a hefty Spanish-English dictionary, Penfield and Dockrill replicated the Spaniard's methods and managed to obtain several visually clear images of interstitial cells. Interpretation of these images, however, proved more elusive. What exactly were they looking at? What was the significance of these cells and what insight could they provide in terms of epilepsy therapy? Penfield thought that he needed to consult with the Spanish histologists themselves in order to understand the importance and the implications of his microscopic preparations. He secured the necessary funding, and in the spring of 1924 he arrived in Madrid to work with Don Pío del Río-Hortega, one of Cajal's students. Penfield was not at all certain that this was time well spent, given that his ultimate concern was therapy, not basic bench science. As he confessed in an anxious mid-Atlantic letter to his mother, "there is not the slightest guarantee that any guiding clue lies ahead in the direction I am taking. . . . If I do get this last weapon in Madrid, shall I be able to see how to use it? Or, will it be the wrong weapon?"[25]

Over the next few months in Madrid, Penfield learned Río-Hortega's silver carbonate technique, a variation on Cajal's methods. He managed to stain the obdurate "third element" and made observations about the structure and functions of interstitial cells. Although this was not well-known outside of Spain, Río-Hortega and his students had already demonstrated that this "third element" was not a unitary one; it was made up of two distinct types of cells—a fact that seemed to explain the confusion in the literature.[26] One type, the microglia, was smaller, had irregular protoplasmic expansions and a triangular-appearing nucleus, and acted like migratory phagocytes following injury to the brain, in essence embodying a defense mechanism.[27] The other, oligodendroglia, were neither as small as microglia, nor as large as the astrocytes, and they were most numerous in the white matter of the brain. Their cytoplasmic projections, difficult to stain, were shown by Penfield in the course of his work in Madrid to be of "considerable length and complexity."[28] These projections, he argued, "formed an irregular and incomplete network about the myelin tubes of the central nervous system," which suggested to him that they played a role in "the formation and maintenance of the myelin sheath."[29]

Penfield could now visualize expertly under the microscope the various types of cells present in the brain, both nervous and interstitial. Armed with this "weapon" which was still of questionable clinical potential, Penfield returned to New York, where he was surprised and pleased to realize that in his absence, Dockrill had spent his days and nights tweaking the Spanish staining methods that Penfield had taught him before he left for Madrid. In fact, Dockrill had himself managed to obtain some excellent results. It became evident to Penfield that despite the young man's previous lack of expertise, Dockrill was "a young perfectionist who would learn all I was ready to teach and who might well add something independently."[30]

Over the next few years, the little pathology laboratory expanded, becoming "The Laboratory of Neurocytology." Penfield secured more funding, a larger room, a secretary, and several staff members, including William Cone, an aspiring neurologist who had studied some neuropathology and who would become over the next three decades Penfield's student, protégé, and, eventually, his virtual equal at the neurological institute they would build together in Montreal. Visiting researchers came and went. Dockrill continued to be a fixture in the laboratory, but as the novel he later wrote suggests, he must have realized the lowly social status he occupied and his tenuous identity with respect to the scientific work he performed.[31]

At one point in the novel, for instance, his fictional alter ego, Gerry Armstrong, starts a conversation with Sammy Berman, a young doctor who is doing research in the lab. Armstrong complains to Berman that laboratory technicians don't receive the recognition they deserve, but Berman disagrees, pointing out that as an undergraduate student, he conducted research with a professor, and this work eventually led to a joint publication. "I think genuine ability," Berman claims, "could force a change."[32] Armstrong, however, believes that his position is lowlier even than that of a student and that technicians would not dare to ask for symbolic rewards beyond their salary for fear of losing even that: "Your work leads to bigger things. We fellows work to toe a very rigid economic line. We daren't do anything about it."[33]

Just as in Armstrong's case, Dockrill's work never led to scientific authorship in the same manner in which the work of visiting fellows did. These researchers, who came to Penfield's lab to learn the staining techniques undoubtedly in part from Dockrill himself, published papers with Penfield, while Dockrill's labor remained officially unacknowledged.[34] Like the menagerie keepers Stephen Jacyna describes in this volume, and like the Canadian medical technicians of the first half of the twentieth century whose work the historian Peter Twohig describes as underpaid and invisible,[35] Dockrill made an essential contribution to knowledge, as we will see. Perhaps he was more ambitious and more anxious to publicly receive recognition than most other technicians of his time; perhaps this was so because in his particular case he saw how his scientific contribution began to be used to justify a medical therapy that could, in principle, transform the landscape of medicine.

Dockrill's work in the Laboratory of Neurocytology was centered on Penfield's initial research project: the matter of structural changes in the brain following injury. His work, and that of the other members of the lab, led to increasingly sophisticated techniques for visualizing the interstitial cells of the central nervous system,[36] and it allowed Penfield to describe the structure and the development of scars induced experimentally in laboratory animals. By 1927 Penfield could confidently outline the nature of these scars and what he argued to be their relationship to epilepsy. He noted that astrocytes were the important glial cells involved in the development of scars, with some activity, especially in the immediate aftermath of injury, from microglia. He outlined the cellular structure of astrocytes and the manner in which these "octopus-like" cells,[37] in their attachment to blood vessels and the delicate membrane that encapsulates the brain (the pia mater), "hold the manifold structures of the nervous system within their tentacles."[38] He named this system the vaso-astral framework. From the experimental lesions he inflicted on his laboratory animals, Penfield discovered that if the dura (the outermost membrane of the three that cover the brain) was injured, no adhesions involving the arachnoidea (the middle membrane) occurred. On the other hand, if the pia was breached, "an energetic connective tissue response" took place,[39] and adhesions formed. The adhesions, Penfield saw under the microscope, were the result of the fibrous astrocytes, which projected their expansions "through the pia and into the scar beyond."[40]

Penfield claimed that it was characteristic of the resulting scar, which developed to incorporate increasingly more connective tissue and blood vessels, to contract such that "mechanical traction" was being exerted upon the brain itself by means of the vaso-astral framework.[41] The greater the wound and brain destruction, the stronger this "contractile force."[42] Over time, the tension resulted in the hypertrophy of the astrocyte expansions, and in a pulling of the cortex toward the core of the cicatrix. Although these conclusions were reached in the course of his experimental work with animal models, Penfield did cite clinical evidence from the German surgeon Otfrid Foerster, who had noted a "wandering" of the brain's ventricles toward the side of the brain where the lesion was located.[43] This, Penfield argued, was the result of the cicatricial contraction, and he speculated that "the slow contraction of such a scar, continuing as it does for years, must produce a constant irritation which may well be the starting point for a nervous discharge resulting in Jacksonian epilepsy."[44]

This kind of bench science was important to Penfield, who had studied medicine in an environment in which a particular vision of science was supposed to inform medical practice.[45] In the early 1920s, the discovery of insulin was just the latest spectacular therapy that had come out of the laboratory. As historian Harry Marks demonstrated in his classic study, this period was characterized by a broad movement of reformers whose express goal was to establish a "rational therapeutics"—that is, to discover therapeutic agents whose effects and mechanisms of action had to be first demonstrated in a rational, scientific way in the laboratory.[46] Surgery registered the influence of this movement as well, and in Europe elite university surgeons especially, as historian Thomas Schlich shows in the previous chapter, were anchoring surgical epistemology in experimental physiology and animal experimentation since the last decades of the nineteenth century.[47] Harvey Cushing, one of the first American neurosurgeons, with whom Penfield had very briefly worked and who was an influential figure in the establishment of neurosurgery as a medical specialty, argued that the laboratory was the place where aspiring brain surgeons should practice and perfect their technique on animals first.[48]

Penfield clearly articulated not only a commitment to basing therapy on an understanding of underlying mechanisms, but also on a distrust of therapeutic empiricism. In a 1930 paper on the surgical treatment of epilepsy delivered at a meeting of the Philadelphia Neurological Society, he lamented that "the empirical method in treating this disease has been followed too long."[49] His aim was "to point out the necessity of finding a rational basis for attack on this disease, rather than to follow the 'wandering fires' of empiricism,"[50] and he argued that therapy ought to be based on "a logical hypothesis which bears the inspection of pathological studies and physiological consideration."[51] It was, then, not enough for Penfield to simply provide empirical evidence that, for example, the surgical excision of a brain scar led to the cure or amelioration of epilepsy. He had been trained to look for theoretical justification for surgical intervention—and such theory could be built upon evidence uncovered by basic bench science.[52]

The problem, however, was that histology did not provide unambiguous evidence to inform, in a straightforward fashion, rational clinical practice. The arrow of discovery did not lead unidirectionally and in an uncomplicated fashion from histology to therapy. Ultimately, in these early years, Penfield wove together evidence, in a back-and-forth effort, from the microscope and the operating table to craft a theory that justified a surgical intervention that he called "radical."[53] The theory of cicatricial contraction, which in turn had been built in conjunction with the histological work that allowed Penfield to visualize the cellular composition of brain scars, was the first step in this process. The second step relied on operating room experience that Penfield translated into a hypothesis for which Dockrill again provided histological evidence. This continuing collaboration between doctor and technician, however, almost never reached this second step. It nearly came to an end in 1928.

That year Penfield was offered a surgical position at the Royal Victoria Hospital in Montreal, and glimpsing the possibility of building his own neurological institute in Canada, Penfield accepted it. As he left New York, he parted ways with his technician, but not with William Cone, whom he convinced to move to Montreal with him. After packing up his laboratory and shipping the instruments, slides, and specimens to Montreal, Penfield decided to embark on an "interlude in Germany,"[54] where he wanted not only to assess the state of the broad field of neurology-neurosurgery-neuropathology,[55] but more importantly, to observe the surgical work of Otfrid Foerster. Foerster had started to operate on his own after years of working as a neurologist and relying on other surgeons to conduct the therapy he thought his patients needed. During the war he had dealt with many brain injuries, but he was now increasingly turning his attention to epilepsy.

Over the course of several months, Penfield watched Foerster operate, and he stained and observed under the microscope the scars that Foerster had removed from the brains of patients suffering from traumatic epilepsy. In a letter to his mother, Penfield expressed again the powerful belief that reductive neuropathology paved the road to rational therapy: "In such tissue," he said, referring to Foerster's preserved scars, "lie hidden some of the secrets of epilepsy, if not the whole story."[56]

While the patient was lying on the operating table under the influence of local anesthesia, Penfield observed that the surgeon could induce an epileptic attack in two different ways: by means of stimulation with an electrode and faradic current, or by mechanically pulling on the scar with a pair of forceps. To Penfield the latter observation was quite remarkable; it accorded so well with his cicatricial contraction theory. Despite the fact that Foerster's surgical technique was much different from his own, the two surgeons collaboratively developed a justification for surgical intervention in these cases. In a joint paper for the journal *Brain*, they laid out a theory about the structural basis of traumatic epilepsy, and they outlined their rationale for a "radical operation."[57] The practice of removing a scar or a compromised section of the brain—the point of origin for focal epilepsy—was certainly not new, stretching back into the late nineteenth century with the work of surgeons such as Victor Horsley in England and Fedor Krause in Germany, as well as neurologists like Moses Allen Starr in the United States.[58] But Penfield and Foerster's rational justification of the operation, the reliance on histology, and their speculations about the underlying mechanisms of traumatic epilepsy certainly contained novel elements.[59] Their model relied on reductionist techniques and a reductionist ethos in the era before the entrenched reductionism of molecular neurobiology, which Brian Casey and Justin Garson describe in subsequent chapters of this volume.

Defining epilepsy generally as "a specific reaction on the part of the central nervous system to a noxious stimulus,"[60] Foerster and Penfield focused on seven cases of focal epilepsy, in which some kind of trauma had created "a circumscribed area upon which the stimulus first acts."[61] They plotted the course of the clinical encounter, from the initial use of visualizing technology (encephalography)[62] to obtain information about the location of cerebral abnormality, to the electrical exploration of the exposed cortex, to the removal of the affected tissue. Their main concern was, however, building a rational case for this kind of surgery: "The radical excision of a lesion," they argued "even though it is obviously the focus for epileptic discharges, can only be a rational procedure if the lesion produced by the excision be a more innocent one than the original focus."[63] The empirical evidence for this rational procedure was provided by Penfield's work with animal models, which showed that a clean cut with the scalpel produced much less scarring than a blunt injury.[64] Penfield's vaso-astral framework was marshaled to explain the increasing tension exerted by the contracting cicatrix, which in turn exerted a pull on the whole brain and furnished the stimulus that resulted in the electrical discharge of the epileptic attack.

But what exactly was causing the epileptic discharge itself? How could non-nervous tissue—the astrocytes and connective tissue and blood vessels of the cicatrix—lead to a seizure? Penfield and Foerster, armed with their experimental and clinical data, posited a mechanism—one which was made possible by a particular view of the brain.

What kind of brain was the brain of the 1920s and early 1930s? Scholars have argued that different conceptions of the brain engender dramatically different ways of conceptualizing diseases of the brain. Before the plastic brain,[65] before even the chemical brain, there was the electrical brain.[66] In this volume, Max Stadler reveals the vast array of idiosyncratic electrical elements and techniques that made up this electrical brain. Certainly, in the 1920s the ground was already being laid for an understanding of the chemical transmission of nerve impulses through the work of Otto Loewi and Henry Dale.[67] And certainly Penfield was well aware that chemical compounds such as potassium bromide and phenobarbital sometimes decreased the frequency and severity of seizures, while other compounds induced seizures.[68] But the epistemic shift that led to the overwhelming understanding of the brain as a chemical machine in the middle of the century was still a couple of decades away, and at any rate, as with all epistemic shifts, the breaks and boundaries are not sharp. In fact, just like different kinds of objectivity can coexist (sometimes amicably, sometimes in conflict),[69] different conceptions of brains continued to coexist as well, sometimes seamlessly, at other times in tension with each other.

In this pre-chemical transmission era, then, Penfield and Foerster argued that "if the stimulus for an epileptic seizure arises in the nervous elements one might expect the attack to begin shortly after the infliction of the wound when the elements are plentiful and undergoing progressive destruction."[70] Because this was not the case—epileptic attacks, according to them, developed months or years after the damage, Penfield and Foerster argued that "the vaso-motor reflex secondary to [the] traction [of the cicatrix] is responsible for the initiation of the convulsive seizures."[71] In other words, the reason why mechanical traction led to an epileptic attack was because it triggered a vaso-motor reflex—the constriction or dilation of a blood vessel caused by the nervous system.[72]

There was however, one problem with this hypothesis. Although some anatomists had demonstrated the existence of vascular nerves on meningeal blood vessels, including on the capillaries of the pia mater, and despite some tenuous evidence to the contrary, it was thought at the time that the vessels in the brain itself did not possess vascular nerves.[73] Because Penfield and Foerster had suggested the vaso-motor reflex as a mechanism for epileptic attacks, and because they had observed repeatedly in the operating room dramatic changes in blood circulation in the brain during an epileptic attack (such as arterial constriction, the cessation of pulsation in the arteries, the appearance of areas in which the brain appeared blanched or anemic), Penfield left Germany with the understanding that he now had to prove the existence of intracerebral vascular nerves in order to buttress the underlying mechanism for epilepsy that he and Foerster had theorized.

From Germany, Penfield traveled directly to Montreal to take up his new position at the Royal Victoria Hospital. Dockrill did not initially accompany him, because at some point in late 1926 or 1927, Dockrill had returned to Edinburgh and had gotten a job as a lab technician at the Royal Infirmary.[74] By the spring of 1928, however, he was writing both to Penfield and to Cone asking for his old job back. Both were reluctant to reemploy him. Although the technician had done excellent work, the neurosurgeons saw him as a difficult person to work with: "My first instinct too was never again," confessed Cone in a letter to Penfield. "In checking the pros and cons I lean in that direction still. However, his loyalty to you and his good silver work make me perfectly willing to have him if you think it is wise. I have written him a non-committal letter saying we could not offer him more than $100. As you say that will decide the matter very likely."[75]

Soon after his move to Montreal, Penfield was shocked to open the door to his own residence one day to find Dockrill waiting patiently for him. Leaving his wife and child in the UK,[76] he had come to Montreal, after all, despite the meager salary that was offered to him in hopes he would decline. He wanted to be part of Penfield and Cone's new Laboratory of Neuropathology, but the fact that Penfield had campaigned for Cone to join him in Montreal, while Dockrill himself had been rebuffed, would have made it plainly obvious to Dockrill just how replaceable he was (see fig. 5.1).

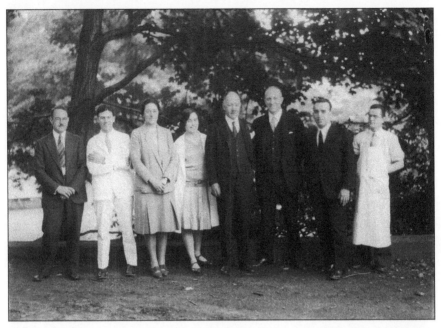

Figure 5.1. The personnel of the Neuropathology Laboratory of the Royal Victoria Hospital, Spring 1929: Ottiwell Jones, Maurice Brodie, Dorothy Russell, Hope Lewis (secretary), Colin Russel, Wilder Penfield, William Cone, Edward Dockrill. Reproduced by permission of the Osler Library of the History of Medicine, McGill University.

In the novel, Armstrong's peripheral position in the economy of the laboratory is evident at the annual "gathering of medical clans" of the "International College of Physicians and Surgeons."[77] Because he is not a doctor, he does not get a pass to enter the "numerous sideshows" where "patients and animals alike, both looking very bored, were brought to parade for the visitors' edification."[78] He is relegated to the laboratory, where he demonstrates his histological techniques to visitors. Nevertheless, from the sidelines, he provides a scathing critique of the commercialization of medicine evident in the various medical products available for sale and the "press representatives" on hand to record the specialists' presentations. He runs into Frank, a technician from the Bacteriology Department, who at this point in the novel is more cynical than Armstrong himself and who quips that the doctors who thronged the meeting "swear an oath to the goddess of Hypocrisy not Hippocrates."[79] Indeed, while inside the hotel miracles are peddled and important-looking doctors claim they work to alleviate human suffering, right outside the doors Armstrong enters a very different world. Outside, "a semi-paralyzed cripple sold newspapers giving full details of the marvelous inventions and cures reported at the meetings."[80] And park benches are full of "destitute humans [who] sat huddled in non-descript attitudes, spitting when an ugly cough moved them."[81] An "indigent blind woman" offers him matches, and Dockrill, troubled, hurries away "from such disturbing contrasts"[82]—the glittering, optimistic world of self-congratulatory medical men on the one hand, and the grim reality of poverty and disease on the other. Over the course of the novel, he moves back and forth between these two different worlds.

One could read Armstrong's fictional experience against the very real gathering of the American College of Physicians, a gathering that was held for the first time outside of the United States in 1933 at Montreal's grand Windsor Hotel.[83] Representing Quebec's premier, the Provincial Secretary Hon. Louis-Athanase David welcomed the hundreds of medical men and expressed an ideal of scientific work as cooperative and international, enthusing that "in the highest spheres of science friendships are easily established and maintained."[84] The newspapers reported the presentations of doctors who outlined various therapies, such as X-rays for goiter. Penfield himself gave a talk about his successful surgical therapy for focal epilepsy, mentioning his theory of the vaso-motor reflex.[85] If Dockrill did attend this meeting, as his fictional alter ego does in the novel, he would have then presided like Armstrong over an exhibit showcasing photographs of nerves, as well as histological preparations, "absolutely beautiful . . . definite . . . irrefutable" evidence of intercerebral nerves (see figs. 5.2 and 5.3).[86]

The problem of the intracerebral nerves was one of the most important tackled by Dockrill in the new Montreal lab. Working in conjunction with Stanley Cobb and J. E. Finesinger from Harvard and George Chorobski (a research fellow at the Royal Victoria Hospital),[87] Penfield and Dockrill

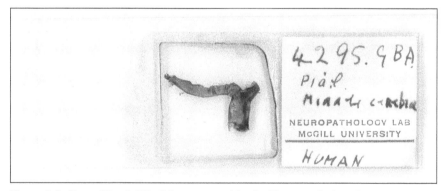

Figure 5.2. One of Dockrill's slides prepared in the Neuropathology Department. Reproduced by permission of the Osler Library of the History of Medicine, McGill University.

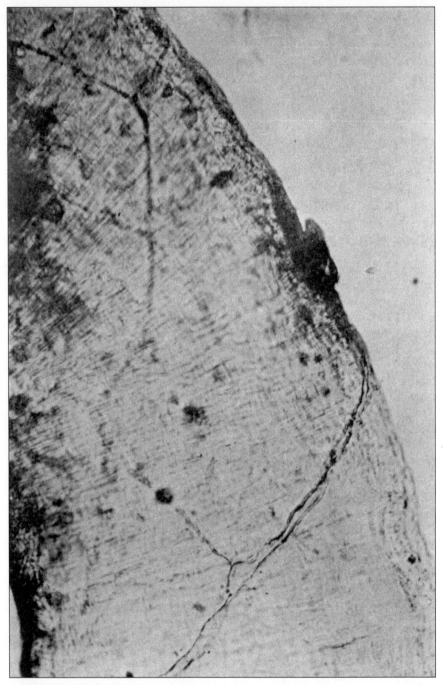

Figure 5.3. Photograph of intracerebral perivascular nerves around an artery. Wilder Penfield, ed. *Cytology and Cellular Pathology of the Nervous System* (New York: Paul B. Hoeber, Inc., 1932), 417, fig. 16.

started out with a modified version of Cajal's silver method but found it unreliable, albeit occasionally successful. Another variation on the silver-nitrate staining method, the Gros-Bielschowsky method, was modified further, and it proved more consistent in visualizing vascular nerves in different parts of the brain of cats, monkeys, and humans. In 1932 Penfield published a short note in his edited volume *Cytology & Cellular Pathology of the Nervous System*,[88] followed by a more detailed and richly illustrated article in the *Archives of Neurology and Psychiatry* in which he announced that the nerve plexus of the pia's blood vessels was continuous with that of the vessels of the brain itself.[89] The brain's vascular system was indeed innervated.

In light of Penfield's theory about the vaso-motor reflex as a mechanism of traumatic epilepsy, the first slides that showed the delicate nerve fibers encircling cerebral vessels must have been a cause of great celebration in the Montreal lab. Penfield chose to begin and end his article with a nod to his theory, concluding that "from a purely morphological point of view, intracerebral vasomotor reflexes are possible."[90] He also took the unusual step of mentioning, in the body of the article, the contribution of his technician: "I have now been able to demonstrate nerve fibers on the intracerebral blood vessels throughout the central nervous system by means of certain modifications in histological method devised by our technician, E. Dockrill."[91] Although the sentence still firmly identifies Penfield as the active discoverer ("I have . . . demonstrate[d]"), the nod to Dockrill's technical achievement was unambiguous ("method devised by . . . Dockrill"). It is quite possible that this unusual public acknowledgment was a result of the vocal technician's lobbying for his own recognition.[92]

At the same time, however, it is likely that Dockrill had in mind something even grander; perhaps he had in mind a coauthorship. His alter ego Armstrong implies the desirability of such symbolic compensation in his own fictional lamentations about the invisibility of technicians. Armstrong idolizes Dr. Meadowes at first,[93] but he soon begins to describe him as more of a shrewd politician than an ideal scientist: "Meadowes came often to the laboratory but never stayed long."[94] Instead, he relied on the work of others:

> Very early, Gerry realised, that the chief, Dr Meadowes, was no scientist although he reaped a good deal of publicity and was honoured as one. He saw how that was effected by cleverly done self advertisement. Dr Meadowes travelled everywhere in the academic world and by a chain letter system of introductory letters, made himself known to every-one of importance. Now, he had men, Research Fellows, he called them, culled from international sources to work in his laboratory. It was a good scheme. Soon, they would give place to others and in their going, would carry Meadowes' fame with them.[95]

On the other hand, Armstrong thought that Dr. Peake, "the other partner in the scheme and co-director of the institution . . . was the ideal scientist."[96] He was present in the hospital and the lab at all hours of the day and night; he appeared to be kind to his patients *and* to the laboratory technicians; he promised Armstrong that he would share the publicity from any discovery they made together. Armstrong appreciated this kindness precisely because he thought it rare. In fact, he was aware of stories like that of Frank's, the laboratory technician in the Bacteriology Department, who had isolated a bacteria responsible for a series of cases of contagious disease, but whose superior announced Frank's discovery as his own, naming the bacteria after himself. Frank did get paid for his work—something to the tune of $100 or $120 a year. His superior, meanwhile, got recognition, fame, *and* a salary of $15,000.

Frank's story is meant to foreshadow what happens to Armstrong himself later in the novel. Peake is studying the role of the kidneys in diabetes, and he wants to use Armstrong's histological expertise to be the first to prove renal innervation. When Armstrong does succeed, Peake takes advantage of Armstrong's short vacation to announce the discovery and take singular credit for it. What is more, Peake claims that this discovery could shed light on the mechanisms of cancer, turning a scientific discovery into a potentially transformative clinical therapy.

Armstrong becomes more and more disillusioned with his life. The daily work at the lab, where he has to constantly hurt and sacrifice animals, becomes slowly unbearable. He is sullen and unfriendly toward the other members of the lab. He increasingly prefers to work in the silence of the night, when everybody else has gone home. Eventually, Meadowes becomes aware of Armstrong's haphazard schedule and antisocial behavior and expresses his displeasure; the chief likes to run a tight ship, organized, efficient, predictable. Meadowes scolds Armstrong and gives him a New Testament for Christmas—part of the ongoing project to make him a better man. But Armstrong is not religious and finds the gesture distasteful. At the root of his alienation is a clash between an ideal of science—and of the scientist's persona—and the reality of contemporary organized science, as he sees it:

> There was no room in modern, organized science for the disreputable scapegoat with his uncouth habits and occasional flashes of inspiration. He was just a relic of the days when men sought Truth because they must have an outlet for the fire that was in them and they diagnosed his genius as a psychosis. He was an individualist, a throwback to those old creators of Van Leeuwenhoek's day who worked secretly because their reward was death instead of fame and their pay was a jail sentence instead of riches. There were still of these men about but they no longer feared death as a reward for their work. Organized science had seen to that. It encouraged them. It bought them up, directed their efforts, and fattened on the results of their labours. And, when they baulked at the wholesale barter of their souls, it threatened them with the terrifying

bogey of economic insecurity. How could they fight economic battles when their whole equipment was designed and trained merely to aid their play with the elements?[97]

Eventually, Armstrong has an outburst in Meadowes' office, accusing the perplexed doctor of "becom[ing] famous with work you never did, paid for by money you never owned," which came from "the industrial barons who stole it and then made donations to salve their conscience."[98] He also accuses Meadowes of profiting financially at the expense of his patients. Scientific discoveries in the laboratory are sacred, Armstrong fervently believes. They can't be patented. They ought not to bring riches and fame to their discoverers.

But of course there is a tension here between the ideal of the disinterested, self-effacing, saintly laboratory worker and Armstrong himself, who, for all his protestations, is often driven by a feeling that he is not receiving enough money and enough recognition for his labors. The writer explores this tension skillfully. Dockrill's characters are not caricatures of the noble and the debased, of the good and the evil; they are complex and subtle. Meadowes, for all of Armstrong's negative evaluation of him, is at his core a kind and decent person. After Armstrong storms out of his office and takes up residence in the city's alleyways, ultimately becoming quite sick, it is Meadowes who rescues him and arranges for medical treatment in a comfortable hospital room. For his part, Armstrong is often portrayed as a deeply flawed character (he behaves abominably toward several women, and he frequents the red light district). When at the end of the novel Dockrill invokes a deus ex machina to allow Armstrong to cure a wealthy donor of his cancer, the fictional technician does not get a happy ending. As punishment for his faults and his hubris, and, simultaneously, as a meditation on the impossibility of happy endings for individuals in his social position, Armstrong watches helplessly as his beloved dies in a senseless car accident in front of the hospital.

It is tempting to read these two lives—the real and the fictional—in parallel. In Dockrill's fictional world, the innervation of cerebral blood vessels becomes renal innervation, while a cure for epilepsy becomes a cure for cancer. For indeed, the innervation of the brain's vascular system was used not only to justify Penfield's theory of the vaso-motor reflex as a mechanism for epilepsy, but it was also employed to suggest a novel surgical therapy for epilepsy: the removal of the sympathetic nerves of the cerebral arteries. Not only was this a new surgical procedure for this particular neurological condition, but in theory it promised to offer a much more widely-applicable solution for epilepsy. Whereas the excision of a cicatricial scar was obviously appropriate only in cases of traumatic epilepsy, this new therapy could be deployed in cases of idiopathic epilepsy in which no gross abnormalities could be detected and which comprised the majority of epilepsy diagnoses.

Starting with the vaso-motor reflex, which had been buttressed by the discovery of the innervation of the brain's vascular system by means of Dockrill's histological work, Penfield built a case for the powerful involvement of the circulatory system during epileptic attacks. Citing the classic observations of neurologists such as John Hughlings Jackson, as well as relying on his direct observations of thirty patients who had seizures while on the operating table, Penfield showed that epileptic attacks led to vasomotor spasms and a host of other changes in blood circulation in the brain, which in turn had effects such as the formation of "focal areas of cortical anemia,"[99] essentially cortical patches and spots where blood circulation ceased for a period during and after an epileptic attack. Since stimulation of the brain of nonepileptic patients did not lead to such vasomotor effects, Penfield concluded that sufferers from idiopathic epilepsy had an underlying abnormality of cerebral circulation, a defect he called "vasolability."[100] He reasoned that since the nerves of the blood vessels of the pia were known to be under the control of the sympathetic and parasympathetic nervous system, one could naturally assume the same about the blood vessels of the brain. In theory, then, a "rational therapeutic attack" that prevented the constriction of these blood vessels by disrupting the nerves that controlled them should have an effect on epilepsy, or at the very least on the postconvulsive paralysis that afflicted the patients.[101]

The surgical procedures that were suggested by this theory consisted in the destruction of the ganglia located near the spinal cord in the region of the seventh cervical vertebrae in the neck (a cervicothoracic sympathetic ganglionectomy), as well as in stripping off the nerves that innervated the arteries supplying blood to the head and neck (a periarterial sympathectomy of the internal carotid arteries and the vertebral arteries). Penfield performed these surgeries on at least four patients, but he had to conclude that "complete removal of all sympathetic nerves entering the skull did not make epilepsy impossible."[102] One patient did get better, but one got worse. Two remained the same. Penfield cautiously concluded that sympathetic ganglionectomy "does not make seizures impossible and is hardly justifiable as a treatment for epilepsy except in the presence of unusual evidence of abnormality of the sympathetic nervous system. In such instances it may be looked on as an aid but not as a cure."[103]

Although it might have seemed like a great promise when Penfield first envisioned it, the sympathetic ganglionectomy never became an accepted therapy for idiopathic epilepsy. In contrast to the fictional world of Gerry Armstrong, the histological methods that Dockrill perfected did not bridge the gap between a "rational therapy" and an empirically successful one—not even partially, as an aid in the management of this neurological condition.

🙦   🙦   🙦

What do these tales—the fictional one in Dockrill's novel and the real story of Dockrill's life and work—tell us about the mind and brain sciences of the 1920s and 1930s? To begin with, they shed light on the epistemology of surgical therapy at the time. Dockrill's histological work was seen as important primarily because of the therapeutic potential it fostered. Mere therapeutic empiricism was dangerous; therapy, surgeons such as Penfield argued, had to be anchored in laboratory science.[104] Penfield was so committed to this ideal that even though his "rational" surgical intervention for idiopathic epilepsy failed to be empirically validated, he continued to maintain that all surgical therapy had to be "directed by rational analysis of the individual etiologic problem" and that neuropathology "should be the sine qua non of [a neurosurgeon's] entrance into the field of epilepsy."[105] This chapter has shown that histological techniques could lead to ambiguous results, however, and that in fact Penfield's rational theories involved a complicated and constant back-and-forth negotiation and mutual justification between scientific evidence, clinical observations, and theoretical speculations. There was no straight, unidirectional, magic arrow from science to therapy, from histology to surgery— despite what both Penfield and Dockrill had hoped. In the coming years, as Penfield soon realized, it was a different technology—electroencephalography—that proved to be a more fruitful approach in dealing with epilepsy.[106]

Dockrill's refinement of specific histological techniques allowed Penfield to both craft and shore up his vaso-motor reflex theory and to conceive and justify surgical therapies for traumatic epilepsy (the excision of the focal area) and idiopathic epilepsy (sympathetic ganglionectomy and periarterial sympathectomy). Dockrill's work as a laboratory technician, while largely invisible both to historians and to many of his contemporaries, appears marginal (in the sense of minor and irrelevant to broader histories of the brain sciences), but this is so only in retrospect: his name is not recognizable and the failed therapy that he helped justify is equally obscure. At the time, however, his work helped provide some of the scaffolding for a "rational therapy" that held enormous, if ultimately unfulfilled promise.

Apart from his histological techniques, Dockrill deployed sophisticated narrative techniques to fight against what he felt to be the invisibility of laboratory technicians such as himself. The story of his fictional alter ego describes the highly skilled work of technicians and the extent to which they were as invested in an ideal of science as the scientific masters they served. But mastery of technique is not enough, Dockrill suggested in his manuscript. The translation of histological knowledge into the humanitarian but also economic enterprise of clinical therapy was the step that mattered most for the medical establishment, organized science, and society at large in the interwar period. In the novel's dénouement the hero conquers cancer by devising a cure, but the novel's lack of a happy ending signals the writer's uneasiness about the popular glorification of science only for its practical results. Dockrill's literary techniques as much as his histological ones gave him a voice and helped him forge an identity for himself in the context of such concerns about the role of science and the epistemic underpinnings of clinical therapy.

❧   ❧   ❧

Edward Dockrill stopped working as a technician in Penfield's lab in the early 1930s. Immigration records and a ship's passenger manifest show that in September 1935, Dockrill returned to Montreal from England, where he had moved the previous year.[107] Interestingly, immigration officials recorded his occupation as "author," although for the rest of his life, official government documents refer to him as a "technician."[108] Perhaps Dockrill undertook this 1935 journey with the express purpose of submitting his novel to a publisher, and in a moment of pride and confidence in the nearly four-hundred-page tome in his luggage, he saw himself as an author. Although it is not clear when Dockrill made the submission, it appears that the publisher recognized Penfield in the story and forwarded the manuscript to him at the brand-new institute he founded, the Montreal Neurological Institute, which opened its doors in 1934. At some point Dockrill must have returned to England, and he settled in Essex. In June 1949, along with his wife and seven children, who ranged in age from nine years to six months, Dockrill boarded the brand-new British Royal Mail Steamer Orcades, with Fremantle, Australia, as his destination. Now forty-nine years old, he was once again poised to start life in another country. He gave his occupation as "technician" and continued to do so until his death in 1969.[109]

"A new technique can help to mold a man or to make him famous or to create a cause,"[110] Penfield wrote a few years later in his autobiography, within a section about Cajal. Dockrill—whose novel's title is in fact adapted from a Cajal quote, and whose fictional hero idolizes the Spanish histologist—had hoped his improved technique would lift his invisibility, if not make him famous. At any rate, it certainly created a cause, which he expressed passionately and articulately in a novel that never found an audience. Penfield himself claimed not to have read it.[111] But, ironically perhaps, if Dockrill's invisibility did eventually lift, it was in no small measure because of Penfield himself, who made possible the reconstruction of Dockrill's stories—the real and the fictional alike.

Notes

For comments on a previous draft of this paper, I am grateful to Stephen Casper, Samuel Greenblatt, Katja Guenther, and the volume's anonymous reviewers. I wish to thank Chris Lyons and Anna Dysert from the Osler Library at McGill University, who have provided invaluable archival support. The initial research that has led to this chapter was supported by the Social Sciences and Humanities Research Council of Canada through a CGS Doctoral Scholarship and by Osler Library through a Research Travel Grant. *Epigraph.* Edward Dockrill, "The Means Are Nothing," Osler Library, McGill University, Montreal, A/N 1a, c. mid 1930s, 23–24.

1. Edward Dockrill, "The Means Are Nothing," Osler Library, McGill University, A/N 1a, c. mid-1930s, 90.

2. Ibid.

3. Ibid., 319.

4. Steven Shapin, "The Invisible Technician," *American Scientist* 77 (1989): 554–63. Shapin noted, in the context of early modern science, that the technicians were invisible not only to Robert Boyle and his contemporaries, but also to historians of science.

5. N. C. Russell, E. M. Tansey, and P. V. Lear, "Missing Links in the History and Practice of Science: Teams, Technicians and Technical Work," *History of Science* 38, no. 120, pt 2 (2000): 238.

6. E. M. Tansey, "Keeping the Culture Alive: The Laboratory Technician in Mid-Twentieth-Century British Medical Research," *Notes and Records of the Royal Society of London* 62, no. 1 (2008): 77–95; Peter L. Twohig, *Labour in the Laboratory: Medical Laboratory Workers in the Maritimes, 1900–1950* (Montreal: McGill-Queen's University Press, 2005).

7. David Alan Grier, *When Computers Were Human* (Princeton, NJ: Princeton University Press, 2005).

8. Jennifer S. Light, "When Computers Were Women," *Technology and Culture* 40, no. 3 (1999): 455–83.

9. Jean-Paul Gaudillière and Ilana Löwy, eds., *The Invisible Industrialist: Manufactures and the Production of Scientific Knowledge* (New York: Macmillan, 1998).

10. Wilder Penfield, *No Man Alone: A Neurosurgeon's Life* (Boston: Little, Brown, 1977), 365n46.

11. Penfield, handwritten note on Dockrill's manuscript, Osler Library, McGill University, Montreal, A/N 1a.

12. Mary E. Fissell, "Making Meaning from the Margins: The New Cultural History of Medicine," in *Locating Medical History: The Stories and Their Meanings*, ed. Frank Huisman and John Harley Warner (Baltimore: Johns Hopkins University Press, 2004). On medical technicians in particular, see Twohig, *Labour in the Laboratory*.

13. Anne Stiles, *Popular Fiction and Brain Science in the Late Nineteenth Century* (Cambridge: Cambridge University Press, 2011); Anne Stiles, *Neurology and Literature, 1860–1920* (Basingstoke, UK: Palgrave Macmillan, 2007).

14. Thomas Edward Dockrill, Apr-May-June 1900 registration, Chorlton, Lancashire, England & Wales, FreeBMD Birth Index, 1837–1915, vol. 8c, p. 959, database accessed through ancestry.com Operations Inc., 2006.

15. Penfield, *No Man Alone*, 364. On Penfield, see Jefferson Lewis, *Something Hidden: A Biography of Wilder Penfield* (Toronto: Doubleday Canada, 1981); William Feindel, "The Physiologist and the Neurosurgeon: The Enduring Influence of Charles Sherrington on the Career of Wilder Penfield," *Brain* 130, no. 130, pt. 11 (2007).

16. On the complex professional identity that Penfield and other neurosurgeons of his era embraced, see Delia Gavrus, "Men of Dreams and Men of Action: Neurologists, Neurosurgeons, and the Performance of Professional Identity, 1920–1950," *Bulletin of the History of Medicine* 85, no. 1 (2011): 57–92; "Men of Strong Opinions: Identity, Self-Representation, and the Performance of Neurosurgery, 1919–1950" (PhD diss., University of Toronto, 2011).

17. At this time, some neurologists were attempting to ground analysis and diagnosis of other neurological diseases in laboratory practices, as Kenton Kroker has shown in his analysis of epidemic encephalitis: Kenton Kroker, "Epidemic Encephalitis and American Neurology, 1919–1940," *Bulletin of the History of Medicine* 78, no. 1 (2004): 108–47.

18. Jean-Gaël Barbara, "Interplay between Scientific Theories and Researches on the Diseases of the Nervous System in the Nineteenth-Century, Paris," *Medicine Studies* 1, no. 4 (2009): 341.

19. For a literature review on work on neuroglia over the past century and a half, see V. Parpura and A. Verkhratsky, "Neuroglia at the Crossroads of Homoeostasis, Metabolism and Signalling: Evolution of the Concept," *ASN Neuro* 4, no. 4 (2012); Emily K. Mathey, Ariel Arthur, and Patricia J. Armati, "CNS Oligarchs; the Rise of the Oligodendrocyte in a Neuron-Centric Culture," in *The Biology of Oligodendrocytes*, ed. Patricia J. Armati and Emily K. Mathey (Cambridge: Cambridge University Press, 2010): 1–18; H. Kettenmann and A. Verkhratsky, "Neuroglia: The 150 Years After," *Trends in Neurosciences* 31, no. 12 (2008): 653–59.

20. L. M. Garcia-Segura, "Cajal and Glial Cells," *Progress in Brain Research* 136 (2002): 255–60.

21. More broadly on the history of histology and microscopy, see, for instance, Brian Bracegirdle, "The History of Histology: A Brief Survey of Sources," *History of Science* 15 (1977): 77–101; L. S. Jacyna, "'A Host of Experienced Microscopists': The Establishment of Histology in Nineteenth-Century Edinburgh," *Bulletin of the History of Medicine* 75, no. 2 (2001): 225–53; Ann La Berge, "The History of Science and the History of Microscopy," *Perspectives on Science* 7, no. 1 (1999): 111–42.

22. See, for example, the technic as described in Ulric Dahlgren and William A. Kepner, *A Text-Book of the Principles of Animal Histology* (New York: Macmillan, 1908), 502–7.

23. On Cajal's techniques, see Joseph D. Robinson, *Mechanisms of Synaptic Transmission: Bridging the Gaps (1890–1990)* (Oxford: Oxford University Press, 2001), 11–12; Richard L. Rapport, *Nerve Endings: The Discovery of the Synapse* (New York: W. W. Norton, 2005); Gordon M. Shepherd, *Foundations of the Neuron Doctrine* (New York: Oxford University Press, 1991).

24. Wilder Penfield, "Alterations of the Golgi Apparatus in Nerve Cells," *Brain* 43, no. 3 (1920): 290–305; Penfield, *No Man Alone: A Neurosurgeon's Life*, 92.

25. Penfield to his mother, quoted in Penfield, *No Man Alone*, 96.

26. The confusion was further heightened by the fact that Cajal refused to recognize these two types of cells because he could not replicate Río-Hortega's stains, a fact to which Penfield obliquely refers in his article, "Oligodendroglia and Its Relation to Classical Neuroglia," *Brain* 47 (1924): 430–52.

27. Wilder Penfield, "Microglie Et Son Rapport Avec La Dégénération Névrogliale Dans Un Gliome," *Travaux du laboratoire de recherches biologiques de l'université de Madrid*

22 (1924): 277–93; Wilder Penfield, "Microglia and the Process of Phagocytosis in Gliomas," *American Journal of Pathology* 1 (1925): 77–89.

28. Penfield, "Oligodendroglia and Its Relation to Classical Neuroglia," 440.

29. Ibid., 440–41.

30. Penfield, *No Man Alone*, 116.

31. Perhaps a sign that he was not content is the fact that by late 1926, Dockrill expressed a desire to return to England. Penfield wrote letters of introduction for him. See Penfield's letter to George Riddoch (London General Hospital), October 29, 1926, Penfield Fonds P142, box 51, C/G 26.27 Osler Library, McGill University, Montreal.

32. Dockrill, "Means Are Nothing," 90.

33. Ibid.

34. See, for instance, the example of Richard Buckley, visiting from Yale: Wilder Penfield and R. C. Buckley, "Punctures of the Brain: The Factors Concerned in Gliosis and in Cicatricial Contraction," *Archives of Neurology and Psychiatry* 20 (1928): 1–13.

35. Twohig, *Labour in the Laboratory*.

36. See, for instance, the extremely refined protocols described here: Wilder Penfield and William Cone, "Neuroglia and Microglia (the Metallic Methods)," in *Handbook of Microscopical Technique for Workers in Both Animal and Plant Tissues*, ed. Clarence Erwin McClung (New York: P. B. Hoeber, Inc., 1929): 359–88.

37. Wilder Penfield, "The Mechanism of Cicatricial Contraction in the Brain," *Brain* 50 (1927): 500.

38. Ibid.

39. Ibid., 501.

40. Ibid.

41. Ibid., 505.

42. Ibid., 511.

43. Ibid., 513.

44. Ibid., 516.

45. For background regarding this question about the relationship between science and medical practice in the preceding period, see John Harley Warner, "Ideals of Science and Their Discontents in Late Nineteenth-Century American Medicine," *Isis* 82, no. 3 (1991): 454–78.

46. Harry M. Marks, *The Progress of Experiment: Science and Therapeutic Reform in the United States, 1900–1990* (Cambridge: Cambridge University Press, 1997).

47. See also Thomas Schlich, *The Origins of Organ Transplantation: Surgery and Laboratory Science, 1880–1930* (Rochester, NY: University of Rochester Press, 2010), 154.

48. Harvey Cushing, "The Special Field of Neurological Surgery after Another Interval," *Archives of Neurology and Psychiatry* 4, no. 6 (1920): 611–12n8. On the surgical epistemology of the first generation of neurosurgeons see Gavrus, "Men of Strong Opinions," 52–54; Samuel H. Greenblatt, "Harvey Cushing's Paradigmatic Contribution to Neurosurgery and the Evolution of His Thoughts about Specialization," *Bulletin of the History of Medicine* 77, no. 4 (2003): 789–822. On Cushing's work, see Michael Bliss, *Harvey Cushing: A Life in Surgery* (New York: Oxford University Press, 2005); Samuel H. Greenblatt and Dale Smith, "The Emergence of

Cushing's Leadership: 1901–1920," in *A History of Neurosurgery in Its Scientific and Professional Contexts*, ed. Samuel H. Greenblatt, T. Forcht Dagi, and Mel H. Epstein (Park Ridge, IL: American Association of Neurological Surgeons, 1997): 167–90.

49. Summary of "The Place of Neurosurgery in the Treatment of Epilepsy," 1, enclosed in a letter from Bernard J. Alpers to Wilder Penfield, March 15, 1930, Wilder Penfield Fonds P 142, box 52, C/G 30.31, Osler Library, McGill University, Montreal.

50. Answers to questions in the discussion period following Penfield's paper "The Place of Neurosurgery in the Treatment of Epilepsy," 5–6, enclosed in a letter from Bernard J. Alpers to Wilder Penfield, March 15, 1930. Wilder Penfield Fonds P 142, box 52, C/G 30.31, Osler Library, McGill University, Montreal.

51. Summary of "The Place of Neurosurgery in the Treatment of Epilepsy," 1, enclosed in a letter from Bernard J. Alpers to Wilder Penfield, March 15, 1930, Wilder Penfield Fonds P 142, box 52, C/G 30.31, Osler Library, McGill University, Montreal.

52. Historian Ellen Dwyer has shown that starting in the 1930s, other epilepsy specialists were increasingly using experimental protocols to investigate and justify various kinds of invasive medical and surgical interventions. Ellen Dwyer, "Neurological Patients as Experimental Subjects: Epilepsy Studies in the United States," in *The Neurological Patient in History*, ed. L. S. Jacyna and Stephen T. Casper (Rochester, NY: University of Rochester Press, 2012): 44–60.

53. Wilder Penfield, "The Radical Treatment of Traumatic Epilepsy and Its Rationale," *Canadian Medical Association Journal* 23, no. 2 (1930): 189–97.

54. Penfield, *No Man Alone*, 154.

55. On the importance of this mission and its consequences, see Gavrus, "Men of Dreams and Men of Action: Neurologists, Neurosurgeons, and the Performance of Professional Identity, 1920–1950."

56. Penfield, letter to his mother quoted in Penfield, *No Man Alone*, 164.

57. Otfrid Foerster and Wilder Penfield, "The Structural Basis of Traumatic Epilepsy and Results of Radical Operation," *Brain* 53, no. 2 (1930): 99–119. On their collaboration and on Penfield's continuing work with electrical stimulation, see Katja Guenther, *Localization and Its Discontents: A Genealogy of Psychoanalysis and the Neuro Disciplines*, Chicago: University of Chicago Press, 2015, ch. 6; Katja Guenther, "Between Clinic and Experiment: Wilder Penfield's Stimulation Reports and the Search for Mind, 1929–55." Canadian Bulletin of Medical History 33, no. 2 (2016): 281–320.

58. See, for instance, S. Shorvon, "The Evolution of Epilepsy Theory and Practice at the National Hospital for the Relief and Cure of Epilepsy, Queen Square between 1860 and 1910," *Epilepsy & Behavior* 31 (2014): 228–42; William Feindel, "History of the Surgical Treatment of Epilepsy," in *A History of Neurosurgery in Its Scientific and Professional Contexts*, ed. Samuel H. Greenblatt, T. Forcht Dagi, and Mel H. Epstein (Park Ridge, IL: American Association of Neurological Surgeons, 1997): 465–88.

59. Feindel, "History," 468–69, in his description of the German surgeon Fedor Krause's work on epilepsy, notes that around 1912, Krause had developed a similar theory of the mechanism of epilepsy, whereby cicatricial traction led to an epileptic attack. Penfield and Foerster did not cite Krause, and it seems very likely that Penfield developed this theory independently.

60. Foerster and Penfield, "Structural Basis of Traumatic Epilepsy," 99.

61. Ibid.

62. Most likely ventriculography, although Penfield and Foerster did not describe exactly the technique they employed.

63. Foerster and Penfield, "Structural Basis of Traumatic Epilepsy," 101.

64. Penfield, "Mechanism of Cicatricial Contraction."

65. Tobias Rees, *Plastic Reason: An Anthropology of Brain Science in Embryogenetic Terms* (Berkley: University of California Press, 2016).

66. The brain "became electrified" in a world in which much of everyday life became electrified as well. See Cornelius Borck, "Electrifying the Brain in the 1920s: Electrical Technology as a Mediator in Brain Research," in *Electric Bodies: Episodes in the History of Medical Electricity*, ed. Paola Bertucci and Giuliano Pancaldi (Bologna: Universita di Bologna, 2001): 239–64.

67. See "Otto Loewi and Henry Dale: The Discovery of Neurotransmitters," in *Minds behind the Brain: A History of the Pioneers and Their Discoveries*, by Stanley Finger (Oxford: Oxford University Press, 2000), chap. 16, 259–80.

68. The discovery of the effectiveness of phenytoin (Dilantin), which had a great impact on the treatment of epilepsy, did not take place until 1938. See Lewis P. Rowland, *The Legacy of Tracy J. Putnam and H. Houston Merritt: Modern Neurology in the United States* (Oxford: Oxford University Press, 2008).

69. Lorraine Daston and Peter Galison, *Objectivity* (New York: Zone Books, 2007), 28.

70. Foerster and Penfield, "Structural Basis of Traumatic Epilepsy," 118.

71. Ibid.

72. On Penfield and the vasomotor mechanism for epilepsy, see also William Feindel and Richard Leblanc, *The Wounded Brain Healed: The Golden Age of the Montreal Neurological Institute 1934–1984* (Montreal: McGill-Queens University Press, 2016), 64–69.

73. Changes in blood flow in the brain were explained in terms of changes in overall blood pressure; see Wilder Penfield, "Intracerebral Vascular Nerves," *Archives of Neurology and Psychiatry* 27, no. 1 (1932): 30–44. On the complicated history of the vasomotor reflex, see Greenblatt, "Harvey Cushing's Paradigmatic Contribution," 799n28.

74. Dockrill to Penfield, (May?) 24, 1928, Penfield Fonds D-C/D 21-9 D, Osler Library, McGill University, Montreal. See also, F. E. Reynolds to Wilder Penfield, October 24, 1931, C/G 30-31, box 52 folder R.

75. William Cone to Wilder Penfield, March 26, 1928, Penfield Fonds, C/D 15-1, box 29, Osler Library, McGill University, Montreal. See also, Penfield, *No Man Alone*, 565n46.

76. William Cone to Wilder Penfield, June 10, 1928, C/D 15-1, box 29, Osler Library, McGill University, Montreal.

77. Dockrill, "Means Are Nothing," 163.

78. Ibid., 166.

79. Ibid., 167.

80. Ibid., 168.

81. Ibid.

82. Ibid., 169.

83. It is not clear whether Dockrill attended this meeting. He may have left Montreal in 1931. It's possible that he could have based his fictional description on other medical gatherings.

84. "American College of Physicians in Convention Here," *Montreal Gazette*, February 7 1933.

85. "Montreal Centre for Treatment of Epilepsy Victims," *Montreal Gazette*, February 10 1933.

86. Dockrill, "Means Are Nothing," 169. In this passage, Dr. Laflamme, a Quebec general practitioner, admires Armstrong's histological slides that showed beautifully stained nerve cells.

87. Wilder Penfield, "Report of Sub-Department of Neurosurgery," *Royal Victoria Hospital 38th Annual Report*, 1931, 89.

88. Wilder Penfield, ed. *Cytology and Cellular Pathology of the Nervous System* (New York: Paul B. Hoeber, 1932), 416–19.

89. Penfield, "Intracerebral Vascular Nerves."

90. Ibid., 4.

91. Ibid., 32. Dockrill was not mentioned in Penfield's edited volume, *Cytology and Cellular*.

92. There were other technicians in the laboratory. For instance, in 1929 a certain A. Goddard is listed as assistant technician. Penfield Fonds, Osler Library, McGill University, Montreal, A/M 1–3 (Faculty of Medicine, 1928–33), list of staff belonging to the Department of Neurosurgery, October 17, 1929.

93. Note that Meadowes is a play on Pen*field*, just as Peake is a play on Cone.

94. Dockrill, "Means Are Nothing," 84.

95. Ibid., 109.

96. Ibid.

97. Ibid., 286.

98. Ibid., 319.

99. Wilder Penfield, "The Evidence for a Cerebral Vascular Mechanism in Epilepsy," *Annals of Internal Medicine* 7 (1933): 303–10.

100. Wilder Penfield, "Epilepsy and Surgical Therapy," *Archives of Neurology and Psychiatry* 36, no. 3 (1936): 460.

101. Ibid.

102. Ibid., 462.

103. Ibid., 462–63.

104. As I mentioned earlier in the paper, Penfield was certainly not the first to argue for the importance of the laboratory in solving practical problems related to brain surgery; Cushing had made a similar argument—see Samuel H. Greenblatt, "Harvey Cushing's Paradigmatic Contribution to Neurosurgery and the Evolution of His Thoughts About Specialization," *Bulletin of the History of Medicine* 77, no. 4 (2003): 789–92. However, Penfield's point was inflected by a further nuance: he was arguing that what constituted a rational therapy was only that therapy which could be anchored in a solid underlying *mechanism* (physiologically, pathologically, etc.) that could only be investigated in the laboratory. This was the reason why it was not enough to suggest that an epileptic scar should be removed; the surgeon had to first prove experimentally, as Penfield in fact did, that the incision of the surgeon's scalpel was less likely to lead to the kind of damage produced by an indiscriminate

injury to the brain (such as the one that had resulted in the formation of the scar in the first place).

105. Penfield, "Epilepsy and Surgical Therapy," 450.

106. On the EEG, see Cornelius Borck, "Recording the Brain at Work: The Visible, the Readable, and the Invisible in Electroencephalography," *Journal of the History of the Neurosciences* 17 (2008): 367–79.

107. Departure August 15, 1935, Ship: Glitrefjell, UK Board of Trade: Commercial and Statistical Department and Successors: Outwards Passenger Lists, 1890–1960, BT27; Arrival September 10, 1935, Passenger Lists, 1865–1935, Library and Archives Canada, Microfilm Publications. Both accessed on-line through ancestry.com.

108. See, for instance, Australia Electoral Rolls, 1903–80, Western Australia, Swan District, Belmont Subdistrict, 1954, accessed on-line through ancestry.com.

109. June 21, 1941, *UK, Outward Passenger Lists, 1890–1960*; Australia, Electoral Rolls, 1903–80; Australia Death Index, 1787–1985, Thomas Edward Dockrill, 1969, Registration no. 1727/69. All accessed on-line through ancestry.com.

110. Penfield, *No Man Alone*, 109.

111. Handwritten note by Wilder Penfield, July 1971, A/N 1a, Penfield Fonds, Osler Library, McGill University, Montreal.

Chapter Six

"What Was in Their Luggage?"

German Refugee Neuroscientists, Migrating Technologies, and the Emergence of Interdisciplinary Research Networks in North America, 1933 to 1963

Frank W. Stahnisch

Introduction

Technique and technologies in the neurosciences and psychiatry are not only locally developed, but have been historically subjected to the political, contingent, and adaptive living and working contexts of their bearers: neuroscientists and psychiatrists themselves. This essay will explore the particularly disruptive context of the forced migration of neuroscientists from Central Europe under Nazi and Fascist occupation—including the migration of things and technologies and their often marginality and liminality. I map several developments related to this mass exodus in order to assess some of the influences that the forced migration process had on the formation of new neuroscientific networks that transformed existing neurological and psychiatric research communities on the other side of the Atlantic. In this way, we can gain insight into intricate relationships among the techniques, technologies, and diagnostic "repertoires as techniques of manipulation,"[1] which stimulated the development of neuroscientific research in the postwar period, a phase in which the modern neurosciences increasingly became an interdisciplinary technical field.[2] The processes of "mobilization," "transfer," and "(re)integration" of research and diagnostic technologies were crucial for enabling researchers to work in new neuroscientific laboratories and clinical settings. Yet at the same time, such processes also threatened the security of researcher identities.[3]

In the 1930s, hundreds of German-speaking refugees trained in neurology, psychiatry, and neuropathology integrated into preexisting neuroscientific communities in Canada and the United States.[4] The year 1933 in particular marked a time when groundbreaking political changes occurred with the Nazis' rise to power in Germany. The Law for the Reestablishment of a Professional Civil Service (*Gesetz zur Wiederherstellung des Berufsbeamtentums*), enacted on April 7, 1933, deeply affected the scientists working in the mind and brain sciences. The situation further deteriorated with the establishment of the Nuremberg Race Laws on September 15, 1935, when thousands of medical doctors and scientists—mostly of Jewish descent—were driven from their government-supported offices.[5] While the escape from Germany and its neighboring countries makes for a staggering story, I wish to focus here primarily on the narrower question of the roles of technological objects and practical techniques, which were literally mobilized in Central Europe and then transferred to the United States and Canada—what might be called the "parallel migrations" of book collections, instruments, methods, and artifacts. These "migrating things" altered their meanings after crossing the Atlantic. The "luggage" of such individuals as neurohistologist Martin Silberberg (1895–1969) from the University of Breslau, neurologist and psychiatrist Kurt Goldstein (1878–1965) from Moabit Hospital in Berlin, neurophysiologist Otto Loewi (1873–1961) from the University of Graz, and many others—luggage made of books, brain slides, and microscopes—needs to be unpacked.[6]

The methodology of my research is based on previous studies on forced migration,[7] while it also integrates elements from more recent science-in-culture approaches.[8] This allows an exploration of the range of techniques and technologies in the modern neurosciences at a time when historians of science have predominantly focused on the dichotomy of "knowledge and practice" rather than on the material level of "science and technology."[9] An analysis of the influences of German-speaking émigré neuroscientists allows many enriching answers to the question, "What Moves When Scientific Instruments Migrate?"[10]

Art historian Walter W. S. Spencer Cook (1888–1962), the director of the New York School of Fine Arts, made a striking observation when he reflected on the fate of émigré German-speaking art historians arriving in Manhattan: "Hitler is my best friend. . . . He shakes the trees and I gather the apples."[11] Cook's rather positive outlook about the forced migration of German-speaking intellectuals, scientists, and physicians as a "brain gain" phenomenon for North America has been often thought to capture the essential consequence of their expulsion: the addition of intellect and the spread and developments of new ideas and methods, most notably in the United States and Great Britain.[12]

In contrast, I challenge these earlier accounts provided by historians of science,[13] or by scholars of Jewish academic culture.[14] According to this universalist view, it made no difference where the refugee neurologists and psychiatrists went, since they were assumed to have found the same conditions in their new host countries—universities, medical schools, and research institutions—in which they were to continue their work. Personal factors (such as the refugees' age, gender, or reputation), social conditions (for example, local collaborators or family supporters), and physical objects like the necessary laboratory and diagnostic instruments are assumed to have been irrelevant with respect to the development of the scientific endeavor itself. However, this overtly positive view does not apply equally to different groups of émigrés, since numerous less-prominent individuals did not succeed with their emigration from Central Europe at all.

The conventional way of understanding the forced migration of scientists and intellectuals has also led to a neglect of contingent factors in the historiography of scientific emigration.[15] That is, examination of cultural modes, enriching scientific interactions, and evolutionary patterns of techniques and practices has not been a priority. But the intertwining of marginality and technique in the neurosciences during this period can be seen as a particular historical product of the disruptive movement of forced migration. In their new host countries, scientists as well as their knowledge, techniques, and objects had to find a new practical, working context in which they could function and be adapted again. Techniques do have a place of origin, and practices and objects—despite their traveling together with their bearers—need to find new and receptive cultures to be received and taken up following such forced migration.

Scientific Objects and Research Instruments as Contingent Factors in the Knowledge: (Ex)changes of Modern Neuroscience

It is a well-observed element of German history that after the Nazi Party's takeover in January 1933, numerous anti-Semitic laws were passed that aimed at the expulsion of Jewish scientists from German universities and state-funded research institutions.[16] The field of the mind and brain sciences, which included clinical neurologists, psychiatrists, and neuropathologists, was one of the area's most profoundly affected by the inauguration of the Law for the Re-establishment of a Professional Civil Service.[17] As a result of their often socially motivated and holistic approaches, which encompassed neurological, psychiatric, psychological, and philosophical elements alike, many of the protagonists of the early neurosciences in Germany—such as the group surrounding the neurologist Kurt Goldstein in Frankfurt, the Munich neuro- and psychopathologists around Felix Plaut (1877–1940), or the private neurologists and rehabilitation specialists in Berlin and Breslau, including Frederic Lewey (born Frederic Lewy) (1885–1950) and Ludwig Guttmann (1899–1980)—not only faced imminent expulsion from academic working circles, but were prohibited from pursuing their medical careers. After 1935 they were further excluded from journal editorial boards and scientific publishing venues.[18] Those who had been well-connected and privileged—such as Berlin neuropathologist Carl Stern (1906–75), who had international acquaintances with Montreal neurosurgeon Wilder Penfield (1891–1976)—were able to react quickly when the political conditions deteriorated. A considerable number decided between 1933 and 1935 that it was better to leave Germany before things worsened, while the second-largest wave occurred from 1938 to 1939, shortly before the outbreak of World War II.

Jewish and politically oppositional psychiatrists and neurologists emigrated often with nothing more than suitcases filled with clothes, a little seed money, and the addresses of international colleagues in their pockets—such as Frankfurt neurochemist Otto Loewi, who brought a personal card of introduction from pharmacologist George B. Wallace (1874–1948) at New York University with him.[19] Others were able to bring a little more with them—but not much more. Prague-trained psychiatrist Robert Weil (1909–2002) described his arrival in North America in a way that mirrors the experience of many other émigrés: "[I was] parachuting from Europe into the new world of North American psychiatry at the very brink of WWII with nothing in my backpack other than Emil Kraepelin's [1856–1926] and Eugen Bleuler's [1857–1939] guides to the diagnosis of the major psychoses, manic depressive disorder, and schizophrenia."[20]

Such objects received a new place, quite often new users, and became rearranged with other objects that were already "in place." For example, Lothar B. Kalinowsky (1899–1992) continued his work in electroshock therapy at the Mount Sinai Hospital in New York, where he introduced his prototype apparatus brought with him from Europe to a predominantly psychoanalytic clinical setting. He also sought advice and support from the first-generation German immigrant engineer Walter E. Rahm (b. 1914) in the mechanics shop at the New York Psychiatric Institute in order to build a new electroshock therapy apparatus. Through this collaboration, they integrated Kalinowsky's clinical work with the wider technological and engineering know-how present at the New York Psychiatric Institute. Another case from biological psychiatry is the pathologist Franz Joseph Kallmann (1897–1956), who brought with him hundreds of photographs, graphic tables, and large data sets to introduce genetic twin studies to the American

Society of Human Genetics. Such rearrangements led to new relationships among scientists and physicians, as well as contingent patterns of adaptation into the scientific working groups of the refugees in their new home countries. In Kallmann's case, based on the reception of both his work and his imported techniques and data sets, he was also able to resume his former role as a major international player in human psychiatric genetics. This was further solidified when he acted as a cofounding member and later president (1950–51) of the American Society of Human Genetics and also assumed the directorship of the New York State Psychiatry Institute in 1955. Kallmann's research program was prominently supported by the director of the National Institute of Mental Health, Seymour S. Kety (1915–2000), who sought to use Kallmann's work and findings to underpin his strategy to redirect American psychiatry toward biology and somatic treatments.

Some of this luggage was intellectual. Austrian American neurophysiologist Eric J. Kandel (b. 1929), the son of a shopkeeper, was born into the intellectually vibrant culture of the former Austro-Hungarian Empire.[21] But the triumphal march of Adolf Hitler (1889–1945) into Vienna on March 12, 1938, brought annexed Austria the same race laws that had been established in the German Reich.[22] Kandel's parents eventually made up their minds that the situation had become too dangerous and that more suppression of Jews would occur. So in 1939 the family left for New York, only months before the outbreak of World War II. Kandel portrayed the time of his arrival in the United States as a liberating experience: "Arriving in the United States was like starting life anew. Although I lacked both the prescience and the language to say 'Free at last,' I felt it and I have ever felt it since. . . . [And] my father was undeterred. He loved America. Like many other immigrants, he often referred to it as the golden Medina, the land of gold that promised Jews safety and democracy."[23] In his autobiography *In Search of Memory* (2007), Kandel repeatedly emphasized how much he felt that the experiences of these last years in the vibrant cultural city of Vienna helped him to determine his later research interests in the human mind and human memory. In addition, Kandel traced his own interest in the biochemical and physiological aspects of memory functions to his exposure to Vienna psychoanalysis. This is not a link that is usually made by early twenty-first century neuroscientists, and this remarkable in that it points to the parallel origins of late nineteenth-century neuropathology and psychoanalysis and the early interdisciplinary origins of the emerging field of neuroscience connected with this forced scientific migration. Kandel received the Nobel Prize in Physiology or Medicine in 2000.[24]

After German-speaking émigré neuroscientists had moved past the gates and customs offices of New York, Halifax, or Quebec City,[25] their lives in the new scientific environments often depended on continued institutional support. When this support emerged, it took the form of a reciprocal relationship defined by the ability of émigrés to interest regular staff members in their projects, gain the favor of higher-ranking officials, and obtain assistance through fund-raising activities in support of their research programs. The description of émigré artists in Hollywood as "strangers in paradise" is equally valid for the situation of émigré neuroscientists in North America: "After all, they had to live somewhere, and on something. They had to deal with local shopkeepers, converse with neighbors, have some sort of social life. And they had to earn a living."[26]

Even senior neuroscientists were not given as much institutional support as they had previously been used to receiving in Europe. Successful individuals had the necessary aptitude to convince greater audiences as well as the social competency to negotiate budgets with their new administrators. The possession of such skills was far from trivial. Many émigré neuroscientists had to first pass North American medical relicensing in order to practice medicine.[27] They then had to find work in research institutes or medical faculties and often held low-paying or nonsalaried positions. A most instructive example is the émigré pathologist couple of Ruth (1906–97) and Martin Silberberg (1895–1966), who started out at Dalhousie University in Halifax, then went back and forth between Washington University in St. Louis and Rockefeller University in New York. Eventually, they settled in St. Louis, though Ruth, a professional pathologist, continued to travel to the University of Zurich every year, where she had held an adjunct position.[28] In an interview, Ruth described how when they left Europe, they had packed into their luggage a number of textbooks, some instructive brain slides stored in a padded case, and a carefully wrapped microscope from their courses at the University of Breslau.[29] After arrival, however, Ruth Silberberg worked for four years without any salary at all, while Martin, a histologist, was forced to move from one low-paying position to the next: first at Dalhousie in Canada on a Carnegie fellowship, then in the United States on Rockefeller grant money.[30] In one of Martin's letters from 1938 to his mentor Leo Loeb (1869–1959), he wrote plaintively about turning down a possible job in Massachusetts: "I am sick and tired of moving around, unless it means a definitive step forward. . . . I cannot risk any more adventures."[31] Their subsequent move to the Rockefeller University, however, did not prove to be much of an improvement on their financially constrained living circumstances, as Martin wrote to Loeb in 1943:

> Nothing has been heard of promotion or salary raises since Dr. Graef's departure. I am pretty (!) sure that no changes will take place. It is the policy of the school to exploit everybody and to make use of everybody's plight. The school has the highest percentage of jewish (!) students, who are glad to pay fees that

are about 30% higher than Yale's or Harvard's. On the other hand, the salaries paid to the Faculty (!) are ridiculous.[32]

The Silberbergs are but one example of many that illustrate the pragmatic and social challenges that the newly arrived émigrés frequently faced in North America. An extraordinary pathologist in her own right, Ruth Silberberg had to change her main research interests into general pathology during their time in St. Louis, as she could not find a research niche and position as a specialized neuropathologist. This process also downgraded her former brain slide collection, which she had put together as a morphological research collection, to the level of a teaching and training collection for medical students and residents.

The Frankfurt neurologist Kurt Goldstein (1878–1965) and his wife, Dr. Eva Rothmann-Goldstein (1878–1960), eventually reached New York in 1934. Kurt Goldstein wanted to continue working in his field and his wife wanted to establish a professional position as a physician. But the Goldsteins' emigration story illustrates well what French critical theorist Michel Foucault (1926–84) calls the "historical contingency of . . . (technological and scientific) things" and the scientist's "insecurity of identity."[33] Such contingency emanates from émigré neuroscientists' disruption of access to those techniques that they had used in their home countries.

Kurt Goldstein was known for his neurological theory as expounded in his well-known book *The Organism* (1939) (*Der Aufbau des Organismus* [1934]),[34] which was holistically oriented and renounced the reductionist assumptions of the influential cortical reductionists, the advancement of clinical and experimental psychology, and the development of the early neurorehabilitation tradition in Germany.[35] Before his arrival in the United States— which was facilitated through the help of the British Assistance Council of neurophysiologist Archibald V. Hill (1886–1977)—Goldstein contacted the Rockefeller Foundation bureau in New York:

> Prof. Goldstein called today on his way to America. He leaves from Cherbourg by the "Berengaria" on the 29th [September 1934]. I reviewed his whole situation with him. He feels there is practically no chance of an opportunity either in the University of Amsterdam or in practice in Holland, for himself as well as for other Germans. . . . G. expects to call on you shortly after his arrival, and hopes he may have the chance of discussing with you any openings that might occur. He has been invited to stay with [Smith Ely] Jelliffe [1866–1945]; he knows a few people about New York and is planning to visit them.[36]

To earn a living once he arrived, Kurt Goldstein opened a private practice in neurology and psychiatry. He was by then already fifty-eight years old. He divided the rest of his time between an appointment as clinical teacher in psychopathology at Columbia and the running of a small laboratory of neurophysiology at the academic Montefiore Hospital in Brooklyn. Yet even with the help he received from his new East Coast network—Harvard scholar of comparative education Robert Ulrich (1890–1977); the phenomenologist Aaron Gurwitsch (1901–73); the experimental psychologist Martin Scheerer (1900–1961); and his own brother-in-law, Ernst Cassirer (1874–1945), who all actively fostered Goldstein's intellectual exchanges with American neuroscientists, psychologists, and sociologists—it was still far from clear how this process would play out in the long run. Apparently, at this time in the United States, Goldstein's work was known only by psychologists and rehabilitation specialists rather than by clinical neurologists. An exception was the behavioral neurologist Norman Geschwind (1929–84) at the Boston Veterans Administration Hospital, of Jewish descent himself and surrounded by a group of German-speaking émigrés, such as Fred A. ("Quad") Quadfasel (1902–81) from Berlin. It certainly was a major advantage in this situation that Geschwind worked in the innovative neurological aphasiology field, developing the "disconnection syndrome" to a full-fledged structural and functional model into which Goldstein's concept of the catastrophic cortical reactions fit in quite well.

Another problem Goldstein faced was that the Rockefeller Foundation had originally recommended him to the Institute for Advanced Studies in Princeton, which would have been a position in line with his academic standing in German clinical neurology. The Foundation inquired whether the Institute was able to offer an adequate position for him as a principal investigator so that he could build a new interdisciplinary holist group there. With the help of Abraham Flexner (1866–1959), this plan appears to have been close to acceptance in late 1939 but then faced a serious setback when the costs for the necessary biomedical research technology and personnel were found to be too high. As Princeton responded, "He knows that the answer is 'No.' The institute is not in a position to add a new department. AF [Abraham Flexner] advises me to speak frankly with G. on the question of his family obligations—that he must not expect this or any other organization to provide extra funds."[37]

Moving also created many contingencies for the objects these scientists brought with them. Here the Goldstein story is also illustrative. Soon after the Nazis seized power, Goldstein was arrested while working in his neurology clinic at the Moabit hospital in Berlin. He was only released after signing a document stating that he would leave Germany forever. Goldstein then passed through Switzerland, where he took time to cofound the Emergency Society for German Scholars in Exile (Notgemeinschaft Deutscher Wissenschaftler im Ausland) with the Budapest pathologist, Philip Schwarz (1894–1962), and Carl Zuckmayer (1896–1977), the novelist from Mainz. Goldstein then found refuge in Amsterdam, where he finished his seminal publication, The Organism (Der Aufbau des Organismus), in 1934.[38] Yet even the completion of this major work was overshadowed by the difficulties of moving things around during the process of forced migration; for instance, when switching trains in Bavaria and later in Austria, Goldstein lost significant parts of his bibliographic notes and was only able to hold on to the offprints that he brought with him to Zurich and Amsterdam.[39] This aspect of his sudden flight from Germany is reflected in the group of well referenced chapters on one hand—all based on previous publications—and the errors he made in chapters written after his exile had commenced, on the other. Due to a lack of access to the German literature at the University of Amsterdam, he had had to construct his bibliographies often based on his memory alone.

Goldstein's arrival in New York then began a long quarrel with the customs officials about his research library and film collection. After he had fled from Germany, he left his films in Zurich; he could only take a small library of textbooks with him to Amsterdam, the intermediary location of his exile. Most of these books, however, remained stored, unpacked, in his apartment. Before traveling to America, Goldstein had made calls to the Customs Office and told them that he intended to bring most of his and his wife's belongings with him. However, once he arrived in New York with these things, the affair concerning his collection dragged on for more than a year, since US Customs could not see the importance that objects such as a library and a neurological film collection might have for a brain scientist who sought an academic position in America. In fact, the US customs officers thought that the films, which Goldstein had officially identified and declared before he embarked in Normandy, were for commercial purposes. Thus, the customs duty he was initially charged was astronomically high. Goldstein therefore urged the New York Bureau of the Rockefeller Foundation to call the customs office and send letters of support. In response, Rockefeller Foundation officer Robert A. Lampart wrote, "Doctor Goldstein, a distinguished German Professor of Psychiatry, arrived recently in this country, bringing a collection of books and cinematographic films, the latter ones to be used to illustrate lectures before learned societies, that is, for purely scientific purposes. The books and the films have no commercial value. We are sure that Doctor Goldstein's lectures will promote the advancement of psychiatry in America and as the books and films referred to are essential for his addresses, it will be appreciated if their entry can be facilitated."[40]

Even after this letter of support had arrived, it took another six months before the complete collection of Goldstein's belongings were cleared, but at last he received back all the items that he had missed so dearly and for such a long time and which had played such an essential part in his research activities in Germany. Another example of this close alignment of the scholar with his books, films, and scientific things can be found, for example, with his office photographs, which he had put up to alleviate the emotional burdens from the forced migration process. Goldstein's international renown in the scientific world had not spared him from quarrels with US Customs, from problems in finding a placement with an adequate income, or from the difficulties his wife experienced in obtaining a physician's license in the United States.

Not even Nobel Prize winners were free from such petty problems, as the example of well-known neurochemist Otto Loewi from the Austrian University of Graz shows. With some of his electrophysiological equipment in his suitcase, packed in together with books and clothes, and cautiously having informed New York University about which ship he would be arriving on from his previous exile at Oxford University, Loewi still nearly failed to reach the other side of the Atlantic.[41] In order to immigrate to the United States, he was required to apply for an entry visa from the American consulate. While he conscientiously attended to all the necessary paperwork, Loewi ran into serious trouble when a government official in London asked him for written proof that he had taught courses at the University of Graz rather than having been only a research professor there. At this time, previous teaching experience at international universities was a formal prerequisite to finding academic employment at comparable postsecondary institutions in North America. However, Loewi had lost most of his own papers when fleeing from Austria, and he no longer had his university employment letter. In fact, his flight from Austria was so hasty, taking place as it did under police pressure, that he even had to hand over the entire sum from his Nobel Prize to Nazi officials.

His adventures were not over yet. Before he embarked in England, he was given a sealed envelope, containing an immigration officer's note and a doctor's physical exam, that he was to present to the immigration agencies following the Atlantic crossing. What happened during his entrance to the United States can best be related in Loewi's own words:

> Upon my arrival in New York harbor, a clerk prepared my papers for the immigration officer. While he was busy doing this, I glanced over the doctor's certificate—and almost fainted. I read: "Senility, not able to earn a living." I saw myself sent to Ellis Island, and shipped back to Mr. Hitler. The immigration officer fortunately disregarded the certificate and welcomed me to this country. I arrived here June 1, 1940.[42]

And what "excitement of a life in science" this must have been for Loewi! Fortunately, his path into the country had been smoothed behind the scenes by a cable from the New York University president's office as well as by a copy of the international *Who's Who* shelved in the immigration office. The relevant entry meticulously described to the officer exactly who this

Mr. Loewi was: "Loewi, Otto, Prof. Dr., Universitaet Graz, Oesterreich. . . . Nobel Prize Winner in Physiology or Medicine in 1936."

Other émigré psychiatrists and neurologists were not so lucky and lost almost all of their belongings. Among this group were Herta Seidemann (1900–1984), a doctor who had trained with eminent psychiatrist Karl Bonhoeffer (1899–1957) at the Charité Medical Faculty and who established herself in New York as a consultant psychiatrist to Goldstein's working group at the Montefiore Hospital, and the Leipzig-based neurophysiologist and Nobel Prize laureate of 1970, Bernard Katz (1911–2003). During his emigration first from England to Australia, where he worked in the library of John Carew Eccles' (1903–97), Katz could not take much more than his clothing and some articles. At the time, he had been a naval physician on a yearlong reconnaissance voyage aboard a military ship facing the ever-present threat of Japanese submarine attacks. Katz still continued to write research articles on board the ship, basing them on his previous neurophysiological findings at the University of Oxford and his alma mater, the University of Leipzig.[43] In 1945 he traveled back from Australia to England, this time with a number of electrophysiological devices, to become assistant director of research in the unit led by neurophysiologist Archibald Vivian Hill (1886–1977). Katz was also appointed to a prestigious research fellowship by the British Royal Society and lectured as a reader in physiology at University College London, becoming professor in biophysics in 1952. During his postwar research on the physiology of nerves and muscles, and particularly the structural and functional mechanism of neuromuscular transmission, he also passed an extended visiting period with neurophysiologist Stephen W. Kuffler (1913–80) at the University of Chicago. They had met in Eccles's laboratory in Australia and now continued their investigations of muscle fibers in the frog and the innervation of mammalian muscles—a development made possible by the contingencies of the forced migration process.[44]

Conclusion: Looking at Emigrating Things and Technologies with Historical Hindsight

Most of the newly arriving émigré neuroscientists made landfall in North America with nothing but their luggage to call their own.[45] Often, their "migrating things"—their scientific instruments and diagnostic technologies—were delayed and arrived only after many frustrations: being lost on a train; not being allowed to be shipped; sent back by customs officers; or after all the hardships of their journey, simply being converted into quick cash by émigrés eager to make the bare beginnings of a new life in exile possible. Still, for the newly arriving émigré neurologists and psychiatrists, books, photographs, and instruments assumed an immense scientific, social, and personal meaning when they reached North America. Certainly, neuroscientists and physicians, who can be included with lawyers, teachers, and artists among the "illustrious immigrants" moving from Europe at this time,[46] were fortunate to be traveling in ship cabins on the higher decks of the transatlantic liners. Many of their compatriot émigrés populated the lower decks in large numbers, where guards abused them, stole their jewelry, or ransacked their bags.[47] Still, neuroscientists, like all other German-speaking émigrés, had to answer the existential question that Russian émigré writer Sergeij Donatowitsch Dowlatow (1941–90) had raised during his own exile in *The Suitcase: A Novel* (1996): "What shall I put in my luggage?"[48]

The variety of answers to this question mirrored that of other illustrious émigrés—from Belgian playwright and essayist Maurice Maeterlinck (1862–1949), who brought thirty-two pieces of luggage, two Pekingese lap dogs, and his whole library after the German *Wehrmacht* invaded Belgium, to Communist author Stefan Hermlin (1915–97), who escaped with basically two books that held sentimental value for him.[49] The Silberbergs managed to get most of their belongings across the Atlantic, including a collection of histological objects and a Zeiss microscope they used for pathology teaching purposes in America.[50] Kurt Goldstein lost parts of his manuscript for *The Organism*, yet most of his books and films arrived safe and sound.[51] Otto Loewi came with a single electrophysiological device in his luggage, which was otherwise stuffed mostly with personal belongings.[52] Herta Seidemann and Bernard Katz brought virtually nothing. They relied solely on the affidavits of friends and colleagues to make their emigration possible.[53] The items that had to be left behind were significant as well. One example was the long-delayed publication of the thesis of historical sociologist Nina Rubinstein (1908–96), which finally took place when she was eighty-one years old because the author had to abandon her original manuscript in Europe when she fled. Its title was "In Search of Exile, 1880–2000."[54]

For émigré academics, their belongings conveyed a strong sense of connection. A poignant recollection of their home (*Heimat*), figured strongly in their autographical writings and scholarly papers. In their *Kaffeekraentzchen*, salons, and *Gespraechsrunden*, concepts of identity and belonging were socially exchanged among many Jewish and other refugees from Nazi Germany.[55] As journalist Renate Rauch wrote in a review of the book by German writer Richard Wagner (b. 1952) book, *Habseligkeiten*:

> When Richard Wagner named his novel *Belongings*, it was still unknown that shortly after the book's appearance, the word *belongings* would come to be identified as the most beautiful German word. . . . [However], it is hardly possible to join the word to a perception of blessed pathways and possessions. Instead, unspeakable grief has been attached to the word as it represents the loss of everything that had to be left behind over and beyond the reach of material things.[56]

One of the items Goldstein had brought with him was a portrait of the experimental psychologist Adhémar Gelb (1887–1936), his collaborator and friend, who had tragically died of tuberculosis in 1936 before he was able to complete his emigration. Gelb had lost his position as the chair of experimental psychology at the University of Halle following the Nuremberg Race Laws of the previous year and had just been offered a professorship in experimental psychology at the University of Kansas.[57] As MIT psychologist Hans-Lukas Teuber (1916–77) later recorded, "A portrait of Gelb hung above Goldstein's desk, together with his Goethe portrait, throughout the period of his exile.[58]

There have been other kinds of loss as well surrounding this transition. Former historiographical approaches have frequently reduced the achievements, modifications, and innovations of refugee researchers to circumscribed individual contributions and have been centered on a product-oriented approach to the process of emigration-induced change.[59] But the actual experience of émigrés—and their scientific "things"—was often fragmented. This is reflected, for example, in the unequal cultural reception of Goldstein's ideas in America, which was paralleled by the disintegration of the holistic and interdisciplinary program of neurology. Goldstein himself had to split his holistic interests back into various separate disciplinarily organized areas, such as rehabilitation psychology, social psychology, laboratory experimentation, clinical neurology, and empirical sociology in order to continue his career. These research programs also had to be pursued at very different institutions. On the other side of the Atlantic, the loss of most of the practitioners of holist neurology, with the exception of the Tuebingen psychiatrist Victor von Weizsaecker (1886–1957), caused the practice to altogether cease to exist in the neuroscientific communities of the German-speaking countries.

Of course, it is a case of *esprit d'escalier* that for many neuroscientists, the political and human catastrophe instigated by Nazi and Fascist rule in Central Europe created the unanticipated prospect of working in new scientific settings in fields that Nazi politicians and doctors had sought to destroy forever.[60] Yet this generalization does not apply to all groups of émigré individuals. Many of the less prominent physicians and researchers did not succeed with their emigration from Central Europe at all. For women, entry was possible only in a few disciplines and often at the cost of giving up their previous profession. Some tried and failed or chose not to adapt to local norms. For other émigrés, the emotional trauma of the experience could not be overcome. One tragic example is the suicide of the Vienna psychiatrist and psychoanalyst Paul Federn (1871–1950), whose family was not able to receive visas to follow him to New York after he had received privileged landing papers for the United States and hoped that his loved ones could soon join him. Neuropathologist Carl Stern, who had been born in Bavaria, became so appalled by Canadian biological psychiatry through his holist understanding of neurology that he deliberately turned away from McGill University to take up a position as clinical psychoanalyst at the Catholic University of Ottawa, where he began working on end-of-life treatments for the chronically ill, engaging with questions of psychoanalysis and religion. Still other émigrés had to learn the hard lesson that aid organizations could make negative as well as positive decisions; the financial support available in no way rose to meet the human and scientific catastrophe at hand.[61]

Few could have predicted the scientific changes in neurology and psychiatry following the forced migration wave after 1933, such as the creation of many new training programs in psychiatry (e.g., in Halifax, Toronto, and Saskatoon in Canada), the development of genetic psychiatric research programs (such as in New York and Baltimore in the United States), or the increasing introduction of psychoanalytic therapies in the clinical psychiatric system of the US Army's Veterans Administration. Objects, processes, and techniques became integrated into the new sciences of the brain and mind in émigrés' new home countries in North America with their refugee inventors and proprietors after so many physicians and neuroscientists of Jewish origin from Central Europe saw their personal and professional lives disintegrate. Scientific things such as the holist neurological therapies, the histopathological analyses in neuro-oncology, or the neurophysiological synapse research with electrical stimulation devices could be newly organized during the transatlantic transfer of the forced migrants with their research objects. This laid the foundations for new personal and professional identities in Canada and the United States. And the bigger the wave of forced migration grew, the more chances the émigrés had not only to succeed in developing a new scientific and personal life but also to transform North American medicine and neuroscience.[62] Some scholars, such as Edward Shorter, have gone so far as to argue that the twentieth century was actually "brought in the luggage" of Austrian émigrés.[63]

While the luggage of émigré neurologists, psychiatrists, and neuropathologists may appear to be an unfamiliar lens into the historiography of the forced migration in twentieth-century neuroscience (see Katja Guenther's coda in this volume), it is nevertheless a very fruitful one from both a material and an intellectual history perspective on the state of techniques in the neurosciences. In this sense, émigré neuroscientists also established their professional identities and cohesion as a group based on their "transitory objects" and their relationship to previously learned techniques carried with them from their homelands to their life in exile. Émigré neuroscientists then sat on the margins until they were relicensed, readjusted, and reintegrated into North American research communities together with their techniques, objects, and practices. The resulting hybrid objects and technologies also helped to underwrite different epistemic virtues, for some as masters of scientific cultures previously unknown to the United States and Canada and

178   FRANK W. STAHNISCH

for others as experts in cutting-edge techniques only then coming into use in North America. Focusing on the contributions of the forced migration wave of Central European émigré researchers and clinicians in neurology and psychiatry will contribute to a much broader and more nuanced understanding of technique in twentieth-century neuroscience among both historians and practitioners.

The exodus of large numbers of neuroscientists from German-speaking Europe often resulted in significant changes in their research orientation, the abrupt end of medical and scientific careers, and other tragic personal outcomes. But in trying to adapt to North American scientific and professional cultures, these individuals gradually and steadily enriched them, giving rise to hybrid states of knowing in the neurosciences during and after World War II.[64] The year 1963 was a watershed in the history of neuroscientific research in the United States and Canada: the year when American-born and St. Louis–trained biophysicist Francis O. Schmitt (1903–95) laid the foundation for the postwar research endeavor by creating the Neuroscience Research Program at the Massachusetts Institute of Technology.[65]

Notes

The author gratefully acknowledges the support of the Mackie Family Collection in the History of Neuroscience, the Hotchkiss Brain Institute, and the O'Brien Institute for Public Health, all at the University of Calgary. He also wishes to thank Delia Gavrus (Winnipeg), Stephen Casper (Potsdam, NY), Bob Brain (Vancouver), and Elizabeth Neswald (St. Catharines, ON) for their comments on previously presented parts of this essay, as well as the Social Sciences and Humanities Research Council of Canada for an Insight Development Grant (SSHRC No. IDG 430-2013-001068) award, which made the research for this article possible. Finally, the author is indebted to Mr. Stephen Pow (Calgary, AB) and Ms. Christine Wenc (Potsdam, NY) for the meticulous adjustment of the English language of the manuscript.

1. For the concept, see Ian G. Simmons, "Environments, Ecologies, and Cultures across Space and Time." In *A Companion to World History*, ed. Douglas Northrop, 143–55 (Oxford: Wiley Blackwell, 2012), 143.

2. Theodore M. Porter, "How Science Became Technical," *Isis* 100, no. 3 (2009): 292–309.

3. On the issue of the newly received authority of the modern neurosciences since the turn from the twentieth to the twenty-first century, see also the introductory chapter to this volume by Delia Gavrus and Stephen Casper, esp. 2ff.

4. For the wider research project, see Frank W. Stahnisch, "Transforming the Lab: Technological and Societal Concerns in the Pursuit of De- and Regeneration in the German Morphological Neurosciences, 1910–1930," *Medicine Studies* 1, no. 1 (2009): 41–54; Frank W. Stahnisch, "German-Speaking Émigré Neuroscientists in North America after 1933: Critical Reflections on Emigration-Induced Scientific Change,"

Oesterreichische Zeitschrift fuer Geschichtswissenschaften 21, no. 3 (2010): 36–68; or Frank W. Stahnisch and Thomas Hoffmann, *Kurt Goldstein and the Neurology of Movement during the Interwar Years*—Physiological Experimentation, Clinical Psychology and Early Rehabilitation," in *Was bewegt uns? Menschen im Spannungsfeld zwischen Mobilitaet und Beschleunigung*, ed. Christian Hoffstadt, Franz Peschke, and Andreas Schulz-Buchta (Bochum, Germany: Projektverlag, 2010), 283–311.

5. Cf. Mitchell Ash and Alfons Soellner, eds. *Forced Migration and Scientific Change: Émigré German-Speaking Scientists after 1933* (Cambridge: Cambridge University Press, 1996), 1–19.

6. For example, see Frank W. Stahnisch, "Zur Zwangsemigration deutschsprachiger Neurowissenschaftler nach Nordamerika: Der historische Fall des Montreal Neurological Institute," *Schriftenreihe der Deutschen Gesellschaft fuer Geschichte der Nervenheilkunde* 14, no. 1 (2008): 414–42.

7. Klaus Fischer, "Identification of Emigration-Induced Scientific Change," in *Forced Migration and Scientific Change: Émigré German-speaking Scientists and Scholars after 1933*, ed. Mitchell G. Ash and Alfons Soellner, 23 (Cambridge: Cambridge University Press, 1996). See also Hans-Peter Kroener, "Die Emigration deutschsprachiger Mediziner im Nationalsozialismus," *Berichte zur Wissenschaftsgeschichte* 12, no. 1 (1989): 1–35.

8. Cf. D. Heward Brock and Ann Harward, *The Culture of Biomedicine* (Newark, DE: 1984), 10; Peter Galison, Stephen R. Graubard, and Everett Medelsohn, *Science in Culture* (New Brunswick, NJ: Transaction Publishers, 2001), v–vii; Henning Schmidgen, Peter Geimer, and Sven Dierig, *Kultur im Experiment* (Berlin: Cadmos, 2004).

9. Francesca Bray, "Science, Technique, Technology: Passages between Matter and Knowledge in Imperial Chinese Agriculture," *British Journal for the History of Science* 41, no. 3 (2008): 319–44.

10. Nicolas Rasmussen, "What Moves When Scientific Instruments Migrate? Software and Hardware in the Transfer of Biological Electron Microscopy to Postwar Australia," *Technology and Culture* 40, no. 1 (1999): 47–73.

11. Quoted in *Meaning in the Visual Arts*, ed. Erwin Panowsky (New York: Penguin, 1970), 380.

12. Uwe-Hendrik Peters, "Emigration deutscher Psychiater nach England. (Teil 1)," *Fortschritte der Neurologie und Psychiatrie* 64, no. 5 (1996): 161–67.

13. See Jean Medawar and David Pyke, *Hitler's Gift: The True Story of the Scientists Expelled by the Nazi Regime* (New York: Arkade Publishing, 2001), 231–40; Linda Hunt, *Secret Agenda: The United States Government, Nazi Scientists, and Project Paperclip, 1945 to 1990* (New York: St. Martin's Press, 1991), 217–39; or Eric Koch, *Deemed Suspect: A Wartime Blunder* (Toronto: Methuen, 1980), 230–54.

14. See Sulamit Volkov, "Jewish Scientists in Imperial Germany (Parts I and II)," *Aleph: Historical Studies in Science and Judaism* 1, no. 1 (2001): 1–36; Howard M. Sachar, *A History of the Jews in America* (New York: Knopf, 1992); or Giorgio Israel, "Science and the Jewish Question in the Twentieth Century: The Case of Italy and What it Shows." *Aleph: Historical Studies in Science and Judaism* 2, no. 1 (2004): 191–261.

15. It can be argued that this "neglect of contingent factors" in the historiography of emigration science followed a similar trend in general history of science, where

the role of instruments and research technology came only recently into focus. Allan Franklin, *The Neglect of Experiment* (Cambridge: Cambridge University Press, 1989), 103–37.

16. Peter Longerich, *Holocaust: The Nazi Persecution and Murder of the Jews* (New York: Oxford University Press, 2010), 38.

17. Cf. Mitchell Ash and Alfons Soellner, eds. *Forced Migration and Scientific Change: Émigré German-Speaking Scientists after 1933* (Cambridge: Cambridge University Press, 1996), 1–19.

18. Frank W. Stahnisch and Peter J. Koehler, "Three 20th Century Multi-authored Handbooks Serving as Vital Catalyzers of an Emerging Specialization—A Case Study from the History of Neurology and Psychiatry," *Journal of Mental and Nervous Diseases* 200, no. 12 (2012) 1167–75, esp. 1070.

19. A very important role as a networking protagonist for the émigré German-speaking psychiatrists and neurologists was filled by the Johns Hopkins psychiatrist Adolf Meyer (1866–1950). Meyer had himself been a German-speaking émigré from Switzerland and had already arrived in the United States in 1892.

20. From the presidential address of Robert Weil to the Canadian Psychiatric Association (CPA) in 1953; citation taken from his manuscript from the folders on the Robert Weil Correspondence (Ms 2–750, call # 2003–47, box 6, file 15, 10 pp.) in the Dalhousie University Archives & Special Collections, Killam Memorial Library, Halifax, NS.

21. Brian Robertson, "An Interview with Eric Kandel," *Journal of Physiology* 588, no. 5 (2010): 743–45.

22. Eric R. Kandel, *The Age of Insight: The Quest to Understand the Unconscious in Art, Mind, and Brain, from Vienna 1900 to the Present* (New York: Random House, 2012), 16–17.

23. Eric R. Kandel, *In Search of Memory: The Emergence of a New Science of Mind* (London: W. W. Norton, 2006), 33–35.

24. Ibid.

25. Bat-Ami Zucker, "Frances Perkins and the German-Jewish Refugees, 1933–1940," *American Jewish History* 89, no. 1 (2001); Irving Abella and Harold Troper, *None Is Too Many: Canada and the Jews of Europe: 1933–1948* (Toronto: University of Toronto Press, 1982), 26–40.

26. John Russell Taylor, *Strangers in Paradise: The Hollywood Émigrés 1933–1950* (New York: Holt Rinehart and Winston, 1983), 9.

27. Kathleen M. Pearle, "Aerzteemigration nach 1933 in die USA: Der Fall New York," *Medizinhistorisches Journal* 19, no. 1 (1984): 112–37, esp. 117.

28. Anonymous, "In Memoriam: Martin Silberberg, 1895–1969," *Gerontologia* 16, no. 4 (1970): 199–200.

29. Ruth Silberberg, interview by medical librarian Estelle Brodman (1914–2007), January 16, 1976, Washington University School of Medicine: *Oral History Project*, Washington University in St. Louis, accessed December 6, 2013, http://beckerexhibits.wustl. edu/oral/interviews/silberberg.html.

30. See, e.g., Archives and Rare Books Division of the Becker Library, Washington University School of Medicine (Loeb, Leo; FC0002; corr. C-Ha, box 2).

31. Martin Silberberg (St. Louis), to Leo Loeb (staying at Woodshole), April 4, 1938, Archives and Rare Books Division of the Becker Library, Washington University

School of Medicine, St. Louis (FC0002, Leo Loeb, correspondence R-S, box 5, folder: Silberberg, Martin and Ruth).

32. Martin Silberberg (New York City), to Leo Loeb (St. Louis), December 2, 1943, Archives and Rare Books Division of the Becker Library, Washington School of Medicine, St. Louis (FC0002, Leo Loeb, correspondence R-S, box 5, folder: Silberberg, Martin and Ruth).

33. Michel Foucault *The Order of Things: An Archaeology of the Human Sciences*, trans. Richard Howard (London: Pantheon Books, 1970), 170.

34. Thomas Hoffmann and Frank W. Stahnisch, eds., *Kurt Goldstein: Der Aufbau des Organismus: Einfuehrung in die Biologie unter besonderer Beruecksichtigung der Erfahrungen am kranken Menschen*, foreword by Anne Harrington (Munich: Wilhelm Fink, 2014).

35. For example, see Anne Harrington, *Reenchanted Science: Holism in German Culture from Wilhelm II to Hitler* (Princeton, NJ: Princeton University Press, 1996), 103–9.

36. Rockefeller Foundation officer Daniel P. O'Brian (1894–1958) to medical officer Robert A. Lambert (1902–92), September 27, 1934, Rockefeller Archive, refugee scholars collection—Kurt Goldstein, record group 200, series 1.1, box 78, folder 939, 17. Rockefeller Archive Center, Sleepy Hollow, NY. Hereafter RAC.

37. Brief Record of the Rector of Columbia University in New York, Nicholas Murray Butler (1862–1947), November 6, 1939, about a telephone conversation of Dr. Abraham Flexner at Princeton with Kurt Goldstein in New York City, RAC, refugee scholars collection, record group 200 (Columbia University; Goldstein, Kurt—refugee scholar, neurology, 1937–40), series 1.1, box 9, folder 939, pp. 65–6.

38. Thomas Hoffmann and Frank W. Stahnisch, "Einleitung," in *Kurt Goldstein—Der Aufbau des Organismus: Einfuehrung in die Biologie unter besonderer Beruecksichtigung der Erfahrungen am kranken Menschen*, ed. Thomas Hoffmann and Frank W. Stahnisch (Munich: Fink, 2014), 284–87.

39. Ibid.

40. Rockefeller Foundation officer Robert A. Lambert to the US Collection of Customs House, New York City, January 3, 1935, RAC, refugee scholars collection—Kurt Goldstein, record group 200, series 1.1, box 78, folder 939, 18f.

41. Stanley Finger, *Minds Behind the Brain: A History of the Pioneers and their Discoveries* (New York: Oxford University Press, 2000), 259–62.

42. Otto Loewi, "The Excitement of a Life in Science," in *A Dozen Doctors: Autobiographical Sketches*, ed. Dwight J. Ingle, 126 (Chicago: University of Chicago Press, 1963).

43. Bernd Sakmann, "Sir Bernard Katz: 26 March 1911–20 April 2003," *Biographical Memoires of the Fellows of the Royal Society* 53, no. 1 (2007): 185–202.

44. Finger, *Minds Behind the Brain*, 233–36.

45. Laura Fermi, *Illustrious Immigrants: The Intellectual Migration from Europe, 1930–41* (Chicago: Univeristy of Chicago Press, 1968), 1–15.

46. Ibid., 407–8.

47. Ibid., 57–75.

48. Sergeij Donatowitsch Dowlatow, *The Suitcase: A Novel*, trans. Antonia W. Bouis (Berkeley, CA: Counterpoint, 1990), 5.

49. Taylor, *Strangers in Paradise*, 185ff.

50. Ruth Silberberg, interview by medical librarian Estelle Brodman.

51. Kurt Goldstein, *Preliminary Manuscript* for the Introduction to "*Der Aufbau des Organismus*" (July 1934), RAC, archive group 1.1, series 200, box 78, file 939.

52. Loewi, *Excitement of a Life in Science*, 130.

53. Wenda Focke, *Begegnung: Herta Seidemann, Psychiatrin-Neurologin 1900–1984* (Konstanz, Germany: Hartung-Gorre, 1986), 110–13; Sakmann, *Sir Bernard Katz*, 185–202.

54. Nina Rubinstein, *In Search of Exile, 1880–2000* (New York: Bard College, 1989).

55. See, for example, the recollections of the essayist Leslie Sachs (1952–2013), in Leslie Sachs, "Advice from the Midwest," in *Hitler's Exiles: Personal Stories of the Flight from Nazi Germany to America*, ed. Mark M. Anderson, 229–32 (New York: The New Press, 1998).

56. Renate Rauch, review of *Habseligkeiten: Roman*, by Richard Wagner (Berlin: Akademie Verlag, 2004), *Berliner Zeitung*, October 28, 2004, 36.

57. Aron Gurwitsch, "La Science biologique d'après K. Goldstein," *Revue Philosophique* 129, no. 3 (1940): 244–65.

58. Hans L. Teuber, "Kurt Goldstein's Role in the Development of Neuropsychology," *Neuropsychologia* 4, no. 4 (1966): 299–310.

59. Ash and Soellner, *Forced Migration and Scientific Change*, 1–19.

60. Cf. Waltraud Strickhausen, *Kanada*, vol. 3, in *Handbuch der deutschsprachigen Emigration 1933–1945*, ed. Krohn Claus-Dieter (Darmstadt: Wissenschaftliche Verlagsbuchhandlung, 1998), 284–97, and Claus-Dieter Krohn, *Vereinigte Staaten von Amerika*, vol. 3 of *Handbuch der deutsch-sprachigen Emigration, 1933–1945*, ed. Claus-Dieter Krohn, 284–97, 446–66 (Darmstadt, Germany: Wissenschaftliche Verlagsbuchhandlung, 1998).

61. John Fawcett, "Networks, Linkages and Migration Systems," *International Migration* 23, no. 6 (1989): 638–70.

62. Horace Winchell Magoun, *American Neuroscience in the Twentieth Century: Confluence of the Neural, Behavioral, and Communicative Streams*, ed. Louise H. Marshall (Lisse, The Netherlands: A. A. Balkema, 2002), 405–10.

63. For a similar view, see Kandel, *Age of Insight*, 68–73.

64. On the blurred boundaries between psychiatry, neurology, and neurosurgery, see Delia Gavrus, "Men of Dreams and Men of Action: Neurologists, Neurosurgeons, and the Performance of Professional Identity, 1920–1950," *Bulletin of the History of Medicine* 85, no. 1 (2011): 57–92.

65. Francis O. Schmitt, *The Never-Ceasing Search* (Philadelphia: The American Philosophical Society, 1990), 214–17.

Chapter Seven

Dualist Techniques for Materialist Imaginaries

Matter and Mind in the 1951 Festival of Britain

Stephen T. Casper

For the past three centuries, the aim of biological studies and of medicine has been the understanding of the physiology and pathology of the body proper. The mind was out, largely left as a concern for religion and philosophy, and even after it became the focus of a specific discipline, psychology, it did not begin to gain entry into biology and medicine until recently.

—Antonio Damasio, 1994

Introduction

We can say that the power to learn to refrain from attacking lies in this uppermost part of the brain. This power is clearly very like the memory of higher animals or man. The interest of the experiment is that it opens some hope for finding what changes go on in the brain when animals learn. We now know where to look in the Octopus brain and we hope that by comparing this part with those regions of our own brain that are connected with learning, we may be able to find the common fact that makes memory possible.[1]

Thus wrote physiologist J. Z. Young in a script solicited by the Committee for Science and Technology for the 1951 Festival of Britain and for which Young proposed a novel exhibit focused on memory in the octopus. Describing the natural history and behavior of this marine animal, Young explained to his readers those reasons that rendered the invertebrate a model organism for the science of physiology. Noting that octopuses proved to be particularly clever creatures, Young claimed they were highly amenable to training. "The experiment consisted," he wrote, "in training the Octopus not to attack a crab if a white square was also present" in their aquarium. When the square was not present the octopus could feed on the crab. By presenting the crab and the white square together to the octopus, the animal could be trained to associate the white square and the crab with painful experiences.[2] "This was done by dangling the crab on a thread in front of the square to which a pair of electric wires were attached. When the Octopus came out and attacked the crab, it received an electric shock, dropped the crab and retreated home."[3] Over time the octopus connected the white square with the noxious stimulus, but this was not the only technical achievement: "Some progress has been made," Young observed, "in finding the part of the brain that stores" memory in the octopus. "The brain of the Octopus has many lobes, arranged on a plan very differently from our own. The uppermost lobe of all consists of a mass of small cells. When this was removed from one of the trained Octopuses, the animal immediately 'forgot' that the white plate was connected with a painful stimulus."[4]

Like many of the scientists solicited for expert advice by the Committee for Science and Technology for the 1951 Festival of Britain, J. Z. Young had both to explain to the organizers the significance and interest such experiments would generate and also to suggest ways they might communicate that scientific knowledge to a public looking for entertainments—no small task indeed. Pondering this dimension of his remit, Young observed that

> Octopus in good condition feed regularly. This would be a very great attraction, but probably too difficult to achieve. . . . Before deciding the problem, consult the Zoo. They will advise on the difficulty of maintaining the sea water in a suitable condition. It would mean elaborate backstage tanks. The Zoo have kept Octopuses for some months but have found them not very good subjects. . . . I would very much welcome the live aquarium but must advise that the risk of failure is serious. If successful it would make a very attractive exhibit.[5]

Any number of elements from Young's experiment make for fascinating fodder for the history of neuroscience and physiology, not least the seemingly materialist interpretation that although the model organism's lobes were profoundly different from human neuroanatomy, a fact common to both human beings and octopuses would be found, ultimately establishing and unifying the mechanism by which nervous systems made memories possible. In this particular instance, however, the experiment itself is less striking than the audience for whom it was intended. Increasingly in postwar

Britain, the physiology of the nervous system in animals and in human beings was finding its way out of the laboratory and the clinic and into urban spaces. Radio programs, science fiction stories, magazine articles, and more than a few Nobel Prizes, as well as splashy cures for nervous diseases and mental disorders, intimated both of growing public interest and a public sphere for such ideas.[6]

In some sense, of course, as Cornelius Borck has observed, the city had already conquered the imagery of the nervous system; the "urban brain," for example, had already by the interwar period incorporated into its scientific design the city's "technopolis economy" which detailed its functional metaphors of wiring, telephone exchanges, railroads switches, and those myriad electrifications essential to mind and brain (a point more fully discussed in Max Stadler's contribution in this volume).[7] Yet as Young's experiment with the octopus also suggests, a reversal of sorts was underway as well. Where before the brain had been made more material through choice cosmopolitan metaphors, now such traditional spaces of exhibition settings could make the brain and nervous system material for audiences.[8] Like L. Stephen Jacyna's menagerie discussed earlier in this volume, these were spaces of particular 'show techniques'; invisible as they were, marginal as they now seem, these techniques ensured the creation of knowledge in audiences.

For historians of science and medicine, exhibits and expositions of this order have long been sites of interest from which to view the defining intellectual and cultural features of scientific and medical work.[9] The presentation of science at the 1951 Festival of Britain, a celebration of British society and culture intended to bolster the morale of the public following two terrible world wars, indeed offers such an opportunity. The festival contained numerous exhibits exploring arts, crafts, textiles, music, literature, manufacturing, history, as well as people and places of the British Isles, but such topics as science, technology, and medicine were especially prominent in the London-based festival.[10] Planners of the festival had arranged not one, but two large public exhibit halls dedicated to those fields. Science and technology, the organizers speculated, were topics most expressive of the enduring modernity of Britain's cultural accomplishments and national status. On London's South Bank of the Thames, the organizers of the festival developed plans for the construction and organization of a "Dome of Discovery" focused on the practical benefits of the progress of science in Britain. That gigantic exhibit was augmented by an equally impressive exhibit at the South Kensington–based Science Museum which was dedicated to capturing the spirit of scientific discovery. Together, the venues constituted a spectacular vehicle for advancing public and professional understandings of scientific particulars while reinforcing widely held cultural assumptions about the unitary nature of scientific knowledge.[11] In some sense, these tasks were also the greatest challenge; the exhibit organizers struggled to balance the rigor of their scientific messages with equal desires to make the scientific work as culturally accessible for the public as possible.[12]

Among the sciences represented in the Dome of Discovery and the Science Museum at the Festival of Britain were exhibits pertaining to the function of the brain and nervous system in animals and human beings. In recent historical scholarship, such topics might well be regarded as early contributions to the emergence of the new discipline of neuroscience, a field that started to take shape in the 1930s, received growing attention in the 1950s, became programmatic in the 1960s and 1970s, and ultimately achieved distinction in the 1990s. Scholars Nikolas Rose and Joelle Abi-Rached have argued that the emergence of neuroscience in the second half of the twentieth-century signaled an increasingly reductionistic, neuro-molecular cultural style that cast the brain as the organ of the mind. They claim, moreover, that this style also coincided with the advent of a new scientific materialism in biomedicine and pharmacology.[13]

Superficially, the patterns Rose and Abi-Rached observe are evident at the Festival of Britain, but such a claim must be tempered by situating the brain and mind sciences within the overall fields of science and medicine as they were then represented within the two exhibits. In particular, as I shall explain in this essay, the Science Museum's exhibit promoted what seems, at least in hindsight, an unusually materialistic and mechanistic understanding of the world for 1950s Britain. The reductionist narrative that organized the overall exhibit meant to invoke in the minds of the audience a simplifying unitary conception of nature, one that built from a subatomic universe a whole world of living creatures possessing unique and wondrous structures and, presumably, behaviors too. Yet as I shall also explain, invisible and unacknowledged dualisms, that is, the nonphysical phenomena of a particular historical nervous system, nevertheless haunted in a quite literal sense the imaginary and evocative world of knowledge that the Committee on Science and Technology engineered within the confines of the museum's exhibit. In particular the techniques of persuasion the organizers used to convey their reductionist and materialistic story to the public ironically relied upon intentionally engineered psychotechnic illusions in assembling the physical space of the exhibit. Because the organizers never identified or explained the existence of such psychic phenomena, or indeed even related the existence of such phenomena to the overarching metanarrative of the exhibit, they inadvertently created in material fashion a technical dualism in the space of the exhibit. By ignoring the science that explained the content of these illusions, they created a participatory space filled by an invisible reaction formation, a dualism to haunt their materialist claims—claims, which in the context of the British mind and brain sciences in 1951, stood moreover as a controversial interpretation of the physical basis of life, mind, and behavior.[14]

Science, Technology, and Medicine at the Festival of Britain

The Festival of Britain corresponded to the centenary celebration of the Great Exhibition of 1851. It was an ambitious and expensive event, one that actively sought to construct the public's knowledge of Britain. Imagined by the newly elected government of Clement Atlee as an opportunity to renew national pride and foster patriotism, the festival sought also to celebrate a long history of the British people through its focus on labor, culture, and science in the British Isles. The organizers planned it as an autobiography of a great nation and as a tonic too, as a festival and educational entertainment. Traveling exhibits were planned as well. These would move thematic elements of the festival around the nation by land and sea, thereby offsetting the otherwise metropolitan, and as many pointed out at the time, elitist character of those permanent exhibits developed in the capital.[15] The festival also inspired political discontents, not least among political conservatives who variously attacked it for constituting a colossal waste of public funds, for being inspired by socialist imperatives, or for being plebian in its middle-class aspirations. Years in the making, and intended moreover to be semipermanent, the festival opened in the summer but proved short-lived, having fallen afoul of the newly elected Conservative government which had shut it down by the autumn of that year.[16]

Despite this short life, the Festival of Britain left behind significant material evidence of its impact on British society and culture: The documents and manuscripts associated with the various committees, contractors, and associations form an extensive archive of life and labor in the late 1940s and early 1950s Britain.[17] Bric-a-brac sold in shops celebrated the event in glassware, badges, and textiles.[18] The architectural impact, too, was enormous, especially at the site of the permanent exhibition on the South Bank of the Thames River. Located between Waterloo Bridge and Nelson Pier, the grounds were enormous, providing space for twenty-seven different exhibits scattered across thirteen buildings. There were also restaurants; pubs; teahouses; and park spaces filled with trees, sculptures, murals, and decorative architectural art installations, including the famous floating Skylon tower.[19] No structure dominated the South Bank landscape more impressively, however, than the Dome of Discovery, dubbed in retrospect an architectural achievement of the age and used as an inspiration for the Millennium Dome, which was constructed in London in 2000.[20]

The Dome of Discovery should be seen very much as a prospective site for observing what historians Sven Dierig, Jens Lachmund, and J. Andrew Mendelsohn have called the urban history of science.[21] As a site of local (i.e., nationalistic) scientific practices, it contained several thematic areas, all of which the Committee on Science and Technology intended to showcase British contributions to science and cover "the far reaching practical benefits which have sprung from the British scientific march."[22] Ian Cox, director of science, observed to the organizing Council,

> The Dome is intended to display Discovery in its widest sense, point out that the British propensity to direct enquiry and enterprise into spheres beyond the immediate domestic surroundings, and the achievements that have resulted from this. Thus, at one extreme, we shall show the more outstanding of the researches into the nature and behavior of matter, at the other the development of overseas territories by the application of the many sciences and techniques (e.g. engineering) for which we are famous.[23]

As Cox's language suggested, entrants to the Dome would encounter sections devoted to land, sea, the artic reaches, outer space, and earth's ionosphere. But there was a far wider and compelling rhetorical frame underpinning the presentation of science. Even in otherwise mundane minutes describing those various foci, larger cultural narratives central to Britain's imperial imaginary came to the fore. Land exploration, for instance, was illustrated through reference to the "Opening up of the Dark Continent," a phrase at once conjuring manly virtues and past British confidence in their rightful supremacy over Empire. The passing phrase "ingenuity" appeared there too; through it an imaginary intersection linked maritime exploration and industrialization with discoveries about outer space. It seems that "Cook in the Pacific," the Greenwich Observatory" and Harrison's "famous Chronometer" were all part of the progress of scientific empire.[24]

Had the Dome of Discovery been the only exhibit in London dedicated to science and technology, those special areas of society and culture would still have been strongly represented. The additional exhibit at the Science Museum in South Kensington differed in several important respects. While the South Bank exhibit emphasized the practical ends of all science and technology, the South Kensington exhibit focused only on "advances in the understanding of the structure of matter, living and dead."[25] While both exhibits made the ends of science a component of their narratives, the designers of the museum's exhibit only divulged the practical elements of the study of the structure of matter in the final section of the exhibit. In other words, the Science Museum's exhibit—in terms of how visitors were to experience it—emphasized the marvelous dimension of disenchanting nature through discovery firstly, and only afterward came to speculate about the ends of such knowledge. Like at South Bank, the South Kensington one contained a metanarrative. The designers, however, did not emphasize the virtues of science for Empire. Instead, they focused on developing a very clear narrative which claimed that the structure and function of the subatomic world ultimately explained life and reality. Moreover, they sought to shape that narrative in such a way as to make such reductionism seem inevitable, logical, and natural to the audience.

In this exhibit, protons and neutrons were linked in a compelling chain of being to the miracle of life itself.[26]

In retrospect, the most surprising dimension of science in the Festival of Britain was the manner with which the Council for the Festival in general and the Committee on Science and Technology in particular solicited expertise on science, technology, and medicine. Even at the time, the arrangement struck many organizers and designers as novel. In a summary of the work, the director of science, Ian Cox, elaborated:

> The preparation of a science exhibition along such novel lines is in the hands of a small central staff of highly trained scientists, working in collaboration with artists and specialists from the entertainments industry. And this compact organization, and standing for rigorously accurate presentation, are the celebrated scientists, the learned institutions, and trade associations of manufacturers the length and breadth of Britain, who are giving voluntary and skilling help in making South Kensington a worthy tribute to British Science.[27]

The organizers courted up-to-date scientific, technological, and medical expertise by soliciting hundreds of "scripts" from renowned British scientists. These scripts, which ranged in length from three to as many as thirty typed pages, described the state of scientific knowledge in a variety of subfields across the biological and natural sciences.[28] Initially, the authors of the scripts received a formal contract for their work. Typically, they were paid £25 for each script. The contracts specified the place, the section, and the subject for which the script was intended. From today's perspective, the terms of contract are maddeningly vague. For instance, a contract to physiologist and Nobel laureate E. D. Adrian explained only that the festival officer and festival designer desired for the Health Section on the South Bank a synopsis "script of approximately 3,000 words, with suggestions for visual display where possible, on 'The Physiology of the Nervous System'" due in March 1950.[29] By contrast, a contract for a script on crystallography for the Science Museum's section titled Chemical Structure provided many details both about the setting of the exhibit and the specific foci the author should address. The contract explained the ways that visitors would encounter knowledge of the exhibit and then stipulated that the officer and designer required

> an annotated detailed list of suggestions for inclusion in the Crystallography and Petrology sections, so that items may be followed up and converted into story form. The items should preferably but not necessarily concern British work, but bear some relation to the overall theme of the exhibition, which may be summarized as follows: "Advances in the understanding of the structure of matter, living and dead, special attention being given to the application of such knowledge to human and technological problems." Any suggestions as to visual presentation would be very welcome.[30]

Most of the scripts functioned as extensive literature reviews of their subject, albeit ones ostensibly written for a popular audience. As the sample from J. Z. Young cited at the beginning of this essay suggests, the authors of many of these scripts also attempt to make the science attractive to the public without sacrificing accuracy and rigor. In other words, these scripts as an archive form an important if idiosyncratic time capsule for the history of science and medicine, and inform us now about the ways past elite scientists and physicians understood their areas of expertise and also imagined translating that expertise for public consumption and entertainment in 1951. For the scientists and physicians, the technique of communication demanded of them was simultaneously synthetic and thespian.[31]

There are, however, only few hints indicating the ways in which the officers and designers selected experts or about the ways in which the designers incorporated the information in the solicited scripts into their various exhibitions. At an administrative level, it seems clear that administrators treated expertise on science, technology, and health as emanating from related spheres of endeavor. Although health received its own exhibit hall at the Festival, the scripts for that exhibit were compiled in volumes alongside scripts for the biological and natural sciences as well as engineering fields. Only one terse minute from 1949 sheds much light on the ways designers attempted to merge expertise and science into a seamless narrative: "The designer said that what they needed before they could start work was a detailed script, with the 'stories' in correct sequence, for the whole exhibition. It was agreed that the Festival Office should simplify the advisers' scripts where necessary and integrate them into one story."[32]

The Story of Matter and Mind in the Festival of Britain

There were hundreds of stories underpinning that singular sequence. Topics in health, the biological sciences, and physiology, for example, considered a wide array of subjects, including the properties of genetic units, the evolution of hominids, the structure and hypothesized function of cortisone, the history of nursing, the development of plastic surgery, and discoveries in British surgery and anesthesiology. While some topics clearly lent themselves more easily to the health exhibit or the thematic exhibits in the Dome of Discovery than they did to the Science Museum exhibit, it is unclear for which exhibits and for which sections specific scripts were intended.[33]

Perhaps the most striking feature of these scripts was the popularity of certain subjects over others. Scripts on geology, geophysics, oceanography, astronomy, zoology, and genetic and cell biology were extremely common, and most of the fields of medicine had one or two lengthy scripts as well. The chairman of the Council for Science and Technology remarked in passing in the minutes that he was "surprised and delighted" by "how complete a coverage of science had been effected on the South Bank and in South Kensington."[34] As a representation of the whole of science, technology, medicine, and engineering, the scripts therefore can be construed as providing a rather robust measure of trends, fashions, and paradigms in scientific research before the discovery of the structure of DNA.[35] By the same measure, absent topics are also instructive. One seems particularly noteworthy: scripts wholly devoted either to psychological or psychiatric topics—that is, the mind sciences—are almost entirely absent from this historical record and are only mentioned in the most superficial way in other scripts. For instance, in his script *What Is life?*, Erwin Schrödinger made no reference at all to the phenomenon of mind—chromosomes and probabilities determined everything that mattered:

> To all appearances, each region or part or district of the huge chromosome molecule plays an individual role in directing the sequence of marvelously well-determined events that takes place from the moment of the fertilization of the egg, until the phase, thus inaugurated, ends by so-called death—an individual role, one of statistical contribution, as that of molecules in inorganic processes. In this respect (and also by being solid structures) the chromosomes and their several parts are more analogous to a driving gear and its cog-wheels than to the molecules of inorganic matter.[36]

There were some prospective exceptions. For example, scripts on the physiology, biochemistry, and medicine and surgery of the central nervous system were relatively common and gestured occasionally at processes of mind. Not only was J. Z. Young's script on memory in the octopus present in the collection, he had also penned a short, lively essay describing the mechanism of nervous transmission.[37] E. D. Adrian augmented that discussion with a short analysis of the history of discoveries in the physiology of the nervous system.[38] Hamilton Hartridge wrote about the reductive processes in sensation and perception in the organs of special sense (i.e., the eye, nose, and ears).[39] Leonard Harrison Matthews dealt with echo location in the bat.[40] And one even moved from the physical nervous system to contemplate mind in humans, albeit very briefly. In his long essay titled "Neurology," S. F. Dudley summarized trends in the science of neurology and concluded by observing that

> the relationship between neurology and disease of the mind is somewhat confusing and highly controversial. But we have only to consider the effects of such poisons as alcohol, opium, etc., such diseases as poliomyelitis, G. P. I. (syphilis) and trypanosomiosis, such hormone deficiencies as cretinism, and diabetic coma, such vitamin deficiencies as pellagra, and the sequels of injuries on the mind, to realise how there is no hard and fast line between psychiatry

and neurology. Certain forms of madness or mental disease are now answerable to surgical treatments as the division of certain nerve tracts in the brain may cure or improve cases of schizophrenia among other mental diseases. Some of these conditions have been dealt with elsewhere [in other nations], most of them cannot be claimed to have been discovered or elucidated by British scientists but they need mention to show that they have not been forgotten and that psychiatry, as medical psychology is closely related to neurology and neurosurgery.[41]

Dudley appears—the record is unclear—to have been one of those charged with summarizing and synthesizing scripts from experts to aid exhibit designers in their attempt to produce a seamless narrative. In any case, he was the author of many health scripts, and there is significant similarity between his essay on neurology and those others that focused on the function of the nervous system. His essay, it may also be inferred, further supplemented the Health Exhibit on the South Bank.[42] Like Young, Dudley observed in the margins of his essays the ways designers might create thematic narratives. It was unclear to him, however, how the designers might represent the relationship between neurology and diseases of the mind. He observed that perhaps some final illustration indicating that much of this work of discovery had been done by foreign schools of psychiatry was at least necessary.

Thus, the composite picture of the nervous system easily inferred from these scripts created a biophysical, biochemical, physiological, and pharmacological picture of the function of single neurons or intact nervous systems in animals and human beings. Only J. Z Young was so strident as to intimate that such reductionism would lead ultimately toward better understanding of the function of minds (recall his adroit remark implying a translatable commonality between memory in octopuses and memory in human beings). Insofar as any mention of mind was made, it was consequently subordinated to an overwhelmingly reductionist program; insofar as there was any mention of psychology or psychiatry, those fields were subordinated to neurology and neurosurgery. The result, if a weak materialist turn, was nevertheless a turn, not least because such thinking moved against a long-standing idealist tradition in the British mind and brain sciences.

It is clear that the Science Museum exhibit, more than the South Bank ones, focused on the reductionist mechanistic paradigm. By 1949 the general details of the exhibit had been planned. Five thousand square feet of space would introduce the average attendee to the main story which asked "What is life?" and answered that question by navigating attendees through a series of rooms beginning in subatomic worlds and passing to worlds of organisms. The audience would walk through 6,650 square feet dedicated to atomic structure, 6,450 square feet on chemical structure, 4,000 square feet on the living world, and 7,000 square feet devoted to nuclear structure.

At the end of the exhibit, a space termed "Stop Press" would offer approximately 1,500 square feet on such "culminating feature[s]" as a "mock-up atomic power station."[43]

In a later report, Ian Cox further described the design: the first room of the exhibit showed such natural objects as diamonds in their natural size. The second room showed the diamond crystal at ten times its size, the third at one thousand times its size, and the fourth at another thousand times its size, "opening out its structure so that the atoms appear as stars arranged in a regular pattern in three dimensions."[44] By the fifth room, the crystal structure had been "enlarged by ten-thousand million times its natural size." Thereafter, the exhibit would move from illusion to a more detailed discussion of atomic structure, the Bohr atom, radioactivity, and the mechanism of nuclear fission, and then segue into a description of the ways that atoms become such substances as metals or organic compounds: "The final sequence displays modern knowledge of the chemistry of substances associated with life, starting with proteins, which are the basis of the animal and vegetable body and leading onto enzymes, those substances which in living organisms are responsible for joining together great numbers of pairs of molecules with but little change to themselves. Herein is a great part of the secret of life."[45]

From there the exhibition passed to a discussion of the structure of the living cell from whence single-celled organisms became multicellular animals and plants. Stop Press, almost an epilogue to whole exhibition, finally summarized modern understanding of matter and life and indicated future directions for research in the natural and biological sciences.[46] The final chamber included, among other things, three small robot tortoises created by physiologist W. Grey Walter that moved in response to light stimulus. In a reference to the tortoises, Jacob Bronowski, author of the museum guidebook, observed, referencing Pavlovian conditioning, that "a mechanical 'animal' can be constructed to steer itself towards the light in this automatic way."[47] While the exhibit was thus silent on the ultimate question of the animating principle underpinning life and behavior qua mind, such final spectacular demonstrations hinted that the reductionist science would in time disenchant both.

Materialist Narratives, Dualist Techniques

Whether the designers and festival organizers really intended to spin so positivist and materialist an account of matter, life, and mind is unclear. The emphasis on matter was not, of course, bizarre, especially given the concluding events of World War II. The message of the newly born atomic age was clear: matter mattered.

At the same time, the reductionist narrative offered more than a compelling story. It indicated at once a story of progress in discovery and also the steady disenchantment by reductionist British scientists of nature through the elaboration of nature's unity and harmony. Not only did reductionist science explain the properties of crystals; their chemical and physical properties could be extended toward complex macromolecular domains. The kinetics of simple chemical reactions mimicked such more complex chemical reactions as enzyme metabolism. There was, too, a promise that such materialist knowledge would ultimately resolve the defining dialectics of the Enlightenment—that is, body and soul, brain and mind, normal and abnormal, and even life and death.

Some of the scripts that underpinned the Science Museum's exhibit positioned themselves strongly within this materialist imaginary. M. F. Perutz, for example, described the molecular aspects of living processes in strictly anti-vitalist terms: "We now know that under suitable conditions isolated organs can be kept alive and that many 'living' processes can be performed in glass vessels. Scientists find it useful to leave out the idea of a vital force and to think of a cell as a complex system of chemical, mechanical, and electrical devices, a kind of clockwork of great complexity."[48] Perutz explained the living cell, then, in terms of chemical messengers, enzymes, electrical signals, and self-regulation. There was no material explanation for the reproduction of an organism, he admitted, but planetary motion and the action of pendulum clocks, Perutz claimed, gave singular examples of complex mechanisms that might be equivalent.[49] Death, meanwhile, resulted from the universal law of entropy; it was caused by the "universal tendency to chaos. Life was a complex and unstable form of order maintained by solar energy. Life is like a man trying to keep level on a descending escalator."[50] Perutz's script very much embodied the tone of the narrative; council minutes describing the structure of proteins in the exhibit echoed language appearing in his script: "The body is in some ways like an engine, but like an engine which grows its own spare parts and replaces them."[51]

The exhibit's concluding section, Stop Press, took these points toward sciences and medicines of the mind and brain. Some wall diagrams described "how we know" and detailed the structures of the organs of special sense, making clear that sensation and perception, at the least, made some forms of knowledge possible and could be understood as material processes. The inclusion, furthermore, of W. Grey Walter's machine tortoises, mechanical robots that responded to light and touch stimuli, added that further behavioral dimension to the overall argument.

While it would thus be tempting to claim that the narrative of matter had moved through subatomic worlds to offer a materialist account of holistic worlds of mind and behavior, to do so would be to exaggerate the connection of the final section to the rest of the exhibit. Stop Press was very much oriented toward imagining futures—it was fictive whimsy. Even if audiences understood the narrative of the exhibit as continuous and seamless, the exhibit's finale did represent a rupture within the exhibit's narrative. Physically speaking, there was only a small space allocated for grand promises. At the same time, the emphasis on matter invited attendees to attend to reductionist progress; those promises were also in a privileged position that was more likely to make an impact on visitors' minds.

Dualisms nevertheless haunted the materialist imaginary contrived within the heart of the exhibition. When director of science Ian Cox described the ways the techniques of the exhibition would transcend classical curation, he wrote,

> The South Kensington Science Exhibition will not be arranged in the usual museum fashion, with small specimens laid out on benches and in glass cases. Often explanations will be cut to a minimum, and the demonstrations will be very largely visual. Every device of show technique has been considered. Motion pictures, animated diagrams, stereoscopic photographs, electric signs, moving three-dimensional models—as well as actual examples of historical apparatus—will all be used. The atomic models are being specifically designed for the exhibition with the collaboration of leading experts in wave mechanics and will employ cathode ray tubes similar to those used in television screens.[52]

On the surface, such museum bric-a-brac denoted a very material basis for the reductive and materialist argument. But the technique of designing an experiential narrative required that the organizers and designers fashion the exhibit's environment in such ways as to induce a state of knowledge in attendees. Cox explained:

> Entry to the exhibition will be through a series of chambers in which ordinary objects are successively magnified until the spectator, narrowing on a single crystal, can see the atoms which compose it. Like Alice, nibbling magic toadstool, he will be able to grow smaller at will and finally, a magnification of ten thousand million times, to wander through a Wonderland which the nucleus of the atom and its surrounding electrons are spread all around him.[53]

The metaphor of the magic toadstool, fascinatingly material in Cox's choice language, suggested that visitors would bring their own capacities to suspend disbelief, indeed that the brain provided its own technique of credulity. At the same time, as Cox explicitly recognized, invisible authors had composed these environments in order explicitly to evoke those hallucinatory capacities. The complexity of the exhibition, and the psychotechnics involved, manufactured ultimately the grand staging of the profoundly material universe. As Cox put it:

196 ❧ STEPHEN T. CASPER

A great deal of thought has already been given to the many problems that arise as a result of increasing the apparent size of the object of study to the enormous extent indicated above. Between each pair of rooms will be a passage where much of the progressive condition of the visitor's mind will be effected. It is here that all additional information necessary to the understanding of the displays will be passed verbally by means of recordings, the voices in which become increasingly remote from the everyday. Progressive changes in the acoustics, temperature and smells will also enhance the visitor's impression of penetrating into a new and different world. Light gradually decreases in the series of rooms until in the last there is none except from the nuclei and electron clouds. Correlated with this is the gradual disappearance of the boundaries of the rooms—walls, ceilings, floors—an essential consideration if the illusion of enormous magnification is to be successful.[54]

That different world, silent precisely on the question of the operation of the mind, embedded a notion of each visitor's mechanical agency in the exhibit through these presentation of stimuli. That there were authors engineering those stimuli implied the existence of a self-determining agency directly in conflict with the reductionist and mechanical image of life perpetuated by the experience of the exhibit. There was then, broadly speaking, an irony firmly embedded in the exhibit. It had first manifested when authors of the expert scripts literally divided scientific knowledge and the work of making that knowledge communicable; but it was even more manifested, if invisibly so, in the techniques of illusion deployed by the exhibit's designers. The expert authors of the scripts that underpinned the exhibition divided their knowledge from the techniques that made it presentable; so too did the designers of the exhibition disseminate a materialist account of matter by making invisible their artful designs. To be sure, these were illusions comprised of atoms and work, but they were also illusions ordered by agents. There was a ghost in this machine; in the absence of the Divine, human agency played the role admirably.

Conclusion

The Festival of Britain in 1951 left an indelible and very material mark upon postwar Britain once the exhibits were shuttered and the buildings razed. Like other such grand festivals, world fairs, expos, and sporting events, it relays a very particular cultural history of people, communities, nations, and empires, and like other such events, the festival in retrospect possesses enormous nostalgic charm. There is, too, clearly the making of an urban history of science in this narrative. Clearly science, technology, and medicine appear to have been celebrated as distinctive cultural and economic spheres important in their own right, and there can be little doubt that both the

Dome of Discovery and the Science Exhibition promulgated through "show techniques" other visions of science, medicine, and technology apart from those described in this essay.

Indeed, it seems most likely that few who paid the price of admission thought much at all about either the premises or conceits of either exhibit. Perhaps many were inspired by them, others confused, and still others simply bored. There is, nonetheless, an inescapable sense that after the World War II, a reductive and materialist narrative came to define the conceptual basis of science in ways that really were novel in the longer history of science. The tendencies on display at the 1951 Festival of Britain, if not a wholehearted harbinger of those changes, seem very much indicative of that larger and to large extent cosmopolitan transformation.

❧   ❧   ❧

Looking outward from this particular case, it is worth closing with reflections on the ways it illustrates the rather misleading portrayal of dualisms in the contemporary neurosciences. There is a tendency in certain quarters of the sciences and medicines of the mind and brain to dismiss dualisms of all kinds. Scholars in the humanities and social sciences who study the neurosciences would be wise to eschew this tendency, not because dualisms or materialisms are right or wrong or pseudoscientific, but rather precisely because the epistemology of the mind and brain sciences now ascribes those dualisms the status of its own misguided pasts. It is perhaps salutary to observe that often those dualisms inadvertently entered into very material techniques, technologies, and therapies, sometimes, as this study of the 1951 Festival of Britain showcases, in highly illustrative ways for a materialist turn and often usually as a reaction formation.[55] It is perhaps also important to observe that those dualisms may well have developed to the benefit of the more reductive natural sciences—the very foundation of action potentials, transcription, and enzyme activity. While many physicists and chemists no doubt pondered broader questions about the nature of thought and life, past dualisms may also have allowed past natural scientists to get on with the business of thinking about matter without reference to such imponderables as the existence of mind. It might therefore be worth studying how humans have practiced dualisms before treating seriously contemporary efforts to cast them aside as errors. Sometimes it is worth leaning the other way in order to see what we are leaning on.

Notes

Epigraph. Antonio R. Damasio, *Descartes' Error: Emotion, Reason, and the Human Brain* (New York: G. P. Putnam's Sons, 1994), 273.

1. National Archives, London (hereafter NA), Work 25/23, Festival of Britain 1951: Specialist Scripts Biology Parts 1, 2, 3, Festival of Britain 1951: Script on Learning in Octopus (J. Z. Young, M.A., F. R. S.), 1.

2. Ibid., 1–2.

3. Ibid., 2.

4. Ibid., 1.

5. Ibid., 3.

6. T. P. R. Laslett, *The Physical Basis of Mind: A Series of Broadcast Talks*, ed. P. Laslett (Oxford: Basil Blackwell, 1950); Cornelius Borck and Michael Hagner, eds., "Mindful Practices: On the Neurosciences in the Twentieth Century," Special Issue of *Science in Context* 14, no. 4 (2001); Cornelius Borck, "Communicating the Modern Body: Fritz Kahn's Popular Images of Human Physiology as an Industrialized World," *Canadian Journal of Communication* 32, no. 3 (2007): 495–520; Cornelius Borck, "Electrifying the Brain in the 1920s: Electrical Technology as a Mediator in Brain Research," in *Electric Bodies: Episodes in the History of Medical Electricity*, ed. by Paolo Bertucci and Giuliano Pancaldi (Bologna: Centro Internazionale per la Storia delle Universita e della Scenza, 2001), 239–64; Fabio de Sio, "Leviathan and the Soft Animal: Medical Humanism and the Invertebrate Models for Higher Nervous Functions, 1950s–90s." *Medical History* 55, no. 3 (2011): 369–74.

7. Cornelius Borck, "Urban Gehirne: Zum Bildüberschuss medientechnischer Hirnwelten der 1920er Jahre," *Archive Für Mediengeschichte* 2 (2002): 261, 267.

8. A similar story has been recorded for the city of Berlin through a sprawling and convincing study of German modernity. This study differs chiefly in the sense that its emphasis is on the post–World War II period in Britain and that the expressly secular construction of the nervous system was something altogether new. Andreas Killen, *Berlin Electropolis: Shock, Nerves, and German Modernity* (Berkeley: University of California Press, 2006). See also Sven Dierig, *Wissenschaft in der Maschinenstadt: Emil Du Bois-Reymond und seine Laboratorien in Berlin* (Göttingen: Wallstein-Verlag, 2006); Alexa Geisthövel and Habbo Knoch, eds., *Orte der Moderne: Erfahrungswelten des 19. und 20. Jahrhunderts* (Frankfurt: Campus Verlag, 2005).

9. Historians of science and medicine have largely refrained, however, from exploring the ethnographic dimensions of the museum. Among the most important studies not to be missed and germane to this study is Sharon Macdonald, *Behind the Scenes at the Science Museum* (Oxford, New York, and Berg, Germany: Oxford, 2002). For a thorough and critical analysis of the public understanding of science, see also Alan Irwin and Brian Wynne eds., *Misunderstanding Science? The Public Reconstruction of Science and Technology* (Cambridge: Cambridge University Press, 1996). In addition, see Peter J. Bowler, *Science for All: The Popularization of Science in Early Twentieth-Century Britain* (Chicago: University of Chicago Press, 2009), and for an up-to-date appraisal of trends in the history of science, see Samuel J. M. M. Alberti, ed., "Focus: Museums and the History of Science" *Isis* 96, no. 4 (2005): 559–608.

10. Harriet Atkinson, *The Festival of Britain: A Land and Its People* (London: I. B. Tauris, 2012); Becky Conekin, *The Autobiography of a Nation: The 1951 Festival of Britain* (Manchester, UK: Manchester University Press, 2003); Festival of Britain, *The Story of the Festival of Britain, 1951* (London: Festival of Britain, 1952); The Festival of Britain, 1951, *The Arts in the Festival of Britain, 1951* (London: Arts Council of Great Britain, 1951).

11. For a brilliant study of science at the Festival of Britain and the projection of identity, see Sophie Forgan, "Festivals of Science and the Two Culture: Science, Design, and Display in the Festival of Britain, 1951" *British Journal for the History of Science* 31, no. 2 (1998): 217–40.

12. See, for instance, the related example: Daniela S. Barberis, "Changing Practices of Commemoration in Neurology: Comparing Charcot's 1925 and 1993 Centennials," *Osiris* 14 (1999): 102–17 (the entire issue is an outstanding study of memory and public science). But I'm also drawing on Ludmilla Jordanova, *Defining Features: Scientific and Medical Portraits 1660–2000* (London: Reakton Books, 2000); Thomas Söderqvist, "Neurobiographies: Writing Lives in the History of Neurology and Neuroscience," *Journal of the History of Neurosciences* 11, no. 1 (2002): 38–48; Eric Hobsbawm, "Introduction: Inventing Traditions," in *The Invention of Tradition*, ed. Eric Hobsbawm and Terence Ranger (London: Cambridge University Press, 1983), 1–9; Caroline Jones and Peter Galison, eds. *Picturing Science, Producing Art* (New York: Routledge, 1998); Geoffrey Cubitt and Allen Warren, eds. *Heroic Reputations and Exemplary Lives* (Manchester, UK: Manchester University Press, 2000).

13. Nikolas Rose and Joell M. Abi-Rached, *Neuro: The New Brain Sciences and the Management of the Mind* (Princeton, NJ: Princeton University Press, 2013).

14. For a discussion of the dualisms in the mind and brain sciences, see Stephen T. Casper, *The Neurologists: A History of a Medical Specialty in Britain, 1789–2000* (Manchester, UK: Manchester University Press, 2014).

15. The Festival of Britain, *Catalogue of Activities throughout the Country* (London: The Festival of Britain, 1951).

16. Conekin, *Autobiography of a Nation*, introduction.

17. NA Work 25 Records of the Festival of Britain Office, 1948–52.

18. Bill Tonkin and George Simner, *Post Cards and Related Collectibles of the Festival of Britain* (West Wickham, UK: Exhibition Study Group, 2001).

19. For discussion, see Henrietta Goodden, *The Lion and the Unicorn: Symbolic Architecture for the Festival of Britain, 1951* (London: Unicorn Press, 2011).

20. Charles Knevitt, *Dome: Ralph Tubbs and the Festival of Britain* (London: Chelsea Space, 2012).

21. Sven Dierig, Jens Lachmund, and J. Andrew Mendelsohn, "Introduction: Toward an Urban History of Science," *Osiris* 18 (2003): 1–19.

22. NA Work 25/44 A5/A6, Council of Festival of Britain 1950, The Council of the Festival of Britain 1951, Science Exhibition, South Kensington—Summary.

23. NA Work 25/47 Presentation Panel Minutes of Meetings: Presentation Panel (48) 11th Meeting, December 20, 1948, 3.

24. Ibid., 3–4. For a discussion of the relationship between Empire and Neurology, see Stephen T. Casper, "An Integrative Legacy: History and Neuroscience" *Isis*, 105, no. 1 (2014): 123–32.

25. NA Work 25/44 A5/A6, Council of Festival of Britain 1950, Annexure II.

26. Festival of Britain, *Exhibition of Science, South Kensington: A Guide to the Story It Tells* (London: H. M. S.O., 1951).

27. NA Work 25/44 A5/A6 Council of Festival of Britain 1950, The Council of the Festival of Britain 1951 Science Exhibition, South Kensington—Summary.

28. NA Work 25/23 contains representative bound volumes of these scripts, but they are also scattered throughout the whole collection. It is not clear why some were bound and others were not.

29. NA Work 25/255 Festival of Britain 1951, Requisition No: 10061, C. L. No 0/2/368 Contract between E. D. Adrian and N. B. Clayton.

30. NA Work 25/255 Festival of Britain 1951, Requisition No: 472, C.L. No. 0/2/395 Contract between unspecified and S. W. Smith. Further correspondence indicates that the authors were W. H. Taylor and Audrey M. B. Douglas. See NA Work 25/255 Festival of Britain 1951, Letter from W. H. Taylor to Festival of Britain Office, Contracts Branch, May 17, 1950. Also see in same file Letter from H. O. Aldhous to W. H. Taylor, April 19, 1950.

31. It is worth noting that such professional performances were not unknown to scientists and doctors. See Delia Gavrus "Men of Dreams and Men of Action: Neurologists, Neurosurgeons, and the Performance of Professional Identity, 1920–1950," *Bulletin of the History of Medicine*, 85 (2011): 57–92.

32. NA Work 25/52 Council for Science and Technology Science Exhibition Working Party (Agenda, Minutes and Papers 1948–51, Minutes October 7, 1949, 3.

33. Such a question could be resolved through a diligent exploration of the contracts, but that analysis would be complicated because the Contracts Office did not make strenuous efforts to organize their tens of thousands of contracts in ways representing obvious divisions of labor within the Festival. See NA Work 25/255 Festival of Britain 1951, which is representative of the chaos awaiting a more determined historian.

34. NA Work 25/52 Council for Science and Technology Science Exhibition Working Party (Agenda, Minutes and Papers 1948–51, Minutes, October 19, 1950, 2.

35. They would make excellent primary sources for pedagogically complementing Soraya de Chadarevian, *Designs for Life: Molecular Biology after World War II* (New York: Cambridge University Press, 2002).

36. NA Work 25/23 Specialist Scripts: Biology, parts 1, 2, and 3. Script prepared by Erwin Schrödinger, 5.

37. NA Work 25/23 Festival of Britain: Scripts Medicine and Physiology, Festival of Britain 1951, A2/B2/152 Script on Nervous Transmission, by Professor J. Z. Young.

38. NA Work 25/23 Festival of Britain: Scripts Medicine and Physiology, Festival of Britain 1951: The Physiology of the Nervous System, by E. D. Adrian.

39. NA Work 25/23 Festival of Britain: Scripts Medicine and Physiology Festival of Britain 1951, A2/B2/155 Script on the Special Senses, by H. Hartridge.

40. NA Work 25/23 Festival of Britain: Scripts Medicine and Physiology, A2 B7/89, by L. H. Matthews.

41. NA Work 25/23S, volume marked "Scripts A2/B2/106-166," S. F. Dudley, "Neurology: Scripts Integrated, Abstracted, and Extended" (marked A2/B2/138) 1–5, quote on 5–6.

42. For example, one contract makes clear that there was a health section devoted to neurology and neurosurgery. See NA Work 25/255 Festival of Britain 1951, Requisition No: unspecified, C.L. No. c/7/319, Contract between Dr. Dohan and Kenneth Chapman, February 16, 1950.

43. NA Work 25/52, Council for Science and Technology Science Exhibition Working Party (Agenda, Minutes and Papers 1948–51) Minutes, October 7, 1949, 2–3.

44. Ibid., 3.

45. Ibid., 6.

46. Ibid., 9.

47. Jacob Bronowski, *Guide to the Exhibition of Architecture, Town-Planning and Building Research*, ed. Harding McGregor Dunnett (London: H. M. Stationery Office, 1951), 32.

48. NA Work 25/23, Festival of Britain 1951; Specialists Scripts Biology Parts 1, 2, 3, Festival of Britain 1951: A/2/B2/63, M. F. Perutz, "Molecular Aspects of Living Processes," 1.

49. Ibid., 5.

50. Ibid., 11.

51. NA Work 25/52, Council for Science and Technology Science Exhibition Working Party (Agenda, Minutes and Papers 1948–51) Chemical Structure—Proteins. ca January 13, 1950.

52. NA Work 25/44 A5/A6, Council of Festival of Britain 1950, The Council of the Festival of Britain 1951 Science Exhibition, South Kensington—Summary.

53. Ibid., 2.

54. NA Work 25/44 A5/A6, Council of Festival of Britain 1950, Annexure II, 3.

55. I have in mind here parallel but contemporary observations by Nicolas Langlitz, *Neurospychedelia: The Revival of Hallucinogen Research since the Decade of the Brain* (Berkeley: University of California Press, 2013), 23.

Chapter Eight

A *"Model Schizophrenia"*

Amphetamine Psychosis and the Transformation of American Psychiatry

Justin Garson

Introduction

During the early 1950s, dozens of individuals began to show up at London area hospitals with delusions of persecution. Some of them had auditory hallucinations that bolstered their delusional ideas. Clinicians promptly diagnosed them with paranoid schizophrenia and admitted them on an in-patient basis. Within days, their symptoms cleared up and they were discharged.

Further examination revealed that the ingestion of large amounts of amphetamines (or the habitual use of amphetamines over a prolonged period of time) precipitated these individuals' psychotic episodes. In 1953 a medical student at the University of London, P. H. Connell, studied several patients and coined the term *amphetamine psychosis* for this rather infrequent but disturbing effect of amphetamine use. In 1958 he published a short, influential monograph with that title.[1] Connell was not primarily interested in the phenomenon from a biochemical perspective. Rather, he was interested in amphetamine psychosis from a clinical perspective, and also from the perspective of a public health advocate. In coining the term, he was not merely giving clinicians a valuable technique for making a differential diagnosis; he was also framing recreational amphetamine use as a kind of silent epidemic or public health nuisance.

While Connell warned the medical profession about the dangers of amphetamine use, biochemical researchers extracted a very different lesson from his monograph. Could amphetamine psychosis be used as a biochemical model of schizophrenia? That is, by studying the mode of action of amphetamines on the brain, could one discover the biochemical basis of schizophrenia itself—and ultimately develop more exacting, pharmacological, treatments?[2] As Solomon Snyder, one of the American architects of the dopamine hypothesis of schizophrenia, later put it, "a drug which could elicit a 'model schizophrenia' would be a boon to psychiatry."[3] To say that it would be a boon to psychiatry was an understatement. Amphetamine psychosis would give researchers a new window into the mechanism of schizophrenia.

Biochemical researchers, however, were slow to adopt the theory that amphetamine psychosis constituted a "model schizophrenia." In fact, from 1959, when the American neuroscientist Seymour Kety suggested it, it took over a decade for the idea to catch on among researchers. On the contrary, by the mid-1960s, the handful of researchers who had investigated the question in any real depth were pessimistic about the ability of amphetamine psychosis to model schizophrenia.[4] Amphetamine psychosis only seemed to mimic some of the more florid symptoms of schizophrenia, such as delusions and, less commonly, hallucinations. It did not mimic Eugen Bleuler's core feature of schizophrenia, the "loosening of associations" or psychic disorganization later known as "formal thought disorder."[5] Nor did amphetamine psychosis induce the bizarre "catatonic" states that define one subtype of schizophrenia, replete with its histrionic posturing or repetition of pointless actions.[6]

There was a second obstacle to the widespread acceptance of amphetamine psychosis as a model schizophrenia. That title belonged to LSD. Before the dopamine hypothesis of schizophrenia, there was the serotonin hypothesis of schizophrenia, so called because many researchers, by the mid-1950s, believed that LSD could induce a state resembling schizophrenia, and that it did so by inhibiting serotonin. LSD would have to be displaced from that position before amphetamines could occupy it.

By the early 1970s, however, everything had changed. Schizophrenia researchers had converted to what I'll call the "mimicry thesis": that amphetamine psychosis is a faithful mirror of schizophrenia, and not just one small part of it, but the illness in its entirety.[7] By 1976 psychiatrists accepted, more or less unproblematically, that amphetamine psychosis was a precise clinical model of schizophrenia. This mimicry thesis was one of the two crucial pillars of the "dopamine hypothesis" of schizophrenia.[8] The second pillar was the perceived effectiveness of dopamine-blocking drugs in relieving schizophrenia, though that is not part of my story here. I will return to this point shortly. In the following, then, I will pose a simple question: what social, historical, and scientific changes took place that rendered the mimicry thesis so plausible, even self-evident, for psychiatric researchers by the mid-1970s?

There were at least three major changes that took place in the 1960s that led researchers to accept the mimicry thesis. First, Scandinavian researchers in the mid-1960s showed that amphetamines could induce stereotypy in laboratory animals.[9] The fact that amphetamines could induce stereotypy, and that stereotypy resembled some of the symptoms of catatonic-type schizophrenia, suggested that amphetamine use could model a broader range of schizophrenic symptoms than merely delusions and hallucinations.[10] The second shift came from the United States. In 1969, the New York clinicians Burton Angrist and Samuel Gershon observed a very small number of patients that showed evidence of thought disorder, based on their rambling and incoherent speech and writing.[11] Their research, like that on stereotypy, helped to close the perceived gap between amphetamine psychosis and schizophrenia.

A third factor in this transition emerged from an unexpected place. The American countercultural revolution of the late 1960s transformed, from outside of psychiatry, the meaning of amphetamine psychosis. Some of the leading figures of the countercultural movement, such as Timothy Leary and Allen Ginsberg, worked tirelessly to invert public perceptions about LSD. They did so, in part, by contrasting the characteristics of the "acidhead" and the "speed freak" (with the "acidhead" coming out favorably in the comparison).[12] Journalists, sociologists, and musicians also adopted and broadcast these distinctions. According to these figures, the use of LSD, along with other psychedelic drugs such as mescaline and peyote, was a cornerstone of a philosophical and spiritual transformation that would reshape the foundations of American society.[13] There was just one hitch: speed. In Haight-Ashbury, Sunset Strip, and the East Village, artists, musicians, writers, and poets issued dire proclamations that speed was antithetical to the progressive values of the counterculture. The speed freak was antisocial, nihilistic, self-absorbed, hedonistic, nomadic, and unpredictable. But more than anything else, the speed freak was paranoid and violent. Speed, in fact, mimicked the paranoia and violence that characterized American society a whole. Speed was madness, because speed was America. Such rhetorical excesses were hardly restricted to American counterculture. As Brian Casey makes clear in his contribution to this volume, they would also become a hallmark technique of the biological psychiatry movement as well.

The American architects of the dopamine hypothesis freely borrowed, and modulated, the new meanings that the counterculture attached to speed. This helped to displace LSD intoxication as an appropriate biochemical model of schizophrenia and install amphetamines in its place. As Angrist and Gershon summarized their results on Bellevue admissions, "Because of . . . their sociopathy and their frankly hedonistic reasons for drug use, [the amphetamine users] resemble heroin addicts as a group far more than the philosophically and religiously preoccupied and less sociopathic hallucinogen users."[14] As the American psychiatrist and researcher Solomon Snyder argued, taking a page from the novelist Aldous Huxley, LSD usage does not mimic schizophrenia; *it merely enhances normal perception*: "The mental state elicited by psychedelic drugs is one of greatly enhanced perception of oneself and one's environment. Similar states occur during mystical and religious introspection and when an individual is profoundly moved by emotions or external events."[15] Snyder was clearly adopting some of the characterizations of LSD use that had become platitudes in the wake of the countercultural revolution. Snyder was eventually able to weave these and other strands of evidence together into support for the "dopamine hypothesis" of schizophrenia.[16]

To begin to tell this story, I first describe the construction of amphetamine psychosis in the late 1950s. By the mid-1960s, researchers and clinicians concluded that amphetamine psychosis was not an appropriate model of schizophrenia. Next, I describe the scientific and social changes that took place in the late 1960s that helped to close the gap between amphetamine psychosis and schizophrenia, including the Scandinavian work on stereotypy and research in the United States that attempted to identify evidence of thought disorder among amphetamine users. The American countercultural revolution waged a kind of war on speed by emphasizing the violent and paranoid qualities of amphetamine users. In doing so, it helped to displace LSD as a "model schizophrenia" in psychiatric research circles. Finally, I'll describe how the American architects of the dopamine hypothesis exploited these new meanings to support the mimicry thesis, and ultimately, the dopamine hypothesis itself. The dopamine hypothesis, in turn, transformed American psychiatry in the 1970s by putatively demonstrating that a major mental disorder could be successfully reduced to neurotransmitter abnormalities. In conclusion, I will suggest some ways that historians and philosophers of science might use this episode to reconstruct the history of biomedical research into other major mental disorders.

Others have recounted parts of this story. Erika Dyck provided an overview of the way that researchers such as Abram Hoffer and Humphry Osmond in Canada converted LSD into a "model psychosis" in the 1950s, and the way that public figures such as Timothy Leary helped to make LSD a symbol of an emerging youth counterculture in the 1960s.[17] I aim to extend her narrative by showing how speed came to replace LSD as a "model schizophrenia" for researchers, and how this came about, in part, as a result of widespread shifts in cultural attitudes regarding speed and LSD in the late 1960s. Nicolas Rasmussen detailed the transformation of amphetamines from the wonder drug of the 1940s to the public menace of the 1960s.[18] He noted, as I do, how early researchers used the threat of amphetamine psychosis to alert a complacent medical profession to the dangers of speed. He also touched upon the tensions in the American counterculture between the speed and acid subcultures. My story homes in much more specifically than does his on the vicissitudes of the concept of amphetamine psychosis, and how researchers came to use it as a stand-in technique for modeling schizophrenia itself.

Finally, David Healy has provided a lucid and masterful narrative of that other pillar of the dopamine hypothesis, namely, the antipsychotic actions of neuroleptic drugs such as chlorpromazine.[19] By the mid-1960s, researchers were beginning to suspect that antipsychotic drugs functioned by acting on the dopamine system.[20] In the early 1970s, Solomon Snyder demonstrated that neuroleptics like chlorpromazine selectively block the D2 dopamine receptor.[21] These two discoveries—amphetamine psychosis and the dopamine-blocking activity of neuroleptic drugs—provided the foundation for the dopamine hypothesis. To put the point simply, amphetamine turns madness "on," and it does so by flooding the brain with dopamine. Neuroleptics turn madness "off," and they do so by depleting the brain of dopamine. By modulating the dopamine levels of the brain, one could effectively generate, or abolish, psychotic episodes.[22] I have nothing to add to Healy's analysis of the chlorpromazine story. Rather, my story complements his by drawing attention to how researchers came to use amphetamine psychosis, and the changing public perception of LSD and speed, to lend additional support to the emerging dopamine hypothesis.

The Constitution of Amphetamine Psychosis

The British psychiatrist P. H. Connell constituted "amphetamine psychosis" as a distinct diagnostic entity in 1958, in a monograph bearing the same title.[23] He based the book on research he had conducted from 1953 to 1956 as an MD thesis for the University of London. He observed forty-eight subjects who had been admitted to four different hospitals with symptoms resembling paranoid schizophrenia but which, on closer examination, were precipitated by the ingestion of large amounts of amphetamines (or the habitual use of amphetamines over a prolonged period of time). Almost half of those individuals had broken open amphetamine or methamphetamine inhalers and consumed their contents,[24] since although amphetamines had been placed on Schedule IV of the Poison Rules in 1955 (which ensured that amphetamine tablets were not distributed without a prescription), the inhalers were still available without prescription. The Benzedrine inhaler, an amphetamine-based inhaler manufactured by Smith, Kline, and French Laboratories, was the prototype for this product and had been on the market as a decongestant from 1934. By the early 1950s, copycat products, including the methamphetamine inhaler, had flooded the market.[25]

For Connell, the concept of amphetamine psychosis performed two different roles: diagnostic and normative-legal. First and foremost, it served to facilitate differential diagnosis. Connell believed that amphetamine abuse, and its psychotic sequelae, were much more widespread than assumed, but that its prevalence was masked because it was easily confused with schizophrenia by unwary clinicians. The clinician's role was particularly vexing as there were "no physical signs diagnostic of amphetamine intoxication."[26] Amphetamine psychosis, however, did much more than describe a syndrome somehow precipitated by amphetamines. The label asserted a direct causal relationship between the consumption of amphetamines and the subsequent symptoms. In so doing, it tied the phenomenon to the normative-legal realm and provoked the question of responsibility and blame. As Connell put the point, "The medical profession as a whole . . . must bear responsibility for the development of a number of cases of amphetamine addiction and amphetamine psychosis."[27] Or, as Burton Angrist, one of the architects of the dopamine hypothesis, was later to put the point, "It seems difficult to say . . . whether the medical profession needs protection from amphetamine users or vice versa."[28]

Prior to Connell's monograph, few clinicians or biomedical researchers had frankly asserted that amphetamines cause psychosis. Connell never claimed to have made a new discovery; he had simply claimed to have reinterpreted the significance of established facts. The first recorded instance of a psychotic episode precipitated by amphetamines occurred in 1938, and several episodes had been reported since that time.[29] Researchers had dismissed such cases in the past by claiming that amphetamine use merely *unmasked* preexisting psychotic tendencies in a handful of disturbed individuals.[30] This was the "latent psychosis" theory. In fact Smith, Kline, and French aggressively promoted this line of defense when the first reports of psychotic episodes associated with the drug became public.[31] One must keep in mind that, during the 1940s, the governments of Germany, Japan, Britain, and the United States, among others, freely dispensed amphetamine tablets to their combat soldiers in an effort to boost morale and vigor.[32] Nobody was eager to think of amphetamines as psychotomimetic agents.

Connell attacked the latent psychosis theory with a fervor unusual for the otherwise dry monograph. The concept of "latent personality traits," he argued, is "specious and dangerous" and promotes "a complacency which stifles further inquiry and shifts attention from the possible disrupting influence of the drug."[33] He attempted to refute the latent psychosis theory by demonstrating amphetamine psychosis in a small number of patients "whose backgrounds and personalities were normal, so far as could be ascertained."[34] Contrary to received medical opinion, amphetamines could induce psychosis in otherwise healthy people.

What exactly *was* amphetamine psychosis? Besides the fact that amphetamine psychosis could provoke symptoms not unlike paranoid schizophrenia, its clinical symptomatology was extremely diverse. Over the next fifteen years, psychiatrists and researchers reconfigured substantially this clinical symptomatology. The malleability of amphetamine psychosis explained both its allure, as well as its weakness, as a research technique qua prototype for schizophrenia.

The clinical profile of the patient with amphetamine psychosis was stable enough: paranoid delusions accompanied by auditory hallucinations. But Connell noted dozens of additional symptoms that may or may not co-occur with paranoid delusions or auditory hallucinations. These included visual hallucinations, grandiose delusions, delusions with homosexual content, homosexual conduct itself, depression, suicidal ideation, anxiety, confusion, mania, catatonia, hyperkinesis, hypertension, insomnia, violent outbursts, thought disorder and logorrhea, increased libido, decreased libido, twitching and spasms, olfactory hallucinations, transvestitism, and a very distinctive tactile hallucination of worms or bugs crawling under one's skin. During the 1960s clinicians added, removed, or corroborated various symptoms on Connell's list.[35] In the early 1970s, researchers such as Solomon Snyder attempted to organize these into a cohesive narrative, that is, to show them to be diverse moments of a complex and multilayered pathological process.

Almost immediately, biochemical researchers such as Seymour Kety recognized that amphetamine psychosis could potentially function as a powerful biochemical model of schizophrenia.[36] That is, by tracing the biochemical mechanisms that are disrupted in amphetamine psychosis, one could perhaps understand the biochemical basis of schizophrenia, too. In fact, an early review of Connell's *Amphetamine Psychosis*, published in 1959, criticized Connell for failing to note the broader theoretical implications of his work.[37]

Yet it would take another decade for Kety's suggestion to grip the imagination of the psychiatric community. One obstacle, as Kety indicated, was that at the time of his writing, researchers widely considered LSD to be the "model of choice" for investigating both the subjective experience and the biochemical mechanisms of schizophrenia. Researchers would have to strip LSD of that title before amphetamines could occupy that role. Another obstacle was that closer examination of the symptomatology of amphetamine psychosis revealed crucial differences between it and schizophrenia.

Breaking the Link between Amphetamine Psychosis and Schizophrenia

Shortly after the publication of *Amphetamine Psychosis*, researchers published a handful of reports that seemed to confirm the clinical similarity of amphetamine psychosis and schizophrenia.[38] A key issue turned on the question of thought disorder. In 1960 the British psychiatrist Edward Marley claimed to have diagnosed the presence of "disconnection of thought" in one of his patients.[39] The fact that amphetamine psychosis could mimic thought disorder *in addition to* delusions and hallucinations suggested that amphetamine psychosis was closely analogous to schizophrenia itself and hence that it shared the same mechanisms. Three years later, another British psychiatrist, W. B. McConnell, also reported thought disorder in several patients with amphetamine psychosis:

> The conversation of all patients, except the patient who had been ill for 10 years, was at times disjointed, incoherent, and irrelevant. Various forms of schizophrenic thought disorder occurred. Thought blocking was common in all the acute illnesses and was associated with marked perplexity. One patient described it thus: "I just can't think of the word to say . . . it is like a light switch going on, it breaks my train of thought . . . maybe it is because I'm not thinking of what I'm saying." Abstract and concrete meanings were confused by two of the patients.[40]

By the mid-1960s, however, further clinical work threw this emerging consensus into question. In 1965 the Australian psychiatrist D. S. Bell published a paper that systematically explored the connection between the two conditions. Bell gathered reports of fourteen patients who had been admitted to different hospitals for amphetamine psychosis. His conclusion was that, contrary to Connell, amphetamine psychosis *could* readily be distinguished on clinical grounds from schizophrenia. First, amphetamine psychosis is associated with both visual and auditory hallucinations, while schizophrenia is typically characterized by only auditory hallucinations.[41] But second, and more importantly, amphetamine psychosis rarely produces the kind of disorganization of thought characteristic of some forms of schizophrenia. The delusions and hallucinations typically take place in an otherwise lucid frame of mind. This alone, he thought, threw into question the "goodness of fit" of amphetamine psychosis as a biochemical model for schizophrenia.[42]

But what about the supposed thought disorder that had been observed by psychiatrists such as McConnell and Marley? Bell conceded that some patients gave outward indications of disordered thought. Patients often spoke quickly, flitting from topic to topic in an apparently disorganized way. But Bell argued that such instances were hardly demonstrative of *actual* thought disorder. This was because such verbal evidence could not discriminate between formal thought disorder, on the one hand, and the mere "flight of ideas in euphoric patients" that could be mistaken for it. In other words, one must distinguish between actual incongruence of thought, on the one hand, and the *acceleration* of thought, on the other. As the amphetamine user's thought speeds up, an outside observer may fail to note the logical connections that are nonetheless present in it, and hence mistakenly make a diagnosis of thought disorder. As Bell put it, the "schizophrenic thought disorder described by McConnell was not convincingly distinguished from the disturbance that may be secondary to elation or paranoid delusions."[43]

This is not to say that genuine thought disorder could not be clinically distinguished from the flight of ideas due to "elation." The two could be easily distinguished simply by asking the patient what he or she meant by a certain utterance. If the patient could adequately reconstruct the inner logic that was incompletely expressed by his or her utterances, then it was not genuine incongruence of thought. In order to confirm or disconfirm thought disorder, one must question the patient: "As an accompaniment of their heightened mood, the thought process of two patients were accelerated leading to rapidity of associations with flight of ideas. . . . However, when persuaded to make the effort these patients were able to explain the logical associations involved in their flight of ideas."[44]

Despite Connell's bold proclamation that amphetamine psychosis and schizophrenia were "indistinguishable," by 1965 medical psychiatry had discovered an important gap between them. Medical opinion quickly followed Bell's assessment. For example, the British physician R. Gardner of Maudsley Hospital also concurred with Bell's judgement,[45] as did American psychiatrist John D. Griffith of the Vanderbilt University School of Medicine.[46] The Swedish psychiatric researchers L. E. Jönsson and L. M. Gunne of the Psychiatric Research Center of the University of Uppsala remarked on what they call "disorganization of thought" in their patients, but also noted that the patient was able to adequately clarify his or her meaning on questioning.[47] Solomon Snyder, one of the founders of the dopamine hypothesis, conceded that the absence of thought disorder marked a crucial difference between amphetamine psychosis and schizophrenia.[48] One of the projects of American psychiatry of the late 1960s would be to close this gap.

A second reason that researchers could not generally accept amphetamine psychosis as a model of schizophrenia is that LSD had already earned that place of pride. By the early 1950s, psychiatrists and medical researchers had begun to appreciate the power of LSD to serve as a model psychosis.[49] At that time, the idea of a model psychosis, a technique really, had two crucially different meanings. Whether or not, however, LSD shared a biochemical mechanism with schizophrenia was not the point. It was enough that it could induce an artificial psychosis in nonschizophrenics that could advance clinical understanding by eliciting a direct, though fleeting, glimpse of the psychotic patient's experiences.

Even before LSD, the idea of using hallucinogens to induce schizophrenia-like experiences was on the table. This phenomenological sense of the term *artificial psychosis* goes back at least to the 1930s, when the German psychiatrist Erich Guttmann, at the Maudsley Hospital in London, encouraged his colleagues to ingest mescaline for the purpose of inducing an artificial psychosis, which would assist in "understanding the mental life of schizophrenics" and ultimately, perhaps, in deriving "hints for the solution of the great problem of psychiatry, that of schizophrenia."[50] Guttmann's longtime colleague, William Mayer-Gross—who had fled Germany with him and Alfred Mayer to take up a post at Maudsley—made the same recommendation about mescaline.[51] Mayer-Gross later oversaw LSD studies as well.[52] The psychiatrists Humphrey Osmond and Abram Hoffer developed this line of research systematically with LSD in the 1950s at the University of Saskatchewan, though they were also aware of the importance of understanding the biochemical mechanisms involved.[53]

In 1954, however, the concept of a model psychosis would come to assume a second meaning: namely, LSD could elicit a model psychosis in a *biochemical* sense. In that year, two research teams, one in the United States and one in Britain, independently concluded that LSD primarily acted on the serotonin system and appeared to inhibit its production or availability. These researchers immediately drew the tentative conclusion that, since LSD intoxication mimics schizophrenia, then schizophrenia, too, probably results from the inhibition of serotonin. This became known, in Kety's words, as the "serotonin hypothesis" of schizophrenia.[54] As the chemists D. W. Woolley and E. Shaw, co-discoverers of the serotonin hypothesis at the Rockefeller Institute for Medical Research, put it,

> The demonstrated ability of [LSD and similar ergot-based agents] to antagonize the action of serotonin in smooth muscle and the finding of serotonin in the brain suggest that the mental changes caused by the drugs are the result of a serotonin-deficiency which they induce in the brain. If this be true, then the naturally occurring mental disorders—for example, schizophrenia—which are mimicked by these drugs, may be pictured as being the result of a cerebral serotonin deficiency. ... Possibly, therefore, these natural mental disorders could be treated with serotonin.[55]

Independently, a chemist at the University of Edinburgh, J. H. Gaddum, arrived at substantially the same conclusion: "It is possible that the HT [5-HT or serotonin] in our brains plays an essential part in keeping us sane and that the effect of LSD is *due* to its inhibitory action on the HT in the brain."[56] Even in the mid-1950s, the dream of mastering schizophrenia was very much alive; LSD would be the key to mastering it.

Stereotypy, Amphetamine Psychosis, and Schizophrenia

The first phase in the transformation of amphetamine psychosis into a "model schizophrenia" came with the work of Axel Randrup and Ib

Munkvad at St. Hans Hospital in Denmark in 1967. They found that stereotypy could easily be induced in laboratory animals through intravenous injection of amphetamines. Somewhat more circuitously, they reasoned that stereotypy resembled certain outward features of amphetamine intoxication in humans, as well as certain features of schizophrenia, namely, the pointless and repetitive actions sometimes associated with catatonic-type schizophrenia. As a consequence, they claimed, amphetamine psychosis, as a laboratory technique, could model a much greater range of schizophrenic symptoms than researchers like Bell appreciated.[57]

To perfect the analogy to schizophrenia, however, they had to argue that stereotypy was not just a somewhat uncommon side effect of long-term amphetamine use (e.g., back and forth jaw movements), but was at the very heart of amphetamine intoxication itself. To this end, they greatly expanded the accepted meaning of "stereotypy" in humans to encompass a much broader range of symptoms and behaviors. For example, they noted that amphetamine users often get "hung up" on the actions they performed. One of the effects of amphetamines, they noted, was a kind of hyperattentive fascination with certain minutiae, such as "sorting objects in a handbag, manipulating the interiors of a watch, polishing fingernails to the point that sores are produced, etc."[58] The Swedish researcher Gösta Rylander coined the term *punding* to describe this particular effect. Randrup and Munkvad cited Rylander approvingly and described *punding* as a kind of stereotypy.[59] In the eyes of Randrup and Munkvad, this *punding* was no different, in principle, from a repetitive mechanical twitch: they are but "more *complicated* forms of stereotypy."[60] In short, the authors associated amphetamine psychosis with stereotypy; schizophrenia was also associated with stereotypy, and therefore, perhaps, the two conditions shared the same biochemical mechanisms.

By the early 1970s, Randrup and Munkvad had entirely abandoned their earlier modesty about the theoretical significance of their work for psychiatry. Their research on stereotypy had blossomed into a firm conviction that amphetamine psychosis was the ideal biochemical model of schizophrenia. As they announced to the American Schizophrenia Association in 1971, "all schizophrenic symptoms have apparently been observed in the amphetamine psychosis," including "thought blocking" and "stereotyped behavior."[61] The use of stereotypy as an animal model for amphetamine psychosis not only helped to close the gap between madness and speed, but provided a crucial clue that amphetamine psychosis was mediated specifically by its effects on dopamine, rather than norepinephrine—a stepping-stone in the evolving dopamine hypothesis of schizophrenia.

Capturing Thought Disorder

There was still a major barrier to the acceptance of amphetamine psychosis as a model of schizophrenia: the problem of thought disorder. To all appearances, amphetamine psychosis, like LSD intoxication, took place in a lucid frame of mind. One of the defining symptoms of schizophrenia, disorganization or incongruence of thought, was absent. To remedy this difficulty, researchers had to demonstrate that amphetamine psychosis could induce thought disorder—precisely the claim that Bell famously denied in his 1965 report. Recall that in Bell's view, amphetamine psychosis did not induce thought disorder but was sometimes mistakenly believed to do so because it led to the acceleration of thought. This endowed the amphetamine user's speech with a fragmentary quality that made it appear very similar to thought disorder.

The second phase of the transition of amphetamine psychosis into a model schizophrenia stemmed from the work of Burton Angrist and Samuel Gershon of the NYU Medical Center, both of whom conducted clinical research at Bellevue Psychiatric Hospital in New York. In particular, they wanted to find evidence of thought disorder. Angrist and Gershon were extremely well-positioned to be able to study, in depth, the symptomatology of amphetamine psychosis, because they had plenty of material for observation. In 1969 they reported a spike in amphetamine-related admissions to Bellevue Psychiatric Hospital that had begun in 1966 and that "rapidly surpassed in frequency the admissions for LSD, marijuana, and all other drugs with the exception of the opiates."[62] In addition to amphetamine admissions, they also administered amphetamines directly to four experienced research volunteers and monitored their behavior closely.[63] In 1969 Angrist and Gershon also published a description of their observations of sixty amphetamine-related admissions.[64] Of those sixty, they reported on one patient, a young man, who seemed to show first-rate evidence of thought disorder: "a formal thought disorder was noted during the acute phase."[65] In particular, the patient gave rambling or incoherent responses to various promptings: "He showed a formal thought disorder some examples of which are as follows: On the day of his transfer, speaking of his brother's drug use, he said, 'My brother has been playing with the fires of hell.' On the same day, when asked what 'a stitch in time saves nine' meant, he said, 'Hurry up with that date and don't be late' (laughs) 'make that first stitch right and the rest will follow.'"[66] The following year, they reported a similar episode, which was to be the crucial bit of evidence for thought disorder in amphetamine users. These observations stemmed from research involving the experimental administration of amphetamines to volunteer subjects. One of the four seemed to exhibit signs of thought disorder and at one point launched into an "agitated philosophical diatribe with riddles that made little sense. For example, 'one man goes to school, the other can't. Then the other "cuts out" say, "fuck you, buddy."' This, he explained, meant that there is no brotherhood in the world. Questions the meaning of gold and source of its value."[67] Later, the same subject began referring to himself as a kind of prophet, "writing and talking excitedly."[68] The latter could have been classed as a delusion of grandeur; this would have represented a somewhat novel clinical insight about the symptomatology of amphetamine psychosis, but it would not have broken from the basic clinical portrait. More importantly, in the absence of a verbal questioning—that is, in the absence of engaging the patient in something like a conversation—the evidential value of such texts were, as Bell observed, dubious. Observation alone would not reveal the difference between formal thought disorder proper and the mere "flight of ideas" due to elation. However, without any further argumentation, Angrist and Gershon interpreted the patient's text as an indication of thought disorder and drew the conclusion that amphetamine psychosis is the ideal model of schizophrenia: "These phenomenologic features [auditory hallucinations and thought disorder] give amphetamine psychosis a greater resemblance to naturally occurring schizophrenia than the states induced by other psychotomimetics. . . . This clinical resemblance of amphetamine psychosis to schizophrenia justifies study of its mechanisms of pathogenesis."[69]

Randrup and Munkvad had expanded the symptomatology of amphetamine psychosis to include stereotyped behavior. Angrist and Gershon expanded it further to include formal thought disorder as well. Amphetamine psychosis was starting to look just like schizophrenia again.

"Drugs That Even Scare Hippies": Acidheads and Speed Freaks

The completion of the transformation of amphetamine psychosis from a disturbing, but uncommon, sequela of amphetamine use, to a biochemical model of schizophrenia, awaited one last step. LSD had to be displaced decisively as the reigning model of schizophrenia in the biochemical researcher's arsenal. There were several reasons that LSD probably lost its allure as a model schizophrenia,[70] but one of those came from an unlikely source. The ideological architects of the American countercultural revolution, such as Timothy Leary, Allen Ginsberg, Gary Snyder, Richard Alpert (Ram Dass), and Michael McClure, worked tirelessly to engineer the public perception of LSD, the kind of experience it induced, and the kind of person who used it.

They did so, at least in part, by contrasting the kind of person who used LSD with the kind of person who used speed: the acidhead versus the speed freak. The use of LSD became, in their teaching, synonymous with a philosophical or even spiritual quest for wholeness and an escape from the alienation produced by a militaristic and competitive society. Speed, in contrast, exacerbated the values of competition and militarism. The speed freak was unpredictable, paranoid, and violent. The ideological clash of the twentieth century, it turned out, was not only between capitalism and communism, or between pacifism and militarism, but between acid and speed.[71] Allen Ginsburg summarized a theme that ran throughout the countercultural literature: "Speed is anti-social, paranoid making. All the nice gentle dope fiends are getting screwed up by the real horror monster Frankenstein Speedfreaks who are going around stealing and bad mouthing everybody."[72]

What prompted the need for these fine discriminations among recreational drug users? The problem was that speed users were beginning to subvert, from within, the countercultural revolution that LSD was poised to bring about. In the eyes of its leaders, speed was undermining the values they sought to promote. As the historian Philip Jenkins put it, "At the end of the 60s, methamphetamine already had the distinction of being one of the very few drugs stigmatized within a drug culture of seemingly limitless tolerance."[73] To exemplify the campaign being waged on behalf of LSD and against speed, I will focus on the events leading up to, and following, the 1967 Summer of Love in the Haight-Ashbury district of San Francisco. I will also focus on the perspective of the leader and founder of the Haight-Ashbury Free Clinic, David Smith. The clinic not only provided free medical assistance for young people affected by drug-related illnesses but also gathered information about patterns of drug use in the area.

By the early 1960s, the recreational use of amphetamines was in full swing in both the United Kingdom and the United States.[74] These were primarily ingested orally, in tablet form or by consuming the contents of amphetamine-based inhalers. However, by the early 1960s there was also a segment of amphetamine users that began administering it intravenously (a form sometimes known as "splash.") According to one sociologist at the time, heroin users began shooting speed intravenously in the United States in the late 1950s "at a time when the heroin market was precarious," and it had become common by the mid-1960s.[75] But speed came to take on a new set of meanings during the Summer of Love.

The first Human Be-In, a gathering of about thirty thousand "hippies" from the San Francisco Bay area, took place at Golden Gate Park's Polo Field on January 14, 1967. It defined not only the counterculture of the late 1960s but enshrined LSD as a kind of sacrament of the movement: this was the occasion on which Timothy Leary, high on LSD, coined the phrase, "tune in, turn on, drop out" shortly before spending the afternoon playing paddy-cake with a little girl.[76] Within weeks, rumors began to circulate that the summer of 1967 would see about one hundred thousand teenagers from around the country descend onto the Haight-Ashbury district of San Francisco.

In response to the impending invasion, pharmacologist David Smith and concerned colleagues at the University of California Medical School began organizing a free clinic that would provide much needed medical assistance, both for drug overdoses as well as problems associated with unhygienic living conditions.[77] In the vision of its founder, the clinic would emphasize "medical treatment free from red tape, free from value judgements, free from eligibility requirements, emotional hassles, frozen medical protocol, moralizing, and mystification."[78] The clinic also provided a crucial alternative to the public hospitals, which likely would have treated drug-related admissions as a criminal problem and thereby deterred young people from seeking help.

The Haight-Ashbury Free Clinic also played a pivotal role in collecting information about drug use in the area. In 1968 David Smith and Dr. Frederick Meyers of the University of California Medical School received a large grant from the National Institutes of Mental Health to study amphetamine use in Haight-Ashbury. This led to the formation of the Amphetamine Research Project, housed in the clinic and led by criminologist Roger Smith, who became known to locals as the "Friendly Fed." The clinic documented the transitions that were taking place within the drug culture of the Haight-Ashbury district.

From 1967 to 1969, the clinic produced several reports on patterns of drug use in the district. The most noticeable trend consisted of a sharp transition, from 1967 to 1969, from the use of LSD and marijuana to the use of amphetamines. According to one of David Smith's reports, the intravenous use of amphetamines was "practically unknown in the Haight" prior to the Summer of 1967; the fall brought "an increasing number of adverse reactions to intravenous amphetamine" at the clinic, and "more moderate users of marijuana and LSD began to dwindle in number as they left the Haight when the two groups began to conflict."[79]

The transition from LSD to speed was not an isolated event, but occurred in other countercultural hubs in the United States. A similar pattern emerged in New York's East Village around the same time period. As noted above, from 1966 to 1968, Burton Angrist and Samuel Gershon documented a sharp increase in amphetamine-related admissions to Bellevue Psychiatric Hospital, one that "rapidly surpassed in frequency the admissions for LSD, marijuana, and all other drugs with the exception of the opiates."[80] The popular press also picked up and broadcast the growing use of amphetamines and labeled it as a "drug that even scares hippies."[81]

Clearly, it was time for some fine ideological discriminations to be made among those who self-identified as recreational drug users. By 1967, a number of artists, musicians, journalists, sociologists, and criminologists had begun to distinguish the characteristics of amphetamine users and LSD users—the speed freaks and the acidheads. Ideologues such as Leary and Ginsberg attempted to convey a simple message: the use of LSD (and other psychedelics such as mescaline and peyote) could become incorporated into a coherent philosophical worldview that emphasized the values of communal living and pacifism over the "mainstream" cultural values of competition and militarism. The speed freaks were another story entirely. The transient and volatile "communities" formed by speed freaks had none of these qualities—no guiding philosophy, no social mandate, and no template for communal organization. Any such speed freak communities would rapidly degenerate in a cycle of paranoia-fueled violence culminating in a hospitalization or criminal investigation.[82]

Like Leary and Ginsberg, David Smith, the founder of the clinic, articulated what he understood to be the chief differences between LSD and speed. Smith (who occasionally used LSD himself) framed the contrast, tellingly, in terms of a clash of two different worldviews, or philosophies. He described the exodus of the LSD user from Haight-Ashbury in the following terms:

> Because of the violent characteristics of the [speed freak], the hippies have moved to the country where they can establish small rural communes which tolerate and reinforce their belief systems. Urban areas such as the Haight-Ashbury can never be a permanent haven for the acid subculture, because in the conflict of *speed freaks* vs. *acid heads*, *speed* always drives out *acid*—as in the broader society the philosophy of violence dominates the higher aspirations of nonviolence, peace and love.[83]

One particular metaphor that seemed to summarize the differences was that the madness of amphetamines reflected, and mimicked, the madness of American culture itself. A lucid statement of this mimicry between speed and America was made by the New York sociologist Seymour Fiddle: "The amphetamine abuser is a burlesque of certain elements of contemporary civilization. First, his hyperactivity is a caricature of urban hustle and bustle. . . . The amphetamine user is an overreacher. One of the models of our day is that of man breaking through boundaries. . . . This underlying purpose of the drug dependent gives us a mock image of the American as a passive consumer searching for stimulation."[84]

As one young user put it, amphetamines mimic the manic velocity of American culture itself.[85] The same theme was summarized by Frank Zappa, in one of many public service announcements promoted by the Do It Now Foundation, an antispeed organization formed in 1968 that solicited the participation of a large number of artists: "I would like to suggest that you do not use speed. And here's why: It's going to mess up your heart, mess up your liver, your kidneys, rot out your mind. In general, this drug will make you just like your mother and father."[86] Just like your mother and father: a generic stand-in for the "old America," everything that the counterculture wished to escape.

Yet madness always wins. In the contest between speed and acid, speed emerged victorious. Though speed won, the acidheads left their distinctive imprint on the state of discourse about LSD and amphetamines in the popular imagination. The madness of speed, and the (relative) sanity of LSD, had been amply demonstrated by a massive social experiment the likes of which seem now unprecedented in psychiatric history. By the 1970s, key schizophrenia researchers freely had borrowed these new meanings in their attempt to demonstrate that amphetamine psychosis, rather than LSD intoxication, was the correct model of schizophrenia itself.

The Dopamine Hypothesis:
Closing the Gap between Speed and Madness

The American architects of the dopamine hypothesis freely borrowed and modulated the new meanings that LSD and amphetamines assumed in the wake of the Summer of Love. They used those meanings successfully to argue that speed, not LSD, is the real model of madness.[87] Since speed was known to produce its effects by amplifying the dopamine system, then schizophrenia, too, must arise from an overproduction of dopamine as well. This was one of the crucial pieces of evidence for the dopamine hypothesis of schizophrenia. The other crucial piece of evidence, as noted above, was the apparent effectiveness of dopamine-blocking agents, such as chlorpromazine, in alleviating schizophrenic symptoms.

The dopamine hypothesis, in turn, was to become the leading biochemical theory of schizophrenia during the 1970s and 1980s, as well as a kind of poster child for the idea that mental disorders, generally, could be successfully "reduced" to neurotransmitter abnormalities. In particular, I will focus on the work of Solomon Snyder of Johns Hopkins Medicine in Baltimore, as he was the author of one of the two canonical papers on the dopamine hypothesis, though I will also describe the way that Burton Angrist and Samuel Gershon borrowed and modified these meanings.

Snyder's own interest in schizophrenia seems to have been prompted by the work of Angrist and Gershon. His primary preoccupation had been, like the Scandinavians Randrup and Munkvad, with amphetamine-induced stereotypy in animals. Prior to 1971, it did not seem to have occurred to Snyder that animal stereotypy would have any special relation with schizophrenia—reasonably enough, as the relation had always represented a somewhat stretched analogy. Instead, Snyder utilized amphetamine-induced stereotypy as a model for Tourette's syndrome.[88] At some point after coming into contact with the work of Angrist and Gershon, however, he submitted an article to *Archives of General Psychiatry*, the first line of which announces that, "amphetamine psychosis appears to be a fruitful experimental model of paranoid schizophrenia or paranoid state."[89] Angrist and Gershon's work rescued Snyder's humble research from oblivion and endowed his work on stereotypy with major research significance.

Before he could defend the dopamine hypothesis, he had to get around two obstacles: the fact that LSD intoxication was still considered a model schizophrenia, and the fact that amphetamine psychosis did not seem to elicit thought disorder, a defining feature of schizophrenia. Regarding LSD, Snyder articulated a set of important disanalogies between LSD and schizophrenia. The most important of these was that LSD usage did not induce madness, *but merely enhanced normal perception:* "The mental state elicited by psychedelic drugs is one of greatly enhanced perception of oneself and one's environment. Similar states occur during mystical and religious introspection and when an individual is profoundly moved by emotions or external events."[90] Solomon was clearly adopting some of the characterizations of LSD use that had become platitudes in the wake of the counterculture.

Like Snyder, Angrist and Gershon also relied on the contrasts between LSD and speed developed by the counterculture during the late 1960s. They used those contrasts to justify their view that amphetamine psychosis is a better model of schizophrenia than LSD intoxication. As Angrist and Gershon summarized their results on Bellevue admissions, "Because of . . . their sociopathy and their frankly hedonistic reasons for drug use, [the amphetamine users] resemble heroin addicts as a group far more than the philosophically and religiously preoccupied and less sociopathic hallucinogen users."[91]

It is crucial to emphasize the importance of these passages: two of the most important schizophrenia researchers of the early 1970s, and two of the strongest advocates for the idea that amphetamine psychosis mimics schizophrenia, clearly adopted the language of the American counterculture in sketching the differences between the kinds of people who take acid and the kinds of people who take speed. LSD users (and the users of other hallucinogens) are "religious," "mystical," "introspective," and "philosophical," and have a "heightened" sense of awareness of self and other. Amphetamine users are "sociopathic" and "hedonistic," mere thrill seekers incapable of authentic relationships.

One final problem remained. This was the problem of thought disorder. To all appearances, amphetamine psychosis, like LSD intoxication, took place in a lucid frame of mind. One of the defining symptoms of schizophrenia, disorganization or incongruence of thought, was absent. To remedy this difficulty, as described above, Angrist and Gershon attempted to demonstrate that amphetamine psychosis does, in fact, possess the power to induce thought disorder, even if it is extremely uncommon. Snyder, however, took a different route to explaining away this disanalogy. Snyder never attempted to demonstrate a relation between amphetamine psychosis and thought disorder. As he put it, "a key aspect of amphetamine psychosis is that it occurs in a setting of clear consciousness and correct orientation."[92]

How, then, did Snyder avoid the apparent implication that amphetamine psychosis was a bad model of schizophrenia? He reasoned that amphetamines do elicit a "pure" schizophrenia, but some of their incidental chemical properties bar the expression of certain symptoms. They produce a true, but hidden, schizophrenia: "It is conceivable that amphetamines possess a "pure" schizophrenia-mimicking action, but that some other effect of the drug transforms the clinical picture into a predominantly paranoid one."[93]

Snyder bolstered this possibility with imaginative deliberations on the inner unity of schizophrenia itself. Paranoid-type schizophrenia, in essence, is no different from disorganized-type schizophrenia (that is, the type associated with thought disorder). The only difference is that paranoid schizophrenics have found a means to consolidate the bizarre and incoherent medley of thoughts, perceptions, and emotions into a rigid system of delusions that endows them with order and significance.[94] Presumably, the disorganized-type schizophrenic is one who has not figured out how to accomplish this feat; all that remains is pure psychic chaos.

Snyder suggested that the dual psychiatric properties of amphetamines—the thought disorder-making component and the paranoid-making component—may be related to its actions on two separate transmitter systems, the dopamine system and the norepinephrine system, respectively. In other words, if amphetamines merely agonized the dopamine system, they would produce "pure" madness in the form of thought disorder. However, amphetamines had the incidental property that they also worked on the norepinephrine system, which elicited the intellectual infrastructure that transforms the incoherence of madness into a meaningful system of delusions. In other words, the norepinephrine agonism "forces the patient to strive for an intellectual framework in which to focus all the strange feelings that are coming over him as the psychosis develops."[95] Amphetamines, then, generated both madness and reason; delusions represent a compromise, or a perverse victory, of reason over madness.

In short, the mimicry thesis—the view that amphetamine psychosis replicates schizophrenia without flaw and thus should be used as a biochemical model of schizophrenia—rested almost entirely upon Snyder's creative imagination and a handful of notes feverishly scribbled by speed freaks. In 1976, partly on the basis of this mimicry thesis, the dopamine hypothesis of schizophrenia was unveiled to the world.

Beyond the Dopamine Hypothesis

Angrist and Gershon's team and Synder's team developed a kind of positive feedback loop, supporting each other's research on the relation between schizophrenia and dopamine.[96] By 1976, with the publication of two influential reviews, the dopamine hypothesis entered mainstream American psychiatry.[97] The fact that Snyder labeled the view a "hypothesis," rather than a "theory" only made the view more seductive, even irresistible, in the eyes of psychiatric researchers. "By definition," announced Snyder, "the dopamine hypothesis is supported by no direct evidence."[98] Though there was ample *indirect* evidence for the hypothesis, American psychiatrists responded to this provocative claim as a kind of taunt.

By the late 1970s, researchers were engaged in a wholesale scramble to find direct biochemical evidence of dopamine abnormalities in schizophrenic patients.[99] Researchers carried out a host of sophisticated research studies involving collection and analysis of urine, cerebrospinal fluid, and blood in order to find heightened metabolites of dopamine.[100] They also carried out postmortem brain studies of schizophrenic patients in search of elevated dopamine receptor concentrations. Although some laboratories were successful in finding elevated dopamine receptor concentrations, these early studies were plagued by the problem of contaminated evidence, as many of the patients had also been taking antipsychotic medications for years.[101] The possibility that elevated dopamine receptor concentrations represented a compensatory response to antipsychotic dopamine blockade could not be ruled out. In the 1980s and afterward, these studies were supplanted by brain imaging studies of schizophrenic patients. Though the biochemical "smoking gun" was never discovered, after a while nobody seemed to care too much. The dopamine hypothesis had become entrenched in the culture of American psychiatry.[102]

The apparent success of the dopamine hypothesis not only triggered a scramble for direct biochemical evidence; it also emboldened biologically and behaviorally oriented psychiatrists in the American Psychiatric Association (APA) in their aggressive campaign to wrest control of American psychiatry from the hands of psychodynamic psychiatrists. Thus, the dopamine hypothesis, as a rhetorical technique, played a particularly strategic role in the years leading up to the 1980 publication of the third edition of the *Diagnostic and Statistical Manual of Mental Disorders* (DSM), which was the first of the DSMs to practically eliminate the old-fashioned psychodynamic terminology. The manuals did so by using theories such as the dopamine hypothesis as leverage for promoting the so-called medical model of psychiatry, according to which mental disorders result from inner or biological "dysfunctions," and thus are analogous to nonpsychiatric medical disorders.[103]

Today, support for the dopamine hypothesis has waned significantly, for two reasons.[104] First, a host of "atypical" antipsychotic drugs developed in the 1990s appeared to achieve their therapeutic effects by engaging a wider profile of neurotransmitters than dopamine. Thus, while dopamine abnormalities were likely implicated in schizophrenia, researchers began to think that they characterized only one small part of a vast puzzle. Second, some evidence suggested that dopamine abnormalities in schizophrenia actually constituted a secondary by-product of other, more "primary," dysfunctions. For example, some researchers actively promoted the view that *glutamate* transmitter abnormalities occupied the privileged role of "primary dysfunction" of schizophrenia. A small number of researchers even advanced the thesis that dopamine abnormalities in schizophrenia actually have the function of *compensating* for hypothesized glutamate abnormalities.[105] If so, this would undermine the foundations of the dopamine hypothesis entirely because it would suggest that, far from being "dysfunctional," dopamine abnormalities have some kind of functional or adaptive significance, much like getting a fever after a bacterial infection.

Apart from the dopamine hypothesis, the analysis undertaken here could be used as a potential "model" or template for writing the history of research into schizophrenia and perhaps other major mental disorders. The above analysis supports the following generalization. Any theory of schizophrenia (e.g., the biochemical or psychological mechanisms at issue) starts with a conception of what the "essence" of the thing is. That is, any attempt to discover a single mechanism underlying the diverse symptomatology of schizophrenia seems nearly hopeless. Therefore, the schizophrenia researcher, in order to make progress, must conceptualize certain symptoms of schizophrenia as "constitutive," "primary," or "essential." Other symptoms must be conceptualized as "derivative," "contingent," or "secondary." Are the so-called positive symptoms of hallucinations and delusions somehow primary, and thought disorder a secondary effect? Is thought disorder the primary effect, and delusions a way of coping with the psychological chaos it brings? And how do the avolition and apathy associated with catatonic-type schizophrenia fit in?

The philosophers of science William Bechtel and Robert Richardson called this sort of work—that is, characterizing the phenomenon at hand as a prelude to biochemical investigation—as "reconstituting the phenomenon."[106] That is, once the researcher or research community has "constituted" or "reconstituted" the phenomenon, then that researcher or research team can begin the "proper" scientific task of building a model to explain these "primary" or "essential" phenomena or describing a mechanism that would generate them. The "secondary" or "contingent" symptoms can be, at least at the outset, ignored. Focusing on certain symptoms and ignoring others forms a strategic handle for "getting a grip" on schizophrenia itself.

But this first task, this reconstituting the phenomenon, is itself, while guided by scientific results, largely driven by imagination and guesswork. It is a "pre-scientific" or, if one prefers, an "extra-scientific" task (assuming that one can distinguish sharply between those aspects of scientific work that are "properly" scientific, such as building and testing models, and those that are not, such as reconceptualizing the phenomenon or publicizing the results). It represents an exercise of the scientific imagination, such as Snyder's deliberations on the nature of schizophrenia. Hence, looking at schizophrenia research at a given moment in time—the models and mechanisms that are considered the most promising avenues of research—is going to reveal what we take schizophrenia to be, at that time. This, in part, will be determined by what we *need* schizophrenia to be at that time: it gives us a window on the way that madness is being collectively imagined.

Notes

1. Philip Henry Connell, *Amphetamine Psychosis* (London: Chapman and Hall, 1958).

2. Seymour S. Kety, "Biochemical Theories of Schizophrenia," *Science* 129, nos. 3362–63 (1959): 1528–32, 1590–96, 598. See also Eliot Slater, "Review of Amphetamine Psychosis by P. H. Connell," *British Medical Journal* 1 no. 5120 (1959): 488.

3. Solomon H. Snyder, "Catecholamines in the Brain as Mediators of Amphetamine Psychosis," *Archives of General Psychiatry* 27 (1972): 169.

4. D. S. Bell, "Comparison of Amphetamine Psychosis and Schizophrenia," *British Journal of Psychiatry* 111 (1965): 701–7; R. Gardner, "Psychotomimetic Effects of Central Stimulants," in *Abuse of Central Stimulants*, ed. Folke Sjöqvist and Magnus Tottie (New York: Raven Press, 1969), 113–39.

5. Eugen Bleuler, *Dementia Praecox or the Group of Schizophrenias* (New York: International Universities Press, 1950).

6. American Psychiatric Assocation, *DSM-5* (Washington, DC: American Psychiatric Publishing, 2013), 88.

7. Solomon H. Snyder, "Catecholamines in the Brain as Mediators of Amphetamine Psychosis," *Archives of General Psychiatry* 27 (1972): 169–79; Burton M. Angrist and Samuel Gershon, "The Phenomenology of Experimentally Induced Amphetamine Psychosis: Preliminary Observations," *Biological Psychiatry* 2 (1970): 95–107.

8. Solomon H. Snyder, "The Dopamine Hypothesis of Schizophrenia: Focus on the Dopamine Receptor," *American Journal of Psychiatry* 133, no. 2 (1976): 197–202; Herbert Y. Meltzer and Stephen M. Stahl, "The Dopamine Hypothesis of Schizophrenia," *Schizophrenia Bulletin* 2 (1976): 19–76.

9. A. Randrup and I. Munkvad, "Stereotyped Activites Produced by Amphetamine in Several Animal Species and Man," *Psychopharmacologia* 11 (1967): 300–10. In humans, stereotypy has been associated with some types of autism spectrum

disorders, such as rocking, tapping, spinning, and hand flapping, and it is also associated with catatonic-type schizophrenia, which may involve holding bizarre postures for long periods of time. See American Psychiatric Assocation, *DSM-5* (Washington, DC: American Psychiatric Publishing, 2013), 88.

10. A. Randrup and I. Munkvad, "Evidence Indicating an Association between Schizophrenia and Dopaminergic Hyperactivity in the Brain," *Orthomolecular Psychiatry* 1 (1972): 2–3.

11. Burton M. Angrist and Samuel Gershon, "The Phenomenology of Experimentally Induced Amphetamine Psychosis: Preliminary Observations" *Biological Psychiatry* 2 (1970): 97.

12. Albert Rosenfeld, "Drugs That Even Scare Hippies" *Life*, October 27 1967, 81–82; Fred Davis and Laura Munoz, "Heads and Freaks: Patterns and Meanings of Drug Use Among Hippies" *Journal of Health and Social Behavior* 9 (1968): 156–64; David Smith, "Speed Freaks vs. Acid Heads: Conflict between Drug Subcultures," *Clinical Pediatrics* 8 (1969): 185–92; Roger C. Smith, "The World of the Haight-Ashbury Speed Freak," *Journal of Psychoactive Drugs* 2 (1969): 77–83.

13. Erica Dyck, *Psychedelic Psychiatry: LSD from Clinic to Campus* (Baltimore: Johns Hopkins University Press, 2008); Peter Conners, *White Hand Society: The Psychedelic Partnership of Timothy Leary and Allen Ginsberg* (San Francisco: City Lights Bookstore, 2010); David Healy, *The Creation of Psychopharmacology* (Cambridge, MA: Harvard University Press, 2002).

14. Burton M. Angrist and Samuel Gershon, "Amphetamine Abuse in New York City—1966 to 1968," *Seminars in Psychiatry* 1, no. 2 (1969): 205.

15. Solomon H. Snyder, Shailesh P. Banerjee, Henry I. Yamamura, and David Greenberg, "Drugs, Neurotransmitters, and Schizophrenia," *Science* 184, no. 4143 (1974): 1252.

16. Solomon H. Snyder, "The Dopamine Hypothesis of Schizophrenia: Focus on the Dopamine Receptor," *American Journal of Psychiatry* 133, no. 2 (1976): 197–202; Herbert Y. Meltzer and Stephen M. Stahl, "The Dopamine Hypothesis of Schizophrenia," *Schizophrenia Bulletin* 2 (1976): 19–76.

17. Erica Dyck, *Psychedelic Psychiatry: LSD from Clinic to Campus* (Baltimore: Johns Hopkins University Press, 2008).

18. Nicholas Rasmussen, *On Speed: The Many Lives of Amphetamines* (New York: New York University Press, 2008).

19. Healy, *Creation of Psychopharmacology*.

20. J. M. van Rossum, "The Significance of Dopamine-Receptor Blockade for the Mechanism of Action of Neuroleptic Drugs" *Archives Internationales de Pharmacodynamie et de Therapie* 160 (1966): 492–94.

21. Snyder, Banerjee, Yamamura, and Greenberg, "Drugs, Neurotransmitters, and Schizophrenia," 1252.

22. Solomon H. Snyder, "The Dopamine Hypothesis of Schizophrenia: Focus on the Dopamine Receptor," *American Journal of Psychiatry* 133, no. 2 (1976): 197–202; Herbert Y. Meltzer and Stephen M. Stahl, "The Dopamine Hypothesis of Schizophrenia," *Schizophrenia Bulletin* 2 (1976): 19–76.

23. Connell, *Amphetamine Psychosis*.

24. Ibid., 65.

25. Rasmussen, *On Speed*.

26. Connell, *Amphetamine Psychosis*, 75.

27. Ibid., 58.

28. Angrist and Gershon, "Amphetamine Abuse," 200.

29. David M. Young and William Scoville, "Paranoid Psychosis in Narcolepsy and the Possible Danger of Benzadrine Treatment," *Medical Clinics of North America* 22 (1938): 637–42.

30. Connell, *Amphetamine Psychosis*. Chapter 1 comprises a literature review. The "latent trait" hypothesis is discussed on p. 60.

31. Rasmussen, *On Speed*, 48.

32. Ibid.

33. Connell, *Amphetamine Psychosis*, 64.

34. Ibid., 63.

35. Edward Marley, "Response to Some Stimulant and Depressant Drugs of the Central Nervous System," *British Journal of Psychiatry* 106 (1960): 7692; Bell, "Comparison of Amphetamine Psychosis and Schizophrenia."

36. Kety, "Biochemical Theories of Schizophrenia," 1528–32, 1590–96; Slater, "Review of Amphetamine Psychosis," 488.

37. Slater, "Review of Amphetamine Psychosis, 488.

38. Marley, "Response to Some Stimulant and Depressant Drugs," 76–92; W. B. McConnell, "Amphetamine Substances in Mental Illnesses in Northern Ireland," *British Journal of Psychiatry* 109 (1963): 218–24.

39. Marley, "Response to Some Stimulant and Depressant Drugs," 82.

40. McConnell, "Amphetamine Substances," 219.

41. Bell, "Comparison of Amphetamine Psychosis and Schizophrenia," 705.

42. Ibid.

43. Ibid.

44. Ibid., 704.

45. Gardner, "Psychotomimetic Effects," 113.

46. See J. D. Griffith, J. H. Cavanaugh, J. Held, J. A. Oates, "Experimental Psychosis Induced by the Administration of D-amphetamine," in *Amphetamines and Related Compounds*, ed. E. Costa and S Garattini, 902 (New York: Raven Press, 1970), which also describes earlier research involving the first experimental administration of amphetamines to human subjects.

47. L. E. Jönsson and L. M. Gunne, "Clinical Studies of Amphetamine Psychosis," in *Amphetamines and Related Compounds* ed. E. Costa and S Garattini, 929–36 (New York: Raven Press, 1970).

48. Snyder, "Catecholamines in the Brain," 170.

49. Dyck, *Psychedelic Psychiatry*.

50. Erich Guttmann, "Artificial Psychoses Produced by Mescaline," *British Journal of Psychiatry* 82 (1936): 220.

51. W. Mayer-Gross, "Experimental Psychoses and Other Mental Abnormalities Produced by Drugs," *British Medical Journal* 2 no. 4727 (1951): 321.

52. Cyril Greenland, "At the Crichton Royal with William Mayer-Gross," *History of Psychiatry* 13 (2002): 469. Both Guttmann and Mayer-Gross note that the ingestion of drugs such as hashish, peyote, or opium specifically for the purpose of gaining theoretical insight about the nature of the mind goes back at least to Emil Kraepelin.

53. Dyck, *Psychedelic Psychiatry*.

54. Kety, "Biochemical Theories of Schizophrenia," 1528–32, 1590–96, 1598, 1593.

55. Dilworth W. Woolley and E. Shaw, "A Biochemical and Pharmacological Suggestion about Certain Mental Disorders *Science* 119, no. 3096 (1954): 577–78.

56. J. H. Gaddum, "Drugs Antagonistic to 5-Hydroxytryptamine," in *Ciba Foundation Symposium on Hypertension: Humoral and Neurogenic Factors*, ed. G. E. W. Wolstenholme and M. P. Cameron, 75–77, 85–90 (Boston: Little, Brown, and Co, 1954).

57. Randrup and Munkvad, "Stereotyped Activities," 307.

58. Ibid.

59. G. Rylander, "Addiction to Preludin Intravenously Injected," *Proceedings of the Fourth World Congress of Psychiatry* (Amsterdam: Excerpta Medica Foundation, 1966); G. Rylander, "Cilnical and Medico-Criminological Aspects of Addiction to Central Stimulating Drugs," in *Abuse of Central Stimulants: Symposium Arranged by the Swedish Committee on International Health Relations, Stockholm, November 25–27, 1968*, ed. F. Sjöqvist and M. Tottie, 251–73 (New York: Raven Press, 1969).

60. Emphasis added. A. Randrup and I. Munkvad, "Biochemical, Anatomical and Psychological Investigations of Stereotyped Behavior Induced by Amephtamines," in *Amphetamines and Related Compounds*, ed. E. Costa and S. Garattini (New York: Raven Press, 1970): 695–713.

61. Randrup and Munkvad, "Evidence Indicating an Association," 2–3.

62. Burton M. Angrist and Samuel Gershon, "Amphetamine Abuse in New York City—1966 to 1968." *Seminars in Psychiatry* 1, no. 2 (1969): 196.

63. Angrist and Gershon, "Phenomenology of Experimentally Induced Amphetamine Psychosis," 97.

64. Burton M. Angrist and Samuel Gershon, "Amphetamine Induced Schizophreniform Psychosis," in *Schizophrenia: Current Concepts and Research*, ed. D. V. Siva Sankar, 508–24 (Hicksville, NY: PJD Publications, 1969).

65. Ibid., 515.

66. Ibid.

67. Angrist and Gershon, "Phenomenology of Experimentally Induced Amphetamine Psychosis," 102.

68. Ibid.

69. Ibid., 106.

70. Healy, *Creation of Psychopharmacology*, 193.

71. E.g., Rosenfeld, "Drugs that Even Scare Hippies," 81–82; Davis and Munoz, "Heads and Freaks: Patterns and Meanings of Drug Use among Hippies," 154–64; David Smith, "Speed Freaks vs. Acid Heads: Conflict between Drug Subcultures, *Clinical Pediatrics* 8 (1969): 185–92; R. C. Smith, "The World of the Haight-Ashbury Speed Freak," *Journal of Psychoactive Drugs* (1969): 77–83.

72. Cited in Rasmussen, *On Speed*, 183.

73. Cited in Frank Owen, *No Speed Limit: The Highs and Lows of Meth* (New York: St. Martin's Griffin, 2007), 104.

74. Rasmussen, *On Speed*, 171–81.

75. J. W. Rawlin, "Street Level Abuse of Amphetamines," in *Amphetamine Abuse*, ed. J. R. Russo, 58 (Springfield, IL: Charles C Thomas, 1968).

76. Conners, *White Hand Society*, 204.

77. Clark S. Sturges, *Dr. Dave: A Profile of David E. Smith, M.D., Founder of the Haight Ashbury Free Clinics* (Walnut Creek, CA: Devil Mountain, 1993), 39.

78. Ibid., ix.

79. Fred E. Shick, David E. Smith, and Frederick H. Meyers, "Patterns of Drug Use in the Haight-Ashbury Neighborhood," *Clinical Toxicology* 3, no. 1 (1970): 43–44. See also see David Smith and Charles M. Fischer, "An Analysis of 310 Cases of Acude High-Dose Methamphetamine Toxicity in Haight Ashbury" *Clinical Toxicology* 3, no. 1 (1970): 117–24.

80. Angrist and Gershon, "Amphetamine Abuse in New York City," 196.

81. Rosenfeld, "Drugs that Even Scare Hippies," 81–82.

82. Ibid.; Davis and Munoz, "Heads and Freaks," 156–64; Smith, "Speed Freaks vs. Acid Heads," 185–92; Roger C. Smith, "The World of the Haight-Ashbury Speed Freak," 77–83.

83. D. Smith, "Speed Freaks vs. Acid Heads," 188.

84. S. Fiddle, "Circles Beyond the Circumference: Some Hunches about Amphetamine Abuse," in *Amphetamine Abuse*, ed. J. R. Russo, 81–85 (Springfield, IL: Charles C Thomas, 1968).

85. Quoted in Lester Grinspoon and Peter Hedblom, *The Speed Culture: Amphetamine Use and Abuse in America* (Cambridge, MA: Harvard University Press 1975), 3.

86. See audio file of Frank Zappa, DoItNow Foundation, accessed April 18, 2012, http://www.doitnow.org/psasounds/zappamomdad11.aiff.

87. Snyder, "Catecholamines in the Brain," 169–79; Angrist and Gershon, "The Phenomenology of Experimentally Induced Amphetamine Psychosis," 95–107.

88. S. H. Snyder, E. Richelson, H. Weingartner, L. A. Faillace, "Psychotropic Methoxyamphetamines: Structure and Activity in Man," in *Amphetamines and Related Compounds*, ed. E. Costa and S. Garattini, 905–28 (New York: Raven Press, 1970), 922.

89. Snyder, "Catecholamines in the Brain as Mediators," 169. This article, unlike S. H. Snyder, E. Richelson, H. Weingartner, and L. A. Faillace, "Psychotropic Methoxyamphetamines: Structure and Activity in Man," in *Amphetamines and Related Compounds*, ed. E. Costa and S. Garattini (New York: Raven Press, 1970), cites an article by Angrist and Gershon to the same effect.

90. Snyder, Banerjee, Yamamura, and Greenberg, "Drugs, Neurotransmitters, and Schizophrenia," 1252.

91. Angrist and Gershon, "Amphetamine Abuse in New York City," 205.

92. Snyder, "Catecholamines in the Brain, " 170.

93. Snyder, Banerjee, Yamamura, and Greenberg, "Drugs, Neurotransmitters, and Schizophrenia," 1245.

94. Ibid.

95. S. H. Snyder, "Amphetamine Psychosis: A "Model" Schizophrenia Mediated by Catecholamines," *American Journal of Psychiatry* 130, no. 1 (1973): 66.

96. Snyder, "Catecholamines in the Brain," 169; Angrist and Gershon, "Psychiatric Sequelae"; Snyder, Banerjee, Yamamura, and Greenberg, "Drugs, neurotransmitters, and schizophrenia"; B. M. Angrist, H. K. Lee, and S. Gershon, "Antagonism of Amphetamine-Induced Symptomatology by a Neuroleptic," *American Journal of Psychiatry* 131 (1974): 817–19.

97. S. H. Snyder, "The Dopamine Hypothesis of Schizophrenia: Focus on the Dopamine Receptor," *American Journal of Psychiatry* 133, no. 2 (1976): 197–202; Meltzer and Stahl "The Dopamine Hypothesis of Schizophrenia," 1976.

98. Snyder, "Dopamine Hypothesis of Schizophrenia," 197–202.

99. R. Walter Heinrichs, *In Search of Madness: Schizophrenia and Neuroscience* (Oxford: Oxford University Press, 2001).

100. See, e.g., D. P. van Kammen, W. B. van Kammen, L. S. Mann, T. Seppala et al. "Dopamine Metabolism in the Cerebrospinal Fluid of Drug-Free Schizophrenic Patients with and without Cortical Atrophy," *Archives of General Psychiatry* 43 (1986): 978–83 and references therein.

101. For example, see Lars Farde, Frits-Axel Wiesel, Sharon Stone-Elander, Christer Halldin et al., "D2 dopamine receptors in neuroleptic-naive schizophrenic patients: a positron emission tomography study with [11C] raclopride." *Archives of General Psychiatry* 47, no. 3 (1990): 213–19.

102. Kenneth S. Kendler and Kenneth F. Schaffner, "The Dopamine Hypothesis of Schizophrenia: An Historical and Philosophical Analysis," *Philosophy, Psychiatry, and Psychology* 18 (2011): 41–63.

103. See R. L. Spitzer and J. Endicott, "Medical and Mental Disorder: Proposed Definition and Criteria," in *Critical Issues in Psychiatric Diagnosis*, ed. R. L. Spitzer and D. F. Klein, 15–39 (New York: Raven Press, 1978), for a particularly clear articulation of this position.

104. See Anthony A. Grace, "Gating of Information Flow within the Limbic System and the Pathophysiology of Schizophrenia," *Brain Research Reviews* 31 (2000): 330–41; Steven R. Pliszka, *Neuroscience for the Mental Health Clinician* (New York: Guilford, 2003).

105. For example Grace, "Gating of Information Flow," 332.

106. William Bechtel and Richard C. Richardson, *Discovering Complexity: Decomposition and Localization as Strategies in Scientific Research* (Princeton: Princeton University Press, 1993).

Chapter Nine

Salvation through Reductionism

The National Institute of Mental Health and the Return to Biological Psychiatry

BRIAN P. CASEY

It has become our mantra at NIMH that mental disorders can be addressed as disorders of brain circuits.

—Thomas Insel, director, National Institute of Mental Health, 2010

The guideline of the institute, to quote the law, is "to provide support of research on the etiology, diagnosis, treatment, prevention, and control of mental illness and the promotion of mental health." This broad mandate contains no restrictions on approaches or disciplines.

—Article encouraging submissions by anthropologists to the National Institute of Mental Health, 1963

Since its founding in 1949, the National Institute of Mental Health (NIMH) has been a major force in shaping America's understanding of mental illness, ushering the shift back toward a biological perspective. This move was not simply the logical outcome of scientific progress, but rather an admission of failure to meet the nation's growing mental health problems and a hope for salvation through reductionism.[1] To facilitate this shift, NIMH modeled, underwrote, and broadcast the new biological revolution in psychiatry.[2] Fulfilling its mission to disseminate mental health information, starting in the 1950s NIMH disseminated press releases, radio spots, television programs, and most recently websites and podcasts to broadcast the message that mental illnesses are fundamentally physical ailments whose cure depends on scientific medicine.[3] The messages NIMH conveyed about how mental illness should be approached had a dramatic disciplinary de facto effect; such messages helped steer psychiatry away from psychosocial and psychodynamic explanations and toward a neurological picture of the mind and mental disturbances.

At the outset, it is prudent to bear in mind Daniel Breslau's cautionary words: "The dramatic reversal of the relationship between the declining psychodynamic orientation and the ascendant biological and nosological approach is inexplicable with reference only to the rhetoric of science."[4] Although this claim is undoubtedly true, it is the argument of this chapter that rhetorical strategies nevertheless did significantly help advance the cause of biological psychiatry.[5] Ostensibly just reporting the latest research, NIMH's messages increasingly suggested that brain science will solve the problem of mental illness.

As the science studies scholar Adam Hedgecoe has noted, NIMH's near total conversion to biological psychiatry has been partly hidden by "a rhetoric of multi-dimensionality." In his 2001 examination of the NIMH-launched publication *Schizophrenia Bulletin* (1968), Hedgecoe detected a "narrative of enlightened geneticization," language that subtly prioritizes genetic explanations while *appearing* to allow a role for nongenetic factors.[6] This alleged bias is significant in light of the original intent of the *Bulletin* (and of NIMH's schizophrenia center), which was to provide "a forum for the exchange of information and eventual rapprochement between mental health professions who hold diverse points of view."[7] Hedgecoe suggested, to the contrary, that this publication developed into a mouthpiece for the biological revolution. In spite of consistently espousing a multidimensional approach to mental illness, NIMH has exhibited an increasing preference for the biological approach, evident in the rising percentage of monies granted to biological research.[8]

Biological psychiatry lends itself to attractively simple mechanical explanations of complex mental and behavioral phenomena. These seductive notions have raised expectations that mental illness is a phenomenon soon to be understood and amenable to engineering. As this chapter will show, NIMH's choice to increasingly favor the biological over the psychosocial was informed by science but constrained by both internal and external forces. In other words, the re-biologization of psychiatry was as much the result of choice—a contingent occurrence in a particular context—as the logical outcome of scientific advance, but rhetoric made it look otherwise.

The Contemporary Understanding of Mental Illness

In the early twenty-first century, both the mainstream of the psychiatric profession and the majority of the American public believe mental illness is primarily a physical condition.[9] According to a MacArthur General Society Survey conducted at the end of the 1990s, 85 percent of American adults believed schizophrenia is caused by a chemical imbalance in the brain, while only 45 percent believed upbringing might contribute to it. In keeping with this understanding, the survey found that the American public endorsed biochemical treatment of depression and schizophrenia.[10] It was not surprising, then, that the Decade of the Brain, the 1990s NIH-led initiative to increase awareness of the importance of brain research for medicine and mental health, enjoyed near universal support.[11] Or that in April 2013, President Obama announced the launch of the Brain Research through Advancing Innovative Neurotechnologies (BRAIN) initiative to help "uncover the mysteries of brain disorders," including depression.[12]

The recent biological revolution in psychiatry has had profound consequences for the mental health field. By considering mental illness primarily a problem of human physiology, the biological revolution has cemented "the medical model of mental illness." Biologizing mental illness has put the responsibility for treatment in the hands of scientific medical experts and, consequently, has narrowed the endorsed approach to mental illness.[13] In this biological paradigm, genetics and brain imaging promised to become the new methods of diagnosis and psychopharmaceuticals and, in rare cases, brain surgery the new favored treatments.[14] By collapsing psychology into biology, the biological revolution has demoted psychosocial factors to mere contributing influences. The biological revolution has even changed mental health researchers' vocabulary. "Environment" takes on a different meaning in the biological perspective; once referring to interpersonal relations, environment now often refers more narrowly to physiological milieu.[15]

The Shift in Mental Health Perspective

The current conception of mental illness reflects a paradigm shift in psychiatric opinion that occurred during the second half of the twentieth century. This shift, which began accelerating in the mid-1970s, replaced psychodynamic explanations and approaches—attention to psychological processes such as unconscious conflicts and defense mechanisms—with biological models and treatments. The new mindset was a return to seeing psychiatry as a branch of neurology.[16] Historians have identified several indicators of this revolution.

Concerning the psychiatric profession, the biological revolution was evident in the fact that in the twenty years following World War II, almost all chairs in psychiatry departments, heads of psychiatric hospitals (including VA hospitals), and heads of the American Psychiatric Association were analysts or psychoanalytically inclined.[17] By the 1970s, few were analysts.[18] The shift was apparent, too, in the professional literature. By the 1990s, dozens of specialty psychiatric journals focused on biological psychiatry.[19]

The revolution was apparent in psychiatric definitions. The first Diagnostic and Statistical Manual (DSM) of the American Psychiatric Association, appearing in 1952, listed schizophrenia as "schizophrenic reaction," a collection of "disorders of psychogenic origin or without clearly defined physical cause or structural change in the brain."[20] At midcentury the analytic description of schizophrenia had been the absence of "significant ego strength."[21] In stark contrast, the DSM IV-TR (2000) described schizophrenia as "a neurodevelopmental disorder characterized by defective neuronal migration."[22]

As mentioned above, the revolution changed psychiatric practice. When NIMH began its work, the certifying body for psychiatry, the American Board of Psychiatry and Neurology, recommended, "psychodynamic psychiatry be the standard of practice, and basis for board certification."[23] Contrarily, a few decades later, Chestnut Lodge, a premier analytic asylum, was very publically sued by a patient denied antidepressant medication.[24] Although the shift toward biology did not entirely eliminate consideration of the psychological or social, it effectively relegated these approaches to a secondary role, one supplementary to physical interventions.[25]

The shift in psychiatry's perspective is reflected in NIMH's own history. NIMH was once a prime supporter of the psychodynamic approach. Through its training branch (pruned off during a reorganization) NIMH had been a major supporter of talk therapies, providing funds for hires and students at institutes and universities throughout America. In fact, NIMH's training division has been credited with making possible the post–World War II rise of psychoanalysis. The largest single recipient of NIMH training funds had been the Menninger Foundation, a flagship psychoanalytic institution.[26]

The research carried out at NIMH was not always premised on a biological underpinning to mental illness. In the years before NIMH's reorganization and reorientation, several NIMH researchers hunted for environmental causes of psychoses. Some of these investigators concluded that dysfunctional family dynamics might account for schizophrenia.[27] These investigators thought they found in their study of discordant twins an important psychosocial clue to the etiology of schizophrenia: twin members with schizophrenia tended to be underweight versus their normal twin, engendering, these researchers speculated, pathogenic fear-based attention on the part of parents.[28] Again, NIMH had supported studies of various sociological aspects of mental illness, most notably the relation between class and mental health and between hierarchies in therapeutic institutions and patient outcomes.[29]

By the 1980s, the biological perspective seemed to dominate NIMH. During the Chestnut Lodge case, the chief of psychopharmacology at NIMH, William Potter, tellingly wondered whether the defendants "ben[t] over backward to see something as psychodynamic that may be physiological."[30] Samuel Keith of NIMH's Schizophrenia Research Branch spoke during that decade of "the grip of psychoanalytic theories of mental illnesses."[31] In the 1990s, NIMH's *Schizophrenia Bulletin* advised against psychodynamic treatment for schizophrenics and almost warned practitioners that such treatment could actually be harmful.[32]

NIMH's Major Contributions to Biological Psychiatry

Both through its intramural and later through its expanding extramural program, NIMH bolstered all five pillars of the biological revolution: drugs, genetics, nosology, brain imaging, and informatics. The research wing of NIMH was in itself an advertisement for biological psychiatry; from the very start, its intramural structure exemplified the basic science model of mental health research. Envisioning NIMH as a premier "brain and behavior" research institute, founding director Robert Felix had the institute's first scientific director establish research sections focused, not on specific illnesses, but rather on neurophysiology, neurochemistry, and pharmacological chemistry.[33]

Although the accepted story of the shift in psychiatry begins in France in the early 1950s with the discovery of the antipsychotic Thorazine, America's NIMH was instrumental in validating and advertising the new pharmacopeia.[34] In the 1960s, its Early Clinical Drug Evaluation Unit program orchestrated the field-testing of nearly two hundred drugs, confirming the safety and efficacy of the tranquilizer phenothiazine for the treatment of acute schizophrenia.[35] NIMH broke ground in the fight against another major class of mental illness, namely manic depression. Dr. William Bunney, acting chief of NIMH's section Psychosomatic Medicine, substantiated the claim that lithium carbonate "checks the intense manic excitement." The repeated observation that mania returned as soon as patients were given a placebo substitute assured researchers that the effect was real.[36] Although many psychiatrists (remembering the crude lobotomies and shock treatments of the past) were skeptical of somatic treatments, the lasting ameliorating effects of drugs (demonstrated through NIMH-coordinated studies) made it more difficult to dismiss the new generation of biological treatments.[37]

What is more, NIMH basic research ostensibly elucidated the mode of action of several of these psychoactive drugs, leading to mechanical models of mental illness. Julius Axelrod, NIMH's first intramural Nobel laureate, discovered that tricyclic antidepressants work by blocking the reuptake of the neurotransmitter noradrenaline.[38] Perhaps even more important for advancing the biological paradigm, Axelrod's NIH mentor, Steve Brodie, established the first connection between a behavior state (sedation) and the neurochemistry of the brain (depletion of the neurotransmitter serotonin).[39] And, as Justin Garson relates in his contribution to this volume, NIMH two decades later contributed to the development of the dopamine hypothesis of schizophrenia.[40]

Although there had been earlier work suggesting a link between genes and mental illness, NIMH's founding intramural director, Seymour Kety, was the first to authoritatively establish that schizophrenia has a significant genetic component.[41] Exploiting Denmark's thorough adoption records, Kety found that adoptees afflicted with schizophrenia (broadly defined) were more likely to have biological parents with the illness than adoptive parents.[42] At the same time, it was clear from Kety's twin studies that genetics was not the whole story; having an identical twin with schizophrenia turned out to give one only a 50 percent chance of also developing schizophrenia. Kety's work, therefore, supported a theory of "genetic transmission of vulnerability."[43] Still, this theory helped topple psychological hypotheses of schizophrenia formation that earlier NIMH work had supported. As the NIMH scientist Solomon Snyder put it, "Clearly something genetic was going on."[44]

By advocating a mental disease categorization scheme, NIMH played a major role in "solidifying" psychiatric categories.[45] In the late 1970s, NIMH employed four hundred psychiatrists to evaluate twelve thousand patients in order to field-test drafts of the radically revised DSM III (1980).[46] Critics of the DSMIII noted that simply through words, the manual transformed behaviors into entities; "schizophrenic reaction" became "schizophrenia."[47] In effect, the DSM III repudiated the search for what is "behind the symptom" (the analytic view) in favor of "the phenomenology of what [is] visible" (the medical model).[48]

NIMH basic science also made possible brain imaging, the most visual and supposedly the most direct evidence of the somatic root of mental illness. The underlying principle of imaging—the tracking of blood flow and the monitoring of metabolic activity (both considered markers of brain function)—rested on the work of NIMH scientists. Seymour Kety, in yet another foundational contribution, invented the use of nitrous oxide to determine cerebral blood flow, a method he trumpeted as a new approach to psychiatric disorders.[49] This technique opened the way to quantitative determination of cerebral blood flow in living animals. Kety hoped his method would yield insight into the major mental illnesses. Preliminary imaging studies, however, failed to detect any significant difference between the cerebral blood flow of "normal" volunteers and schizophrenics. Kety then sought methods to determine *regional* blood flow changes. Kety's NIH colleague (and former postdoc) Louis Sokoloff found a method to measure localized metabolic brain activity. Using an analog of glucose, 2-deoxy-D-glucose, that remains trapped in brain tissue long enough to have its location recorded, exposed regional functional activity.[50]

Finally, to consolidate and mine the new findings about the brain, NIMH helped construct an entirely new field. At the dawn of the public Internet, NIMH harnessed the potential for international information sharing by coordinating a multiagency, neuro-informatics database initiative known as the Human Brain Project, which sought ways to "store, analyze, share, collaborate, integrate, resolve, model, visualize, and interpret the complex experimental data [arising] from basic and clinical nervous system research."[51]

Biological Psychiatry: A Logical Choice?

Given these scientific and technological advances, NIMH's decision to increasingly promote the biological approach is certainly comprehensible. A new generation of drugs could mimic or ameliorate mental disturbances, suggesting the physiological nature of mental illness.[52] Genetics, biochemistry and brain imaging technologies promised to reveal biomarkers of mental illness.[53] Informatics harnessed the power of the computer to accelerate discovery. Moreover, the first coordinated multisite NIMH-sponsored comparison of psychotherapies (cognitive-behavioral and interpersonal) and drugs (imipramine) for effectiveness in treating major depression indicated that, at least for those with severe impairment, drugs might be more effective.[54]

Most fundamentally, biological psychiatry promised diagnostic clarity. NIMH's former intramural schizophrenia researcher Daniel Weinberger remarked that up until the 1970s, the label attached to a mental patient depended on where he or she was admitted; diagnoses were reflective of East versus West Coast training.[55] Similarly, an NIMH biometrician found a significant disparity between countries in rates of diagnosis of schizophrenia.[56] Imaging technologies promised, on the other hand, to become a more objective tool for differential diagnosis.[57] An NIMH annual report announced proof of principle (at least on a gross level): by looking at brain tissue alone, schizophrenia, with its signature ventricular enlargement, wide cortical sulci, and smaller cortical gyri, could be easily distinguished from dementias.[58] It was not surprising, then, that NIMH director Herbert Pardes thought it possible that brain scans would become the X-ray of psychiatry.[59]

The importance of rhetoric for advancing biological psychiatry becomes apparent once one appreciates that the shift occurred despite some serious scientific setbacks. NIMH researchers did not hide the shortcomings of the new battery of drugs. Jonathan Cole, who ran NIMH's psychopharmacology center in the 1960s, sounded a note of caution about the major tranquilizers; they left, he conceded, "an important part of the job undone."[60] Worse, the first generation of drugs for depression did not perform dramatically better than placebo.[61] It soon became clear that a fifth of bipolar patients did not respond to lithium, and medicated schizophrenic patients had a relapse rate of 40 percent in two years.[62] NIMH's Solomon Snyder pointed out that the modus operandi of psychopharmaceuticals was in dispute and that theories reflected disciplinary commitments. Regarding chlorpromazine, neurophysiologists saw important differences in the firing rate of neurons; meanwhile, biochemists focused on the powerful influence on respiration, and cell biologists were preoccupied with the swelling of mitochondria.[63]

In addition to the problems with the dopamine hypothesis of schizophrenia (as discussed by Justin Garson), Seymour Kety was forthcoming about the failure of several other biological theories of schizophrenia.[64] Supposed links between schizophrenia and specific genes did not pan out.[65] As Kety cautioned, to say that something has a "genetic component is a far cry from claiming that the disease is caused only by bad genes."[66] Disputes continued to rage over the essence of mental illness. Snyder wrote, "Despite thousands of scientific publications and innumerable psychiatric theories, no one is yet certain as to what is fundamental to the schizophrenic process."[67] For all the claims of scientific precision, there existed no widely accepted "animal models, biological markers or etiological evidence" for schizophrenia.[68] Brain imaging produced, in the words of another critic, "neuroanatomical findings . . . more notable [for their abundance] than the consistency of the findings."[69]

Biological Psychiatry: A Politically Necessary Choice?

Given these shortfalls, why did NIMH increasingly back biological psychiatry? Historical circumstances heightened the appeal of somatic approaches as political realities rendered alternative methodologies less practicable.[70] The external pressures bearing down on NIMH made the reasonable decision to back biological psychiatry a necessary choice.

First there was economic pressure. With the emergence of third-party payers, the establishment of Medicare and Medicaid in 1966 and HMOs in the 1970s, there came the accounting demand to exclude the "worried well" and to insure efficacy of treatment for those who truly needed it.[71] In 1952 the British behaviorist H. J. Eysenck famously had contended that "insight treatments" were no more effective than no treatment at all.[72] Reinforcing this skepticism, the Johns Hopkins psychiatrist Jerome Frank had concluded in 1961 that no methods of psychotherapy were any more effective than any other and that all such therapies "heal" patients by convincing patients that they are better.[73] In contrast to a community mental health or psychosocial approach, biological psychiatry promised to shorten the length of intervention and to eventually produce a cure.[74]

The public added more economic pressure. Growing public skepticism toward psychiatry in particular and the paternal medical establishment in general (fostered by the antipsychiatry and patient rights movements of the

1960s and 1970s) threatened NIMH budgets.[75] So did the conservative back-lash against the Great Society that elected Ronald Reagan to help get the federal government out of social research.[76] At the same time, NIMH had to placate advocacy groups such as the National Alliance for the Mentally Ill, a grassroots organization made up of family members of psychiatric patients not favorable to the psychodynamic theory that mental disease was caused by pathogenic parenting.[77] The push to restrict the focus of NIMH to crip-pling mental illnesses and to ignore "problems of living" made biological approaches seem the best avenue to attack serious disabilities.[78]

Then there was bureaucratic pressure. Following charges of unproven efficacy, NIMH was looking for a way "to redeem itself within the federal bureaucracy."[79] NIMH was constitutionally bound to listen to overseeing advisory boards like the National Advisory Mental Health Council and the Institute of Medicine, both of which counseled biological approaches.[80] Additionally, there was international pressure to conform mental health research to the rest of modern Western medicine. The US membership in the World Health Organization necessitated that the American Psychiatric Association's classification of mental illness be compatible with the taxon-omy of the International Classification of Diseases. This demand was the immediate impetus for the DSM III.[81]

There were also institutional incentives. Biological psychiatry helped NIMH fit better into NIH. NIMH's nonresearch branches, its training divi-sion that provided the means to increase the ranks of the mental health workforce, and its service division, which funded state clinics and pilot stud-ies, made the institute unique at NIH, a federal organization which saw itself as an engine of scientific medicine. This mismatch was more easily tolerated between 1967 and 1992, when NIMH was officially (if not physically) located outside of NIH as part of an umbrella organization eventually known as ADAMHA, the Alcohol, Drug Abuse, and Mental Health Administration. NIMH's official return to NIH resulted in the elimination of its nonresearch branches, putting the institute in line with the mission of the rest of NIH and sealing NIMH's commitment to biological approaches.

Finally, the sociological force of professionalization undoubtedly played a part in nudging NIMH toward concentrating on biological research. Implicit in NIMH's championing of biological psychiatry was a defense of psychiatry in general. The diagnostic variability alluded to above provoked doubts about the reality of mental illness. A famous field experiment in the early 1970s shockingly found that staff at mental hospitals could not distin-guish between bogus and real patients, leading the authors to conclude that "however much we may be personally convinced that we can tell the nor-mal from the abnormal, the evidence is simply not compelling."[82] By osten-sibly "proving" the biological reality of mental illness, technology like brain scans refuted the thesis of 'the myth of mental illness.'[83] By riding on the coattails of the cutting-edge fields of genetics, molecular biology, and neuroscience, biological psychiatry promised to elevate the status of mental health research.[84] By tying mental illness to the body, NIMH linked psychiatry to more esteemed medical specialties, disciplines such as neurology that were seen as meeting higher scientific standards.[85] By elevating the professional status of psychiatry, biological psychiatry promised to raise the funding priority of mental health research.

Spreading the Gospel of Biological Psychiatry

As other scholars have argued, data and logic alone did not make the biological turn a foregone conclusion, faith in biological psychiatry needed to be "sold." Most scholarship on the selling of biological psychiatry has focused on the DSM III, which marked a conceptual shift from a "clinically-based bio-psychosocial model to a research-based medical model" and the branding and marketing efforts of the pharmaceutical industry.[86]

Numerous critics and historians have dismissed the DSM, the guidebook for mental health professionals, because of the dramatic changes between editions and for the means by which the manual was validated.[87] Needing to place all mental health patients somewhere in its schema, the malleable DSM regularly introduced new (and dropped some old) species of mental illness. In the judgment of detractors, the DSM passed off invented categories as distinct, real diseases.[88] What is more, the evolving DSM altered criteria of mental disturbance in order to increase uniformity and reliability of diagnosis.[89] The field-testing of the DSM III has been deemed a stunt to signal scientific soundness when, in fact, the trials were "methodologically questionable."[90] Nevertheless, despite its shortfalls, the DSM III became the standard reference used not just by therapists but also by courts, prisons, educational institutions, and governments at all levels.[91]

The pharmaceutical industry has been even more sharply criticized. David Healy has argued that drug companies have, through an orchestrated campaign, sought "leverage" to increase the success of their clever marketing. By sponsoring symposia, distributing favorable scientific articles, and wooing patient groups, the pharmaceutical sector has tried to predispose the mental health community to accept drugs as the answer to mental illness.[92] The pharmaceutical firms hired medical communication and public relations agencies to ghostwrite drafts of journal articles that amplified the reporting of favorable results.[93] Others have contended that the pharmaceutical industry has inflated the incidence of specific mental illnesses as a rhetorical trick to expand its markets.[94] And that, having undue influence on the American Psychiatric Association, the pharmaceutical industry has loosened the criteria for mental illnesses; again, thereby expanding markets.[95]

Little attention, positive or negative, has been paid to NIMH's role in the "selling" of biological psychiatry. As a federal expert body with a mandate to disseminate objective scientific information, NIMH was well poised to champion the revolution.[96] As part of its responsibilities, NIMH communicated not only mental health facts and exciting avenues of scientific research, but also its vision of the profitable, humane, and intellectual promise of biological psychiatry.[97]

First and foremost, NIMH sold biological psychiatry as enlightened self-interest. Biological psychiatry could spare society the massive costs of lost worker productivity and long-term psychiatric treatments. As an opinion piece written by an NIMH director baldly stated, "In 1965, thanks to psychoactive drugs there would have been 690,000 hospitalized mental patients instead there were only 470,000 saving two billion dollars."[98] Biological psychiatry, in other words, will justify the public's investment in NIMH even during times of economic retrenchment.

NIMH sold biological psychiatry as salvific. Biological psychiatry promised to spare those afflicted with mental illness "tragic years in institutions" and "help decrease the mass of suffering and suicides associated with depressive illness."[99] Biological psychiatry should improve the social functioning of those struggling with mental illness by freeing them from stigma born of society's ignorance and prejudice. By confirming the physical basis of mental illness, biological psychiatry absolves the patient of responsibility. "Real men have real depression," ran one public awareness campaign. Depression, these posters made clear, is not a problem of character but rather a treatable illness rooted in genetics, brain chemistry, and hormones.[100]

NIMH sold biological psychiatry as revelatory of the real etiology and nature of mental illness. Drugs promised to lead to a nosology that more accurately reflects nature.[101] By dubbing tranquilizers as "antipsychotics" that could treat some of the symptoms of psychosis, NIMH scientists suggested not only that the drugs were effective and specific but, more to the point, that they are effective and specific precisely because mental illnesses have physical loci.[102] Furthermore, biology-based psychiatry is the only psychiatry amenable to "scientific" methodology. NIMH's Jonathan Cole expanded, "Good psychiatric problems ask interesting questions which can be clearly answered. One of the problems of research in psychoanalysis is that it is very hard to make a prediction that could be proven right or wrong, and one of the nice things about drug studies is that the placebo at least gives you a chance of showing that something is different from something else."[103] Indeed, NIMH's "comprehensive study" of antipsychotics helped usher in "a new era of methodological rigor in clinical psychopharmacology," of double-blind studies with placebos.[104]

NIMH's broadcasts have suggested, some more overtly than others, that the ultimate intellectual prize of biological psychiatry will be a mechanical understanding of the mind. The seeds of such reductionism were planted early. Seymour Kety set a reductionist tone for mental health research.[105] In popular periodicals like the *Saturday Review*, he celebrated the pursuit of the biochemical underpinning of mental illness.[106] And, in a *Scientific American* article "Disorders of the Human Brain," Kety enumerated all of the already-known biological causes of mental illness, among them inherited metabolic defects, vascular disease, infections, tumors, and head traumas.[107] Vital to this reductionism is an accurate understanding of how drugs or other brain manipulation techniques bring about their effects. The NIH-supported Swedish pharmacologist Arvid Carlsson explained how antipsychotics work by blocking dopamine receptors, thereby preventing postsynaptic excitation.[108] He offered a molecular explanation of a hitherto psychologically described phenomenon: "Since the world is too much for schizophrenics, phenothiazines might help them to cope by blocking dopamine receptors, thus decreasing the activity of dopamine systems and thereby divorcing sensory perceptions from the internal feelings and memories upon which they normally impinge."[109] In short, "these drugs 'tune down' the onslaught of the impinging world."[110] Such explanations start to make credible the reduction of human behavior to molecular occurrences. "At this point we must start wondering," stated NIMH's Solomon Snyder, "whether or not there is any difference between talking about the patients 'psychological' versus his 'neurological' vulnerability."[111] Another NIH publication's reductionism went further, explaining that "all of your awareness, values, belief and memories appear objectively to be patterns of electrical impulses maintained through the chemicals of your brain cells, and first established through some stimulus from inside or outside your body."[112]

All of these messages, summed up as biological psychiatry equals hope, was most powerfully conveyed in the conversion narratives of NIMH scientists.[113] In numerous lectures and interviews, senior NIMH scientists trained before the 1990s have sharply contrasted their psychodynamic training and the futility of analytical ideas to the progress in understanding and treatment made possible by biological research.[114] Susan Swedo, a striking example, has recounted how she and her colleagues traced some forms of obsessive-compulsive disorder to strep infections, a resounding victory for biological psychiatry as this disorder was once considered the mental illness most explicable through psychodynamic theories.[115] Along these same lines, NIMH director Frederick Goodwin, in "The Legacy of Dr. Heinz Lehmann," a 1999 television documentary about the first trials of chlorpromazine in Canada, commemorated the transformation of Montreal's Douglas Hospital from a desperate seat of analytic reversion therapy, in which mud was manipulated in an attempt to bring patients back to their anal phase, into a beacon of pharmaceutical hope.[116]

NIMH used its directive from Congress to disperse knowledge about research into the causes and treatment of mental illness as an opportunity to mold the public view not only about the merits of biological psychiatry but also about the virtues of NIMH. By pointing to promising NIMH-funded discoveries, these reports justified NIMH's budgetary choices and countered the public's disenchantment with science and government ventures.[117] By absolving the mentally ill and reaching out to their families, these messages aimed to cast NIMH as a responsive, benevolent champion of the suffering.[118] By suggesting that science and technology are gradually revealing the true nature of mental illness, NIMH's messages placed NIMH at the center of a linear, progressive view of psychiatry.[119] Finally, by omitting any reference to politics, these messages made the turn to biology seem to be the result of science alone, concealing the external pressures that compelled NIMH's direction.[120]

One could posit that for the majority of the American public (at certain times more than at others), NIMH's official role as reporter of objective scientific progress made the rhetoric seem disinterested and the rhetoric about itself invisible.[121] Because its messages were more nuanced than pharmaceutical ads, containing caveats cautioning the public about the need for more research, the messages both appeared scientifically sound and further underscored the need for NIMH.

The Need to Dissect NIMH's Messages

On the eve of the new millennium, First Lady Hillary Clinton and NIMH director Steven Hyman reflected on the progress in mental health research. "Not two decades ago," they reminded their audience, "people were taught that dread diseases like autism or schizophrenia were due to some subtle character flaw in mothers."[122]

By calling attention to the role official rhetoric may have played in the rising status of biological psychiatry, I am not arguing against the biological approach or the need for rhetoric to support it. The fact that some biological theories or practices have been abandoned hardly discredits the enterprise. The obsolescence of medical hypotheses or treatments might only support the philosopher of science Karl Popper's contention that science proceeds through falsifications.[123] Moreover, falsified biological theories have been invaluable in stimulating fruitful brain research.[124] The biological approach to mental illness has led to better symptom management and fundamental knowledge about the human brain while demolishing harmful hypothetical explanations for mental illness.[125] Many experiencing mental illness happily embrace the new explanation for their suffering and support NIMH's perspective and objectives.[126]

At the same time, it is for good reason that biological psychiatry contin- ues to elicit educated dissent. "The real story of 20th century psychiatry," one critic has observed, "is how complex mental illness is, how difficult it is to treat, and how, in the face of this complexity, people cling to coherent explanations like power swimmers to a raft."[127] The introduction to the DSM V itself states, "In short, we have come to recognize that the bound- aries between disorders are more porous than originally conceived."[128] On the eve of the millennium, a surgeon general's mental health report warned against jumping to conclusions regarding the biological cause of mental illness.[129]

The hegemony of the biological perspective threatens to overlook the human dimension (the patients' individual history, psychology, and situa- tion), discouraging interpersonal exploration between the client and the therapist and blinding everyone to other (sometimes preferable) avenues of treatment.[130] Meta-analyses of therapies have found that psychological approaches, such as cognitive therapy, appear to be as effective as medi- cation.[131] Talk therapy apparently can have the same biological effects on the brain as physical interventions and without the side effects.[132] Because NIMH is the chief funding agency of psychiatric professions, critics fear that professional expediency creates uncritical audiences eager to echo the gos- pel of biological psychiatry.[133]

This chapter has argued for the centrality of rhetoric for the mission of NIMH. It is a call for fine-grain analysis of NIMH's publications meant for broad consumption to discover the exact messages it has conveyed about the origin of and remedy for mental illness. A more in-depth rhetorical analysis would require addressing questions regarding the form, authorship, con- tent, and reception of NIMH's messages. Regarding form, one needs to ask: What counts as NIMH rhetoric? How many genres did NIMH produce? Can one distinguish between official and unofficial NIMH rhetoric? Regarding authorship, one must determine how many different individual and corpo- rate authors within NIMH can be distinguished. And in whose name are the authors writing? Regarding content, one must consider: Are there quan- tifiable changes over time in mentions of biological approaches? Are non- biological approaches pushed to the background?[134] Are there changes in tone, metaphors, or tropes? In other words, how has technical material been translated into lay language?[135] Regarding reception, it is crucial to ask, how many distinct audiences did these rhetorical messages target (includ- ing Congress, the press, mental health practitioners)? How many people watched, listened to, or read NIMH literature? Finally, how have these mes- sages been echoed in the wider media?

Being the interface between the major authority in mental health research and the American public, the communications of NIMH are wor- thy of closer scrutiny. Such a study would be historically interesting because changes in NIMH's messages must surely have occurred as today's NIMH "resemble[s] only faintly the institute of decades past."[136]

In the meantime it can be said that the rhetoric of the medical model of mental illness fits into the larger themes of this volume of technology and marginality. Rhetoric can be a tool. It can serve as a placeholder, sustaining belief until science fills in knowledge gaps.[137] In the absence of a complete picture of what causes mental illness and despite the failure of many theories, NIMH has kept alive faith in the biological approach. Rhetoric can shape opinions, steer resources, and so make possible the successes it heralds. Spreading the message that "mental illness equals brain disease" has a reinforcing effect: the biological data that is produced as a result of public support soon turns into rhetorical messages that, in turn, appeal for more support.

By placing pharmacological, genetic, and brain science findings front and center, NIMH's communication efforts have served as a kind of stage management. This rhetorical strategy has cast not only light, but also shadows. By shining a spotlight on the promising avenue of biological psychiatry, the "mantra of NIMH" has cast into shadow other approaches to mental illness, including psychosocial interventions.

NIMH research ties into the theme of marginalization in two ways. First, by declaring what is exciting research (biological approaches), NIMH's rhetoric suggests what should be marginalized (sociological or psychological explanations). Second, because this rhetoric can be so guiding, it can be regarded as doing biomedicine on the margins. NIMH's communication and outreach efforts, seemingly secondary priorities and afterthoughts (being located outside NIMH's obvious sites of knowledge generation of laboratories and hospitals), can play a formative role in mental health research. The advertising of the biological approach to mental illness has served as advocacy of the progress it purported to merely report, another way in which biomedicine has been shaped at the fringes.

Notes

Epigraphs. Tomas Insel, "Director's Blog: Tracing the Brain's Connections," National Institute of Mental Health, March 10, 2010, http://www.nimh.nih.gov/about/director/2010/tracing-the-brains-connections.shtml. In his blog, Dr. Insel was referring to the NIH-sponsored Human Connectome Project. Philip Sapir, Julius Segal, and Marcus S. Goldstein, "Anthropology and the Research Grant and Fellowship Programs of the National Institute of Mental Health," *American Anthropologist,* n.s., 65, no. 1 (February 1963): 119.

1. Robert Pasnau has argued that the "remedicalization" of psychiatry began in the 1970s due to many factors, among them the failure of the community mental health movement, the disaster of deinstitutionalization, and the economic need

244   BRIAN P. CASEY

to reduce expenditures. In *Controversial Issues in Mental Health*, ed. Stuart Kirk and Susan Einbinder (Boston: Allyn and Bacon, 1994), 161–62.

2. "To paraphrase Freud, who said that dreams were the royal road to the unconscious, today we can travel the brain as the royal road to the mind," stated another of Insel's blogs, titled "Join the Revolution," National Institute of Mental Health, March 12, 2012, http://www.nimh.nih.gov/about/director/2012/join-the-revolution.shtml.

3. Alas, much, if not most, of NIMH's past public communications have not been systematically archived at NIMH. Published works are available through the Library of Congress and the National Library of Medicine.

4. Daniel Breslau, review of *The Selling of DSM: The Rhetoric of Science in Psychiatry*, by Stuart A. Kirk and Herb Kutchins, *Contemporary Sociology*, 22, no. 4 (1993): 607.

5. One can look at scientific statements through the lens of traditional rhetorical categories. Scientific pronouncements can be regarded as a type of "deliberative oratory" in its directing of future research and as "epideictic" in its celebration of appropriate methods. In its dealing with the character of entities (in this case with mental illness and the brain), NIMH messages can be seen as focusing on the *quid sit*. Alan Gross, *The Rhetoric of Science* (Cambridge: Cambridge University Press, 1996), 10–11.

6. Adam Hedgecoe, "Schizophrenia and the Narrative of Enlightened Geneticization," *Social Studies of Science* 31, no. 6 (2001): 875–911.

7. Loren Mosher, "The Center for Studies of Schizophrenia," *Schizophrenia Bulletin* 1, no. 1 (1969): 4.

8. For the current priorities of NIMH, see the budget proposals of recent years available at "Budget," accessed December 15, 2016, http://www.nimh.nih.gov/about/budget/index.shtml. Comparisons of budget expenditures on biological research is complicated by, in the words of NIMH, "The breadth and heterogeneity of the NIMH research program [which has] posed problems for the meaningful classification and description of projects. Not only do institute studies focus on a wide variety of mental health problems and behavioral phenomena, but a single project often involves several substantive emphases and multiple approaches to the same research question." Julius Segal, editor-in-chief, *Research in the Service of Mental Health: Report of the Research Task Force of the National Institute of Mental Health* (1975), NIMH Rockville, MD DHEW publication No (ADM) 75-236, 41. Nevertheless, in its own estimation, "In the first few years research on mental illness less than 15 percent of all projects were conducted by biological scientists." Ibid., 9.

9. The embracing of the biological perspective by the American Psychiatric Association is clear, for example, in the opening remarks of the 2014 annual meeting: "The very real scientific opportunities before us are unprecedented in human history. We have never before had the capacity to image the brain, to see the impact of genetic abnormalities on neurodevelopment, or begin to understand the complex ways our brains shape our perceptions of the world and in turn are shaped by them." Paul Summergrad, APA Annual Meeting Opening Session Speech, May 4, 2014, http://www.psych.org. A recent survey revealed that mental health care providers, whatever their disciplinary affiliation, consider the shift to the biological perspective as having been one of the most important changes in psychiatry in the post–World War II era. Mark S. Micale, "The Ten Most Important Changes in Psychiatry since World War II," *History of Psychiatry* 25, no. 4 (2014): 485–91.

10. MacArthur Mental Health Module, 1996 General Society Survey, "Americans' View of Mental Health and Illness at Century's End: Continuity and Change," available at http://www.indiana.edu/~icmhsr/docs/Americans'%20Views%20of%20 Mental%20Health.pdf. In this survey, the public rated *stress* (an ill-defined term) as the number one likely cause for all mental illnesses. The survey did not distinguish between immediate and underlying causes. Bruce G. Link, Jo C. Phelan, Michaeline Bresnahan, Ann Stueve et al., "Public Conceptions of Mental Illness: Labels, Causes, Dangerousness, and Social Distance," *American Journal of Public Health* 89, no. 9 (1999): 1328–33.

11. Edward G. Jones and Lorne M. Mendell, "Assessing the Decade of the Brain," *Science* 284, no. 5415 (1999): 739.

12. See White House, "Fact Sheet: Over $300 Million in Support of the President's BRAIN Initiative," September 30, 2014, https://www.whitehouse.gov/sites/default/ files/microsites/ostp/brain_fact_sheet_9_30_2014_final.pdf. Announcement of this initiative can be found at The Brain Initative, https://www.whitehouse.gov/BRAIN.

13. A study of psychotherapy practices over the period from 1998 to 2007 found that expenditures on psychotherapy declined as a greater percentage of clients took psychotropic medicines without any accompanying psychotherapy. Mark Olfson and Steven C. Marcus, "National Trends in Outpatient Psychotherapy," *American Journal of Psychiatry* 167 (2010): 1456–63. A former director of NIMH lamented in a recent address the "decline in depth of psychological discovery and psychiatric care. A tendency to treat superficially, using medication with the goal of symptom relief only, with avoidance of efforts to understand patients more fully by careful interview and assessment." Herbert Pardes, "The American Academy of Psychoanalysis and Dynamic Psychiatry," *Psychodynamic Psychiatry*, 42, no. 2 (2014): 307–18, quote at 310.

14. Regarding the latter, deep brain stimulation has been used to combat severe depression. See "Brain Stimulation Therapies," National Institute of Mental Health, accessed September 15, 2015, http://www.nimh.nih.gov/health/topics/brain-stimulation-therapies/brain-stimulation-therapies.shtml.

15. For example, in "Setting Priorities for Basic Brain and Behavioral Science Research at NIMH," *Report of the National Advisory Mental Health Council's Workgroup on Basic Sciences*, May 2004, six studies on the foundation of social attachment focused on identifying the underlying brain circuitry deemed responsible. National Advisory Mental Health Council's Workgroup on Basic Sciences, 2004, https://www.nimh.nih. gov/about/advisory-boards-and-groups/namhc/reports/bbbs-research_42531.pdf.

16. Tanya Marie Luhrmann, *Of Two Minds: The Growing Disorder in American Psychiatry* (New York: Alfred Knopf, 2000), 223.

17. Gerald Grob, *From Asylum to Community: Mental Health Policy in Modern America* (Princeton, NJ: Princeton University Press, 1991), 100. See also Luhrmann, *Of Two Minds*, 214.

18. Grob, *From Asylum to Community*, 298–300; Bertram Brown, "Life of Psychiatry," *American Journal of Psychiatry* 133, no. 5 (1976): 493.

19. Ross J Baldessarini, "American Biological Psychiatry and Psychopharmacology 1944–1994," in *American Psychiatry after World War II, 1944–94*, ed. Roy Menninger and John Nemiah, 380 (Washington, DC: American Psychiatric Press, 2000).

20. Committee on Nomenclature and Statistics of the American Psychiatric Association, *The Diagnostic and Statistical Manual: Mental Disorders* (DSM) (Washington, DC: American Psychiatric Association Mental Hospital Service, 1952).

21. Jose Brunner and Orna Ophir, "'In Good Times and in Bad': Boundary Relations of Psychoanalysis in Post-war USA," *History of Psychiatry* 22, no. 2 (2011): 215–31. For a side-by-side comparison of DSM II and DSM III descriptions of schizophrenia, see Luhrmann, *Of Two Minds*, 229.

22. "Schizophrenia" DSM IV-TR. American Psychiatric Association, Diagnostic and Statistical Manual of Mental Disorders: DSM IV-TR (Washington, DC: American Psychiatric Association, 2000). One could also notice this shift reflected in the changing theories about antisocial personality disorder. See Martin Pickersgill, "From Psyche to Soma? Changing Accounts of Antisocial Personality Disorders in the American Journal of Psychiatry," *History of Psychiatry* 21 (2010): 294–311.

23. Michael Strand, "Where Do Classifications Come From? The DSM-III, the Transformation of American Psychiatry, and the Problem of Origins in the Sociology of Knowledge," *Theoretical Sociology* 40 (2011): 278.

24. Sandra G. Boodman, "A Horrible Place & A Wonderful Place," *Washington Post Magazine*, Sunday, Final Edition, October 8, 1989, W18. For a discussion of the Chestnut case see Luhrmann, *Of Two Minds*, 233, and David Healy, *The Antidepressant Era* (Cambridge, MA: Harvard University Press, 1997), 245–51. At Chestnut Lodge, as well as at the Menninger Clinic and the McLean Hospital, talking cures were used to treat schizophrenia. See Andrew Scull, "The Mental Health Sector and the Social Sciences in Post–World War II USA, Part 1: Total War and Its Aftermath," *History of Psychiatry* 22, 1 (2011): 3–19, 9.

25. Lamented in Gregory Miller and Jennifer Keller, "Psychology and Neuroscience: Making Peace," *Current Directions in Psychological Science* 9, no. 6 (2000): 212–15.

26. Scull, "Mental Health Sector and the Social Sciences in Post–World War II USA, Part 1," 9–10.

27. NIMH's James Stabenau and William Pollin discovered that in "schizophrenic families (1) emotional tone was over controlled and often inappropriate; (2) control was maintained by the use of guilt and families showed considerable concern about conforming to external standards; (3) communication between family members was fragmented and clarity was seldom reached; and (4) family organization was rigid, with distortion of role differentiation and expectation." At that time, these investigators concluded that the data supported (though admittedly did not prove) the hypothesis that "differing patterns of interaction between parents and child are causally related to the development of psychopathology and the establishment and maintenance of mental health." National Institute of Mental Health, "Comparative Study of Families of Schizophrenics, Delinquents, and Normals," press summary, May 4, 1964, National Institute of Mental Health Science Writing, Press, and Dissemination Branch, room 6200, MSC 9663, Bethesda, MD. See also James B. Stabenau and William Pollin, "Comparative Life History Differences of Families of Schizophrenics, Delinquents and 'Normals,'" *American Journal of Psychiatry* 124, no. 11 (May 1968): 1526–34.

28. They speculated that the underweight twin "would be less able to deal with the stress of everyday life and might well succumb to psychic disintegration." Snyder,

Madness and the Brain, 91–92, referring to W. Pollin and J. R. Stabenau, "Biological, Psychological and Historical Differences in a Series of Monozygotic Twins Discordant for Schizophrenia," in *The Transmission of Schizophrenia*, trans. D. Rosenthal and S. S. Kety (New York: Pergamon Press, 1968), 317–32. A press summary description of this work was released in 1964. National Institute of Mental Health, "Family Studies with Identical Twins Discordant for Schizophrenia," press summary, May 7, 1964, National Institute of Mental Health Science Writing, Press, and Dissemination Branch, room 6200, MSC 9663, Bethesda, MD.

29. Andrew Scull, "The Mental Health Sector and the Social Sciences in Post–World War II USA Part 2: The Impact of Federal Research Funding and the Drugs Research," *History of Psychiatry* 22, no. 3 (2011): 274, 276. On the latter research, see work of Erving Goffman mentioned in text below. It is notable that between 1948 and 1961, NIMH funded 129 projects in anthropology. Sapir, Segal, and Goldstein, "Anthropology and the Research Grant and Fellowship Programs of the National Institute of Mental Health," 117–32. See also Harold Halpert, "Activities of the National Institute of Mental Health Which Affect American Families," *Marriage and Family Living*, 20, no. 3 (August 1958): 261–69.

30. Boodman, "A Horrible Place & A Wonderful Place." In a follow-up study on schizophrenic patients treated at Chestnut Lodge, an NIMH-funded investigator found a high failure rate, ostensibly the consequence of the asylum's reluctance to implement the new standard course of drug treatment. Thomas H. McGlashan, "The Chestnut Lodge Follow-up Study I: Follow-up Methodology and Study Sample," *Archives of General Psychiatry* 41 (1984): 573–601.

31. Constance Holden, "A Top Priority at NIMH," *Science* 235, no. 4787 (1987): 431.

32. Pushback from therapists convinced NIMH to drop this latter warning. Brunner and Ophir, "In Good Times and in Bad," 215–31. An earlier study published in this journal argued for using a combination of drugs and psychosocial intervention with schizophrenic patients, the latter intervention to deal with aggravating stress. Ian R. H. Falloon and Robert Paul Liberman, "Interactions between Drug and Psychosocial Therapy in Schizophrenia," *Schizophrenia Bulletin* 9, no. 4 (1983): 543–54.

33. See "The Lasker Awards," Albert and Mary Lasker Foundation, 1999, http://www.laskerfoundation.org/awards/1999_s_presentation.htm and http://www.laskerfoundation.org/awards/1999_s_interview_kety.htm; Louis Sokoloff, "Seymour S. Kety, 25 August 1915–25 May 2000," *Proceedings of the American Philosophical Society*, 146, no. 1 (March 2002): 101–10. For a discussion of early scientific work at NIMH and its sister NIH institute, see the videocast NIMH/NINDB Intramural Research 1950s, http://videocast.nih.gov/launch.asp?10336. Although Robert Felix focused most heavily on community mental health, historians have credited him with recognizing how mental health tied to biomedicine would have great appeal. Gerald Grob and Howard Goldman, *The Dilemma of Federal Mental Health Policy: Radical Reform or Incremental Change?* (New Brunswick, NJ: Rutgers University Press, 2006), 20–21.

34. David Healy, *The Creation of Psychopharmacology* (Cambridge, MA: Harvard University Press, 2002). NIMH proudly trumpeted its role in validating the new armory in reports such as *Research on Mental Illness and Addictive Disorders: Progress and Prospects*, Institute of Medicine (Washington, DC: National Academy Press, 1984), 44.

In 1967 the World Health Organization asked NIMH to integrate information about psychotropic drugs. Julius Segal, editor-in-chief, *Research in the Service of Mental Health: Report of the Research Task Force of the National Institute of Mental Health*, DHEW publication No (ADM) 75-236 (Rockville, MD: NIMH, 1975), 388.

35. Of treated schizophrenic patients, 75 percent had reportedly much improved, and, indicating a true effect, placebo-treated patients improved only somewhat. Indeed, there were thirteen recognizable differences between placebo effects and the three drugs tested. Judith Swazey, *Chlorpromazine in Psychiatry* (Cambridge, MA: MIT Press, 1974), 253–54.

36. From National Institute of Mental Health, unpublished document, dated March 31, 1967, National Institute of Mental Health Science Writing, Press, and Dissemination Branch, room 6200, MSC 9663, Bethesda, MD.

37. Swazey, *Chlorpromazine in Psychiatry*, 196, 229.

38. Julius Axelrod won the Nobel Prize in 1970 for his pharmacological studies of the stress hormone and neurotransmitter norepinephrine. See his Nobel speech, "Noradrenaline: Fate and Control of Its Biosynthesis," delivered December 12, 1970, http://www.nobelprize.org/nobel_prizes/medicine/laureates/1970/axelrod-lecture.pdf.

39. Alfred Pletscher, Parkhurst Shore, and Bernard B Brodie, "Serotonin Release as a Possible Mechanism of Reserpine Action," *Science* 122 (1955): 374–75.

40. In this volume, see Justin Garson's chapter, "A 'Model Schizophrenia': Amphetamine Psychosis and the Transformation of American Psychiatry." In his conclusion, Garson argues that favored models and mechanisms dictate our view of mental illness. I argue that this collective imagination is in part manufactured by official advertising that champions these favored models and mechanisms. See also S. H. Snyder, "The Dopamine Hypothesis of Schizophrenia: Focus on Dopamine Receptor," *American Journal of Psychiatry* 133 (1976): 197–202.

41. Solomon Snyder touches on the earlier work of Franz Kellman in Solomon Snyder, *Madness and the Brain* (New York: McGraw-Hill, 1974).

42. S. S. Kety, D. Rosenthal, P. H. Wender, and F. Schulsinger, "Mental Illness in the Biological and Adoptive Families of Adopted Schizophrenics," *American Journal of Psychiatry*, 128, no. 3 (1971): 302–6.

43. Seymour S. Kety, "The Syndrome of Schizophrenia: Unresolved Questions and Opportunities for Research," *British Journal of Psychiatry* 136 (1980): 421–36.

44. Snyder, *Madness and the Brain*, 87.

45. Andrew Lakoff, "Diagnostic Liquidity: Mental Illness and the Global Trade in DNA," *Theory and Society*, 34 (2005): 63–92, speaks of the DSM III's "solidification" of psychiatry's objects.

46. Strand, "Where Do Classifications Come From?," 288. John P. Feighner, Eli Robins, Samuel B. Guze, Robert A. Woodruff Jr. et al., "Diagnostic Criteria for Use in Psychiatric Research," *Archives of General Psychiatry* 26, no. 1 (1972): 57–63.

47. Luhrmann, *Of Two Minds*, 227.

48. Brunner and Ophir, "'In Good Times and in Bad,'" 223.

49. Seymour S. Kety, "The Theory and Applications of the Exchange of Inert Gas at the Lungs and Tissues," *Pharmacology Review* 3 (1951): 1–41. Kety made this claim as early as 1948 in S. S. Kety, R. B. Woodford, M. H. Harmel, F. A. Freyhan et al., "Cerebral Blood Flow and Metabolism in Schizophrenia: The Effects of Barbiturate

Semi-narcosis, Insulin Coma and Electroshock," *American Journal of Psychiatry* 104 (1948): 765–70.

50. Sokoloff, Louis. "Mapping Cerebral Activity with Deoxyglucose." *Journal of the American Medical Association* 244, no. 14 (1980): 1612.

51. "The Human Brain Project (Neuroinformatics): Phase I, Feasibility; Phase II, Refinements, Maintenance and Integration," release date December 3, 2002, http://grants.nih.gov/grants/guide/pa-files/PAR-03-035.html.

52. "Tranquilizers can have specific antischizophrenic activity, amphetamine can in low doses activate a quiescent schizophrenic in a fairly specific fashion." Snyder, *Madness and the Brain*, 216. Aarvid Carlsson explored how artificially raising dopamine levels in animals leads to schizophrenic-like dysregulation of motor movement. Deborah M. Barnes, "Biological Issues in Schizophrenia," *Science* 235, no. 4787 (January 23, 1987): 432.

53. NIMH publications celebrated the search for metabolic markers of affective disorders. By the mid-1960s, NIMH scientists were studying the metabolism of catecholamines, hormones made by the adrenal glands, and found an increased level of normetanephrine in the urine of manic patients. And a deficiency of the norepinephrine was found in depressed patients. National Institute of Mental Health, "Norepinephrine Metabolism and Drugs Used in the Affective Disorders: A Possible Mechanism of Action," press summary, May 10, 1967, National Institute of Mental Health Science Writing, Press, and Dissemination Branch, room 6200, MSC 9663, Bethesda, MD. See also Kenneth Greenspan, Joseph Schildkraut, Edna Gordon, Bernard Levy et al., "Catecholamine Metabolism in Affective Disorders," *Archives of General Psychiatry* 21, no. 6 (1969): 710–16.

54. Irene M Elkin, Tracie Shea, John T. Watkins, Stanley D. Imber et al. "National Institute of Mental Health Treatment of Depression Collaborative Research Program: General Effectiveness of Treatments." *Archives of General Psychiatry* 46, no. 11 (1989): 971–82.

55. Daniel Weinberger, interview by Claudia Wassmann, available at the Office of NIH history, accessed on November 1, 2016, https://history.nih.gov/archives/oral_histories.html#w.

56. David Healy, *Creation of Psychopharmacology*, 297. Rick Mayes and Allan Horwitz, "DSM III and the Revolution in the Classification of Mental Illness," *Journal of the History of Behavioral Sciences* 41, no. 3 (2005): 249–67.

57. The general hope for bio-tools for differential diagnosis of mental illness is expressed, for instance, in Barnes, "Biological Issues in Schizophrenia," 430–33.

58. See "Clinical Brain Disorders Branch Report," National Institute of Mental Health, Division of Intramural Research Programs, *Annual Report, NIMH 1987–8*.

59. Robert J. Trotter, "Psychiatry for the 80's," *Science News*, 119, no. 22 (May 30, 1981), 348–49.

60. National Institute of Mental Health, "Drug Use in Schizophrenia," press summary, May 12, 1967, National Institute of Mental Health Science Writing, Press, and Dissemination Branch, room 6200, MSC 9663, Bethesda, MD. "The phenothiazines," Dr. Jonathan Cole explained in this release, "are better at controlling overt psychopathology than they are at producing increases in social effectiveness."

61. National Institute of Mental Health, press release, February 21, 1967, National Institute of Mental Health Science Writing, Press, and Dissemination Branch, room 6200, MSC 9663, Bethesda, MD.

250 BRIAN P. CASEY

62. Luhrmann, *Of Two Minds*, 208, citing Harold Kaplan and Benjamin Sadock, *Pocket Handbook of Clinical Psychiatry* (Baltimore: Williams & Wilkins, 1996), 306.

63. Snyder, *Madness and the Brain*, 239.

64. Garson, *A Model Schizophrenia*; Seymour S. Kety, "Biochemical Theories of Schizophrenia," *Science* 129, no. 3363 (1959): 1590–96. See also Kety, "Syndrome of Schizophrenia, 421–36; Alan Baumeister and Mike Hawkins, "The Serotonin Hypothesis of Schizophrenia," *Journal of the History of the Neurosciences*, 13, no. 3 (2004): 277–91. Kety could be said to have a Popperian approach to scientific failure, embracing failure as the pathway to sounder scientific hypothesis, as I mention in my conclusion. One could also point to problems with the catecholamine hypothesis of depression. For a list of objections to this model see Healy, *The Antidepressant Era*, 155–61.

65. A current critic has commented, "Indeed throughout medicine, the pattern has been that early studies report larger effect sizes for the association of a candidate gene and a disease than do later studies. Often the effect disappears in subsequent studies." Richard McNally, *What Is Mental Illness?* (Cambridge, MA: Belknap Press of Harvard University Press, 2011), 164. McNally has pointed to a study that found no significant association between fourteen candidate genes and schizophrenia and schizoaffective disorder.

66. Kety found that only certain types of schizophrenia (chronic or borderline but not acute) seemed to have a clear genetic tie. Snyder, *Madness and the Brain*, 85–88.

67. Snyder, *Madness and the Brain*, 73.

68. Brunner and Ophir, "In Good Times and in Bad," 226.

69. Robert Rubin, review of *Brain Imaging in Clinical Psychiatry*, ed. K. Ranga Rama Krishnan and P. Murali Doraiswamy, 1125–26, *American Journal of Psychiatry* 155, no. 8 (1998), speaking generally about the field of brain imaging.

70. Regarding the winds of change against community mental health, the defunding of community mental health centers (once more than 50 percent of the NIMH budget, according to Lawrence C. Kolb, Shervert H. Frazier, and Paul Sirovatka, "The National Institute of Mental Health: Its Influence on Psychiatry and the Nation's Mental Health," in *American Psychiatry after World War II, 1944–94*, ed. Roy Menninger and John Nemiah, 219 (Washington, DC: American Psychiatric Press, 2000)), see Phillip Jacobs, "Whither Community Mental Health?," *International Journal of Mental Health*, 3, nos. 2–3(Summer-Fall 1974): 35–43.

71. Strand, "Where Do Classifications Come From?," 273–313.

72. H. J. Eysenck, "The Effects of Psychotherapy: An Evaluation," *Journal of Consulting Psychology* 16 (1952): 319–24.

73. Jerome D. Frank, *Persuasion and Healing: A Comparative Study of Psychotherapy* (Baltimore: Johns Hopkins University Press, 1961).

74. Gerald N. Grob, "Mental Health Policy in Late Twentieth-Century America," in *American Psychiatry after World War II, 1944–94*, ed. Roy Menninger and John Nemiah, 251 (Washington, DC: American Psychiatric Press, 2000).

75. Strand, "Where Do Classifications Come From?, 284; Harry M. Marks, "Trust and Mistrust in the Marketplace: Statistics and Clinical Research, 1945–1960," *History of Science* 38 (2000): 343–55.

76. Lawrence C. Kolb, Shervert H. Frazier, and Paul Sirovatka, "The National Institute of Mental Health: Its Influence on Psychiatry and the Nation's Mental

Health," in *American Psychiatry after World War II, 1944–94*, ed. Roy Menninger and John Nemiah (Washington, DC: American Psychiatric Press, 2000), 223. Earlier, NIMH director Stanley Yolles was effectively ousted over disputes with the Nixon administration over the direction of NIMH. Gerald N. Grob, "Mental Health Policy in Late Twentieth-Century America," in *American Psychiatry after World War II, 1944–94*, ed. Roy Menninger and John Nemiah, 235 (Washington, DC: American Psychiatric Press, 2000).

77. Scull, "The Mental Health Sector and the Social Sciences in Post–World War II USA Part 2," 280.

78. For a brief list of organizations that pushed for focusing on major mental illnesses rather than social problems or problems of living, see Lawrence C. Kolb, Shervert H. Frazier, and Paul Sirovatka, "The National Institute of Mental Health: Its Influence on Psychiatry and the Nation's Mental Health," in *American Psychiatry after World War II, 1944–94*, ed. Roy Menninger and John Nemiah, 222 (Washington, DC: American Psychiatric Press, 2000).

79. Strand, "Where Do Classifications Come From?," 289–90. "In the early 1970s, Congress deeply distrusted the NIMH—in 1976 the dollar amount of funding for the institute was actually lower than it had been in 1969—precisely because there was no way of distinguishing mental health from mental illness." Luhrmann, *Of Two Minds*, 237.

80. Jack D. Barchas, Glen R. Elliott, Philip A. Berger, Patricia R Barchas et al., "The Ultimate Stigma: Inadequate Funding for Research on Mental Illness and Addictive Disorders," *American Journal of Psychiatry* 142 (1985): 838–39. On the establishment of the Institute of Medicine, see Edward Berkowitz, *To Improve Human Health: A History of the Institute of Medicine* (Washington, DC: National Academy Press, 1998), also at http://www.nap.edu/books/0309061881/html. On the establishment of the National Advisory Mental Health Council (and of NIMH itself), see 79th Cong 2d Sess., chs 537, 538 Public Laws-Chs. 538, 539, July 3, 1946. For an example of a push toward the biological, see Samuel H. Barondes, Bruce M. Alberts, Nancy C. Andreasen, Cornelia Bargmann et al., "Workshop on Schizophrenia," *Proceedings of the National Academy of Sciences of the United States of America*, 94, no. 5 (1997): 1612–14.

81. Strand, "Where Do Classifications Come From?," 288.

82. D. L. Rosenhan, "On Being Sane in Insane Places," *Science* 179 (1973): 250–58.

83. Advocates of brain imaging contend that brain scans disprove—and not just ignore—the social construction of mental illness. Fostering drug research that reduced warehousing of the mentally ill kept at bay critics like NIMH's own sociologist-in-residence Erving Goffman, who wrote about the pathological effects of psychiatric institutions. Scull, "Mental Health Sector and the Social Sciences in Post–World War II USA Part 2." See Erving Goffman, *Asylums: Essays on the Social Situation of Mental Patients and other Inmates* (Garden City, NY: Anchor Books, 1961).

84. At the 117th meeting of the American Psychiatry Association, Kety, in the capacity of director of the Department of Psychiatry at Johns Hopkins University, echoed what others had concluded: that the dearth of basic scientific research accounted for the low prestige of psychiatry. Seymour S. Kety, "The Heuristic Aspect of Psychiatry," *American Journal of Psychiatry* 118 (1961): 385–97.

85. In the process, psychiatry had solved its "identity crisis." Robert J. Trotter, "Psychiatry for the 80's," *Science News*, 119, no. 22 (May 30, 1981): 348–49. And, indeed, the controlled clinical trial was introduced into psychiatry via

psychopharmaceuticals. Joanna Moncrieff, "An Investigation into the Precedents of Modern Drug Treatment in Psychiatry," *History of Psychiatry* 10 (1999): 477.

86. Quotation from Mitchell Wilson, "DSM-III and the Transformation of American Psychiatry: A History," *American Journal of Psychiatry* 150 (1993): 399–410. "The important thing now about achieving an indication for a drug is not that pharmaceutical companies get the rights to sell a drug, so much as that they get the power to sell the condition." David Healy, *Mania: A Short History of Bipolar Disorder* (Baltimore: Johns Hopkins University Press, 2008), 227.

87. Some would go so far as to say that biological psychiatry has been bullied into place. Christopher Mallett has argued that the proliferation of youth behavior disorders seen in successive revisions of the DSM has been due largely to the pushing of key individuals through rhetoric resting on paltry data. Christopher A. Mallett, "Behaviorally-Based Disorders: The Historical Social Construction of Youths' Most Prevalent Psychiatric Diagnoses," *History of Psychiatry* 17, no. 4 (2006): 437–60.

88. Strand, "Where Do Classifications Come From?," 299.

89. Critics ridiculed the finished guide as a "Chinese menu" approach to diagnosis, allowing mental health workers to mix and match symptoms. G. Klerman. "The Evolution of a Scientific Nosology," in *Schizophrenia: Science and Practice,* ed. J. Shershow (Cambridge, MA: Harvard University Press, 1978); Strand, "Where Do Classifications Come From?," 289, 296.

90. Breslau, review of *The Selling of DSM,* 607. See chapters 5 and 6 of Stuart A. Kirk and Herb Kutchins, *The Selling of DSM: The Rhetoric of Science in Psychiatry* (New York: Aldine De Gruyter, 1992).

91. As one example of its influence, a study found that almost all social work programs follow the DSM. Jeffrey Lacasse and Tomi Gomory, "Is Graduate Social Work Education Promoting a Critical Approach to Mental Health Practice?, *Journal of Social Work Education* 39, no. 3 (2003): 387. Strand, "Where Do Classifications Come From?," 273–313.

92. David Healy, "Psychopharmacology at the Interface between the Market and the New Biology," in *The New Brain Sciences: Perils and Prospects,* ed. Dai Rees and Steven Rose (Cambridge: Cambridge University Press, 2004), 241.

93. Healy, *Creation of Psychopharmacology,* 311.

94. Allan Horwitz, *Creating Mental Illness* (Chicago: University of Chicago Press, 2002), 212.

95. Alan Schwarz, "The Selling of Attention Deficit Disorder," *New York Times,* December 14, 2013.

96. Following in the footsteps of the Congressional Report *Action for Mental Health* (1961), which called for the dissemination of mental health knowledge, the National Clearinghouse for Mental Health Information was set up in 1963 in response to a "study of communication problems in all fields of science and medicine by the Senate committee on government operations. Moreover, the House appropriations committee had expressed interest in seeing NIMH expand its efforts to disseminate information." From Julius Segal, editor-in-chief, *Research in the Service of Mental Health,* 17. See also Grob and Goldman *Dilemma of Federal Mental Health Policy,* 28–29.

97. In the 1970s and early 1980s, for example, NIMH taped a regular fifteen-minute public service radio program called *Mental Health Matters.* Listeners heard Dr.

Mitchell Balter of the Psychopharmacology Section describe the range of psychotropic medications available and Dr. Carl Merril of the Lab of General and Comparative Biochemistry discuss mental disorders with a demonstrated genetic component. Select recordings of "Mental Health Matters" are available on long-playing vinyl records at the National Institute of Mental Health, Science Writing, Press, and Dissemination Branch.

98. Bertram Brown, "A Brief History of Psychoactive Drugs" (draft of an article for the Alabama Department of Mental Health Bulletin), ca. 1967, National Institute of Mental Health Science Writing, Press, and Dissemination Branch, room 6200, MSC 9663, Bethesda, MD. I hasten to add that Brown was personally exceedingly receptive to other forms of treatment. See my article, Brian Casey, "The Surgical Elimination of Violence? Conflicting Attitudes towards Technology and Science during the Psychosurgery Controversy of the 1970s," *Science in Context* 28, no. 1 (March 2015): 99–129.

99. National Institute of Mental Health, unpublished document, dated March 31, 1967, National Institute of Mental Health Science Writing, Press, and Dissemination Branch, room 6200, MSC 9663, Bethesda, MD.

100. The real men, real depression campaign ran from 2003 to 2005 and is described on the NIMH's website at http://www.nimh.nih.gov/health/topics/depression/men-and-depression/background-on-education-materials.shtml. Depression was defined during this campaign at "Men and Depression," National Institute of Mental Health, accessed December 15, 2016, http://www.nimh.nih.gov/health/publications/men-and-depression/index.shtml.

101. As an example of how biological psychiatry has shaken up nosology, advances in genetics have blurred the boundaries of bipolar and schizophrenia. "A twin study uncovered genes that conferred susceptibility to both disorders as well as genes conferring risk for bipolar disorder but not for schizophrenia and vice versa." McNally, *What Is Mental Illness?*, 159, 171.

102. Swazey, *Chlorpromazine in Psychiatry*, 255–56, quotes from the conclusion of a 1956 NIMH collaborative study group report on chlorpromazine and acute schizophrenia: "The evidence from this study confirms the diverse and generalized effect of phenothiazines on the schizophrenic process. Almost all symptoms and manifestations characteristic of schizophrenic psychoses improved with drug therapy, suggesting that the phenothiazines should be regarded as 'antischizophrenic' in the broad sense. In fact, it is questionable whether the term 'tranquilizer' should be retained." Healy points out that when psychotropic medicines, specifically chlorpromazine, first came out, clinicians regarded their effect to be nonspecific. Healy, *Creation of Psychopharmacology*, 279. The push to see psychopharmaceuticals as agents targeting particular mental illnesses came from the requirements for drug approval. Horwitz, *Creating Mental Illness*, 210–11.

103. Quoted in Luhrmann, *Of Two Minds*, 170.

104. Sketched in a 1964 press release and described in greater detail in Swazey, *Chlorpromazine in Psychiatry*, 235, 245, 246. The patients were given chlorpromazine, flupheniazine, thioridazine, or controls.

105. Kety conveys excitement about the biological approach, and yet he recognizes the legitimacy of other approaches in Seymour S. Kety, "A Biologist Examines the Mind and Behavior," *Science* 132, no. 3443 (December 23, 1960): 1861–70. At the

end of his life, Kety was awarded the prestigious Lasker Award in 1999 for Special Achievement in Medical Science for his "visionary leadership in mental health that ushered psychiatry into the molecular age," http://www.laskerfoundation.org/awards/1999_s_description.htm.

106. Seymour S. Kety, "It's Not All in Your Head," *Saturday Review*, February 21, 1976, 28–32. "There are now substantial indications," the article began, "that serious mental illnesses derive from chemical, rather than psychological, imbalances."

107. Seymour S. Kety, "Disorders of the Human Brain," *Scientific American* 241, no. 3 (1979): 202–14.

108. Snyder, *Madness and the Brain*, 241ff. Arvid Carlsson, "Historical Perspective of the Chemistry and Pharmacological Treatment of Schizophrenia," in *Handbook of Schizophrenia*, vol. 2, *Neurochemistry and Neuropharmacology of Schizophrenia*, ed. F. A. Herm and L. E. DeLisi (Amsterdam: Elsevier Science Publishers B.V., 1987), 1–15. The future Nobel Prize winner was a visiting scientist at the National Heart Institute.

109. Snyder, *Madness and the Brain*, 252; Arvid Carlsson, "The Dopamine Hypothesis of Schizophrenia 20 Years Later," in *Search for the Cause of Schizophrenia*, ed. H. Häffler, W. F. Gattaz, and W. Janzarik (Berlin: Springer-Verlag, 1987), 223–35.

110. Snyder, *Madness and the Brain*, 169.

111. Ibid., 92.

112. *Discovering Yourself in the Brain Age: Journey to the Universe of Inner Space* (US Department of Health, Education, and Welfare Public Health Service National Institutes of Health DHEW publication no (NIH) 72-330).

113. Videos of television spots, interviews, and recorded symposia in which NIMH researchers mention their training and the shift in worldview are available at the National Library of Medicine, Bethesda, MD. This fits an accepted metanarrative. "Psychiatric science is now configured," the anthropologist Tanya Luhrmann has noted, "at least for many of the more senior scientists, as a rejection of the psychodynamic approach to mental illness. . . . Many of the more senior scientists (particularly those who went to medical school when the psychoanalytic model still dominated psychiatry) tell their career story around that turning point." Luhrmann, *Of Two Minds*, 172.

114. A good example is National Institutes of Health, Neuroscience and Mental Illness [electronic resource], R. Wyatt (Bethesda, MD: National Institutes of Health, 2001), https://www.nimh.nih.gov/site-info/citing-nimh-information-and-publications. shtml, a celebration of NIMH "favorite son" Richard Wyatt, a pioneer in bringing neuroscience to the problem of mental illness, http://videocast.nih.gov/launch. asp?10011. See particularly the comments of Daniel Weinberger and the first speaker, http://videocast.nih.gov/launch.asp?10481.

115. See, for example, Swedo's November 2013 testimonial on youtube, http://www.youtube.com/watch?v=jVP0eUjtDnk.

116. Filmmaker's Library, Inc., *Untangling the Mind: The Legacy of Dr. Heinz Lehmann*, videorecording produced in association with Discovery Channel Canada and Green Lion Productions Inc. New York: Filmmakers Library, © 1999.

117. Segal, editor-in-chief, *Research in the Service of Mental Health*, 384, admits that the dissemination of information was partly triggered by public disenchantment and threatened reduction of funds.

118. Formed in 1998, the Office of Constituency Relations and Public Liaison "convenes a series of regular meetings with representatives from over 100 patient advocacy, professional, and scientific community based organizations." "Alliance for Research Progress," National Institute of Mental Health, accessed December 15, 2016 http://www.nimh.nih.gov/outreach/alliance/index.shtml. An overview of this office can be found at NIMH's website, http://www.nimh.nih.gov/health/outreach. At such events, the preference for the biological approach is evident in its focus on the study of brain changes and the hunt for biomarkers.

119. This view of NIMH as leading the way out of the darkness is most clearly seen in the talk by the NIMH director Stanley Yolles, "From Witchcraft and Sorcery to Head Shrinking: Society's Concern about Mental Health" (address, 12th HEW Forum, Washington, DC, May 8, 1968). In this talk, Yolles makes clear his support for community mental health to tackle a broad range of aggravating social problems, but also asks, "By brain stimulation or drug regimen will we erase depression and sedate mania?"

120. In one of its official historical overviews, however, NIMH admits that its priorities have been unavoidably affected by the wider political scene, including the expansive view of the 1960s Great Society and the constrictive backlash of the New Federalism of the 1970s. Segal, editor-in-chief, *Research in the Service of Mental Health*, 18, 26.

121. According to NIMH, it was pushed into becoming a broadcaster. "Both the intramural and extramural programs . . . maintained a low-key attitude toward such dissemination." Ibid.

122. Excerpt from testimony given by Hillary Rodham Clinton and Steven Hyman to the White House Conference on Mental Health, June 7, 1999, Washington, DC, from Tamara L. Roleff and Laura K. Egendof, eds., *Mental Illness: Opposing Viewpoints* (New York: Greenhaven Press, 2000).

123. Karl Popper, *The Logic of Scientific Discovery* (New York: Routledge, 1992).

124. Ross J Baldessarini, "American Biological Psychiatry and Psychopharmacology 1944–1994," in *American Psychiatry after World War II, 1944–94*, ed. Roy Menninger and John Nemiah, 396 (Washington, DC: American Psychiatric Press, 2000).

125. For a list of biological psychiatry milestones see Baldessarini, "American Biological Psychiatry and Psychopharmacology, 1944–1994," 374–75.

126. Simon Cohn, "Disrupting Images: Neuroscientific Representations in the Lives of Psychiatric Patients," in *Critical Neuroscience: A Handbook of the Social and Cultural Contexts of Neuroscience* (Chichester, UK: Blackwell, 2012).

127. The words are Luhrmann's in *Of Two Minds*, 212.

128. *The Diagnostic and Statistical Manual of Mental Disorders*, 5th ed. (Washington, DC: American Psychiatric Association, 2013).

129. US Department of Health and Human Services, *Mental Health: A Report of the Surgeon General* (Rockville, MD: US Department of Health and Human Services, Substance Abuse and Mental Health Services Administration, 1999). There exists, for example, a chasm between genes and behavior. Horwitz, *Creating Mental Illness*, 147–48.

130. One such critic is David Levy; see his comments in Stuart Kirk and Susan Einbinder, *Controversial Issues in Mental Health* (Boston: Allyn and Bacon, 1994), 168–73.

131. Michael E. Thase, Joel B. Greenhouse, Ellen Frank, Charles F. Reynolds III et al., "Treatment of Major Depression with Psychotherapy or Psychotherapy-Pharmacotherapy Combinations," *Archives of General Psychiatry* 54 (1997): 1009–15, reported that psychotherapy was equally as effective in treating minor depression. In a three-year study of 128 depressed patients, investigators found that psychotherapy produced the longest span between depressive episodes. See also J. Shedler, "The Efficacy of Psychodynamic Psychotherapy," *American Psychologist* 65, no. 2 (2010): 98–109.

132. "Effective treatments for obsessive-compulsive disorder, whether the serotonin reuptake inhibitor fluoxetine or behavior therapy, appear to decrease cerebral metabolic rates in the head of the right caudate nucleus." Glen O. Gabbard, "A Neurobiologically Informed Perspective on Psychotherapy," *British Journal of Psychiatry* 177 (2000): 117–22. Similarly, "In a now famous study of obsessive-compulsive disorder, patients were given either medication (Anafranil) or psychotherapy. If a patient improved, his brain scan changed, and the scan changed in the same way regardless of whether drugs or talk was used." Luhrmann, *Of Two Minds*, 209, referring to Lewis Baxter, Jeffrey M. Schwartz, Kenneth S. Bergman, Martin P. Szuba et al., "Caudate Glucose Metabolic Rate Changes with Both Drug and Behavior Therapy for Obsessive-Compulsive Disorder," *Archives of General Psychiatry* 49 (1992): 681–89.

133. Lacasse and Gomory, "Is Graduate Social Work Education Promoting a Critical Approach to Mental Health Practice?," 383–408.

134. Jonathan Shedler, "The Efficacy of Psychodynamic Psychotherapy," *American Psychologist* 65, no. 2 (2010): 98–109, discusses how the psychodynamic research is buried in technical metastudies and not distilled so that even practitioners of psychodynamic approaches are ignorant of them.

135. The concern about such a possible mistranslation was voiced already in the heyday of psychoanalysis. Wilfred Bloomberg, ed., *Psychiatry, the Press, and the Public: Problems in Communication* (Washington, DC: American Psychiatric Association, 1956), 50.

136. Lawrence C. Kolb, Shervert H. Frazier, and Paul Sirovatka, "The National Institute of Mental Health: Its Influence on Psychiatry and the Nation's Mental Health" in *American Psychiatry after World War II, 1944–94*, ed. Roy Menninger and John Nemiah, 208 (Washington, DC: American Psychiatric Press, 2000).

137. Gaps such as the difference between the calculated heritability of a major mental illness and its frequency. Current estimates of heritability are for schizophrenia 50 percent, bipolar 65–90 percent, and anxiety disorder 30–40 percent. McNally, *What Is Mental Illness?*, 160.

Coda

Technique, Marginality, and History

Katja Guenther

As Delia Gavrus and Stephen Casper point out in their Introduction, technique is crucial to the success and prominence of the contemporary neurosciences.[1] In their day-to-day work, the latter rely on an astonishing array of techniques—technologies and practices—to produce, disseminate, and promote their research. Since the early 1980s, scientists have used positron emission tomography (PET) and functional magnetic resonance imaging (fMRI) to correlate mental states such as hunger, love, even religiosity, to physiological changes in specific regions of the brain; these machines provide evidence of the mind "at work."[2] Psychoactive drugs can similarly be seen as technologies for producing changes in both physiological and psychological functions. They thus lend support to the idea that the brain is the ultimate substrate of the mind. In addition, technique plays a central role in neuroscientific funding. To give a recent and extreme example, in 2014 the European Commission awarded the Human Brain Project (HBP) more than one billion Euros to be spent over the next decade. The large sum was justified in part by the need to develop new techniques, including neuromorphic computing and neurorobotics. Technique has thus been instrumental in crowning neuroscience queen of the sciences. It is now a reference point for other academic disciplines from across the social sciences and the humanities, which seek to ground, or at least inform, their work through the results of neuroscientific research.[3]

The close relationship between the neurosciences and technique is not simply a contemporary phenomenon; technique has been important throughout their history. But while in the early twenty-first century, technique seems intimately related to the centrality of the neurosciences, once we shift our attention to the past a curious transformation occurs. It is telling that the essays in this volume relate technique, almost without exception, to the marginal. The relationship between centrality and marginality should not be posed in starkly oppositional terms. As Gavrus and Casper note, the marginal, or "that which . . . appears unusual, unimportant, insufficient, minor, insignificant, on the edge, on the sidelines, [or] flat out wrong" (16), is a shifting category. What appears marginal to us today might well have been central in the past and conversely, what seems central now could well have been marginal earlier. Indeed it is the mismatch between present and past assessments of marginality that can lead to the most egregious of historical sins: teleology, where the historian projects our current understandings of what is central onto a period with very different priorities. Historicizing the marginal thus makes us better historians. The study of technique, I would like to argue, can be helpful in this project.

In "The Question Concerning Technology," Martin Heidegger analyzed technology in a way that draws out its relationships with both history and marginality. Inquiring into the "essence" of technology, Heidegger rejects the conventional "instrumental" understanding, that it is simply a means to an end.[4] Technology is better considered in Aristotelian terms, where four "responsibilities" or causes contribute to the production of an artifact. The four causes together are responsible for "bringing-forth," or "presencing" something: the material cause is the matter out of which a chalice is made; the formal cause provides its shape; the final cause is the rite in which the chalice will be used; and the efficient cause is the force that brings about the finished product, the silversmith. The chalice is thus not "made" by the silversmith; rather, the four causes are co-responsible for the chalice's production, for "revealing" it.[5] In Heidegger's language, technology is a form of revealing.

Heidegger's meditations on technology apply to technique more generally and help us think through its relationship to marginality. If technique reveals, the object on which it works must initially be concealed. But of course to be the object of technique, that object must also exist in some close relationship to the technique being applied and the scientific field applying it. Simultaneously hidden and proximate, the object of technique lies at the outer edges of a scientific field. Stated differently, technique finds its privileged object in the marginal.

The application of technique to the marginal can take two forms, depending upon the particular relationship between what is revealed and the focus of the historical actors doing the revealing. First, technique can work on the marginal *epistemologically*, as a means to learn about something else. In this way, though technique makes the marginal object visible, that object remains subordinate to something else, and thus marginal.

Stephen Jacyna, in his essay, describes the ways in which animals were observed in the menageries of postrevolutionary France. The naturalist

Georges Cuvier and his associates had constructed the modern menagerie in opposition to its prerevolutionary predecessor and emphasized their differences: the Jardin des Plantes and the Natural History Museum in Paris were no longer establishments of luxury, but of utility. Ostentation had been replaced by the systematic and controlled study of nature. The zoo was now an apparatus for making the animals visible and revealing their behavior. This goal informed the structure of the buildings and grounds in the Jardin. It included a variety of structures to house an enormous range of species from across the world: lions, bears, an elephant, a giraffe, a North American bison, camels, zebras, ostriches, cassowaries, and several primates and monkeys. The buildings were designed to be attractive to visitors wishing to observe animals casually, but most importantly they were designed to facilitate observation by naturalists, "mak[ing] the animals as visible as possible" (27). According to Cuvier, it was only in captivity that animals could be systematically observed and experimented upon.

Moreover, at least for Cuvier, in contradistinction to humans, animals were endowed with an immutable essence. Captivity would not sufficiently change their behavior to render, as one might have suspected, the observation useless. That is why for many, the controlled conditions at the Jardin des Plantes produced more reliable accounts of animal behavior than those furnished by "voyagers" traveling to study them in their natural state. The Jardin was thus crucial to a technique that made these animals the objects of scientific observation. It allowed a new set of scientific truths to be tested. For example, the premise that a lion "fears the crow of the cock and the grunting of the pig" was refuted by the experiment of placing these animals near the lion. The lions showed little fear and promptly ate their noisy visitors (28).

What is crucial about Jacyna's argument is that this process of revealing was not structured by the goal of learning more about animals. Animals remained marginal to the true object of knowledge. As Jacyna points out, at each moment "the discourse returned to the question of how the animal mind compared to that of humans" (35). The main motivation for studying "animal intelligence" was the researchers' interest in the human. The exact boundaries between animal and human intelligence were of course contested, but there was agreement over the utility of comparison. Just as the anatomy of the brain was best studied comparatively, so too, the argument went, the brain's product, intelligence, was best made visible when it was placed alongside that of other mammals. The technique of the menagerie was thus not aimed simply at making visible the marginal (animals), but to use them to shed light on what really mattered: the human.

The newly visible animals remain marginal in Jacyna's chapter, but elsewhere in the volume visibility and centrality are closely correlated. This opens a second possibility for the relationship between technique and marginality: technique could affect the marginal in a *transformative* sense. Of course, these efforts toward transformation might not always succeed. In Delia Gavrus's chapter, we learn about Edward Dockrill, a technician in the laboratory of the prominent neurosurgeon Wilder Penfield in the 1920s and 1930s. Dockrill's neurohistological technique offered support for the existence of intracerebral vascular nerves, thus helping to confirm Penfield and Foerster's theory that the vaso-motor reflex was a cause of epileptic attacks. As Gavrus shows, however, the surgical therapies that were based on this technique failed to improve the condition of patients, and this resulted in the sidelining of the theory. In Gavrus's chapter, technique failed in another, less obvious way. Dockrill wrote a semiautobiographical novel that recounted his move from England to North America, his work in Penfield's lab as a young man, and most importantly, his growing disillusion about the lack of acknowledgment for his work. With the novel, the "invisible" (and we should note "marginal") technician set out to "prove his worth" to the world (188). Writing the book thus was a technique aimed at drawing the marginal technician onto center stage. Here the technique failed too; when Dockrill sent the manuscript out to a publishing house, it was rejected.

But in many essays, we can see how the transformation actually succeeds. In Max Stadler's account, for instance, the technique of alternating currents participated in a larger process of moving nerves into the center of investigation for the biophysicists. Previously, researchers with an interest in the properties of "electrical things" (69) used direct currents to investigate them. But direct current stimulation was a fairly blunt tool. It allowed in most cases only the stimulation of different tissues and then the recording of the results, which raised a number of difficult methodological and interpretative questions. Thus, when the "domestication" (73) of alternating currents became possible within the context of the radio age, scientists began to leave direct current behind. Alternating currents allowed the development of techniques that "made salient a range of different electro-physiological effects and properties" that were "different from the typical electrophysiological roster" (74). Using alternating currents of different frequencies, scientists were able to develop a whole range of interventions, therapeutic, diagnostic, and surgical. But in order to make use of these possibilities, Stadler argues, scientists had to consider the objects to which they were applying the alternating currents as a kind of circuit. This brought a whole new range of research objects to light that fit the model. Whereas previously a broad set of materials—including tumor breast cells, algae, and whipped cream—had constituted the arsenal of the biophysicist, those materials were now displaced by nerves, which seemed to resemble better the constituent parts of electric circuits. Alternating-current techniques had made the circuit-like properties of nerves visible, and thus brought this previously marginal object to the center of neurological research.

Similarly, a range of techniques was used to make a "biomedical paradigm" central in neurological research. Thomas Schlich shows how surgeons mobilized the resources of experimental physiology in an attempt to legitimate increasingly radical surgical procedures on a particularly sensitive subject, the brain and nervous system; laboratory methods and techniques—used practically but also rhetorically—thus promoted a new "physiological surgery," which in turn helped turn neurosurgery into a broadly accepted medical specialty. Brian Casey illustrates the means by which NIMH scientists used scientific rhetoric as a technique for establishing the biomedical paradigm at their institution, fending off attacks on the psychiatric profession and moving a newly somaticized psychiatry into the medical mainstream. And Justin Garson shows how medical scientists managed to make schizophrenia more "real" by using the technique of symptom reconceptualization—jigging around which symptoms were "essential" and which only secondary—in a way that allowed doctors to integrate the disease into the biomedical paradigm.

Heidegger's reconceptualization of technique as revelation is, however, only one part of his argument. In his essay he is particularly concerned with modern technology. This has its own mode of revealing, which is not simply "bringing-forth" but rather what he calls "challenging."[6] In contrast to the work of a peasant cultivating and maintaining the soil, the modern technology of mining challenges it "into the putting out of coal and ore."[7] In this process, technological revealing acquires a new dimension, which puts the object into a state that Heidegger calls "standing-reserve."[8] It is this standing-reserve that makes the object appear for us in a different light. We no longer look at the soil with respect and admiration, seeing it as something in its own right, but think of it in terms of efficiency and in relation to its potential use. In this sense, revelation cannot be seen simply as the opposite of concealing; concealment is a constitutive part of revelation. The way in which modern technology eclipses other ways of seeing informs Heidegger's *Technologiekritik*. Modern technology precludes the type of "bringing-forth" that previous forms of technique allowed, and this process has potentially disastrous consequences for humanity, in terms of our relationship to the environment, to each other, and to ourselves. As Heidegger intoned in a famous 1966 interview, "Only a god can still save us."[9]

I am not concerned with this more dystopic aspect of Heidegger's work here. Nevertheless, his attentiveness to the way in which technology can hide as much as it reveals is fruitful for thinking about technology and technique in the brain and mind sciences. Take the example of model building at the 1951 Festival of Britain that Stephen Casper describes in his chapter. The plastic and metal models were designed as a technique for making the physical structure of the universe visible to the spectators, and thus promoted a materialistic worldview. By successively magnifying objects such as crystals as the visitors moved from one exhibition room through to the next, the creators allowed visitors to see the atomic structures of these objects. But it is clear that the process of revelation also required a form of nonvisibility. By casting the atoms of a crystal in a large material model, the scientists allowed great distortions in size, presenting the atoms out of all proportion to their actual existence. To allow "the nucleus of the atom and its surrounding electrons [to] spread all around [the visitor]" (58), the model had to deliberately obscure scale. In fact, it was this process of hiding that led to the Alice-in-Wonderland effect, which the scientists describe.

And because technique can also hide, it can effect a transformation that is the inverse of the one we have described above: it allows that which is central to be marginalized. In Casey's chapter, he shows how the rhetoric of the NIMH scientists allowed them to hide their ignorance about biological mechanisms that were central to the reductionist paradigm. As discussed earlier, Casey outlines a general shift in the 1970s from psychodynamic approaches and explanations—focusing on defense mechanisms and unconscious conflicts—to biological models and treatments. The NIMH helped cement this shift by promoting research at the levels of psychotropic drugs, genetics, psychiatric nosology, and brain imaging. As Casey points out, however, this happened despite the fact that NIMH scientists were acutely aware of and discussed a number of scientific setbacks and doubts about the biological approach. They knew, for example, that early drugs for depression essentially functioned as placebos, that a sizable percentage of bipolar patients did not respond to lithium, and that medicated schizophrenic patients tended to relapse in large numbers. They also knew that the theories regarding the mode of action of these drugs were unfounded. And yet they employed a variety of "rhetorical strategies" (224) to promote the biomedical paradigm: they advertised the biological approach through press releases and media broadcasts and they emphasized the cost-effectiveness of the new paradigm, its potential to destigmatize, and its scientific nature. It was through the technique of rhetoric then, as Casey concludes, that the ignorance of the researchers was concealed: "Rhetoric can serve as a placeholder, sustaining belief until science fills in gaping knowledge gaps" (242). Similarly, in the other two essays on the biomedical paradigm, the ability of technique to obscure or to elide was crucial to its functioning. In the case of neurosurgery, it was used to downplay the radicality and foreignness of this type of surgery, and schizophrenia researchers used their medical expertise to deemphasize previously important symptoms in order to make the disease fit their biomedical hypothesis.

But most importantly, technique also hides itself. Indeed what made the rhetoric of the NIMH scientists so successful was that it was not presented, nor universally recognized, as (mere) rhetoric. Similarly, the Alice-in-Wonderland effect at the Festival of Britain was built upon the momentary forgetting that spectators were actually dealing with a model. In addition to hiding the dimension of space, the model was hiding itself qua model from the visitors.

It is perhaps because of the way in which technique tends to obscure as much as it reveals that history can be important. In the broadest sense, history is itself a technique, revealing what has been lost or forgotten. But in the case of the essays in this volume, history is better considered as a sort of second-order technique: it can reveal what techniques in the past have hidden, undoing techniques or revealing how they worked.

First, history can reveal those things that are hidden by a technique and yet are crucial for understanding its work and function. As we saw, for the scientists at the Festival of Britain, the technique of model building made visible to the spectators the physical structure of the universe. But Casper is able to read the technique of the historical actors to unearth concepts and presuppositions that undergird them. As he argues, such analysis reveals unexpressed dualisms at the heart of their materialist program. The illusionary techniques employed by the exhibition scientists—visual techniques such as motion pictures, animated diagrams, stereoscopic photographs, in addition to the increasingly magnified 3-D models of matter—were techniques of the mind that "induced a state of knowledge in attendees" (57). Because scientists at the festival propagated a reductive materialism, that is, a monist worldview, dualisms for them had the status of the marginal. And yet, as Casper shows, those dualisms nonetheless remained active in their endeavors.

Second, history can recover those things that were central in the past but have since lost their centrality. In fact, one of the curiosities of choosing technique as an analytic focus is that it makes us engage with aspects of the mind and brain sciences that rarely occupy the center of our historical research. The Festival of Britain is an unusual space for historians of the mind and brain sciences, as is the postrevolutionary menagerie; the luggage of émigré scientists is an unfamiliar lens through which to study (neuro) scientific migration (Stahnisch); and bibliography is an uncommon tool to analyze neurological disease (Kroker).

Finally, history can unpick what techniques have achieved to reveal those results as achievements. As Casey's example shows, we need historical analysis to "undo" the move from a psychodynamic to a biological paradigm within psychiatry. By revealing the rhetorical nature of the biological paradigm— revealing, that is, the role it played in transforming the field—it is possible to the historian to reconstruct the move away from psychodynamic approaches and thus help make biological psychiatry appear less absolute than many today take it to be. By revealing the transformative role of technique, it helps us undo teleologies that take these transformations to be natural or inevitable. Similarly, in Stadler's chapter, we learn that alternating currents moved previously marginal nerves into the center of biophysical investigation. The historical study of technique, and the way in which it shifts our understanding of the marginal, can bring to our attention the contingency and the work involved in scientific developments. It thus allows us "to conjure up a different, less brain-centered image of the neuroscientific past" (71).

But if we understand history itself as a technique, we also need to confront the suggestion that it too might be involved in a process of hiding, not least its own status as technique. Understood as a technique, history is a tool used by contemporary actors for particular purposes. That is, while we are never fully bound to the constructions of our age—the historian tries at least to undo certain presentisms (the presentism of biological reductionism, of the immutable and fixed brain, etc.)—the attempt to release ourselves from these constructions is still a contemporary project. Historicism and presentism are not opposed, but inextricably linked. And thus even when we as historians use our discipline's techniques to rescue the marginal from retrospective disdain, we should never lose sight of the fact that we do this in and for the present.

Notes

I would like to thank Edward Baring, Stephen Casper, Delia Gavrus and Erika Milam for their thoughtful comments and suggestions.

1. See the Introduction for a discussion of the terms *technique, technology*, and *techne* and their relationship.

2. Michael Hagner, ed., *Der Geist bei der Arbeit: Historische Untersuchungen zur Hirnforschung* (Göttingen: Wallstein, 2006); Cornelius Borck, "Recording the Brain at Work: The Visible, the Readable, and the Invisible in Electroencephalography," *Journal of the History of the Neurosciences* 17 (2008): 367–79.

3. See especially Nikolas Rose and Joelle Abi-Rached, *Neuro: the New Brain Sciences and the Management of the Mind* (Princeton, NJ: Princeton University Press, 2013); Melissa Littlefield and Jenell Johnson, *The Neuroscientific Turn: Transdisciplinarity in the Age of the Brain* (Ann Arbor: University of Michigan Press, 2012); and Suparna Choudhury and Jan Slaby, ed., *Critical Neuroscience: A Handbook of the Social and Cultural Contexts of Neuroscience* (Chichester, UK: Wiley-Blackwell, 2012).

4. Martin Heidegger, "The Question Concerning Technology," in *The Question Concerning Technology and Other Essays*, trans. William Lovitt, 3–35 (New York: Garland, 1977).

5. Ibid., 11.

6. Ibid., 14.

7. Ibid.

8. Ibid., 17.

9. "Nur noch ein Gott kann uns retten," *Der Spiegel*, May 31, 1976, 193–219. The interview with Rudolf Augstein and Georg Wolff took place on September 23, 1966.

Bibliography

A. and W. Galignani and Co. *Galignani's New Paris Guide*. Paris: A. and W. Galignani and Co., 1839.

Abella, Irving, and Harold Troper. *None Is Too Many: Canada and the Jews of Europe: 1933–1948*. Toronto: University of Toronto Press, 1982.

Abir-Am, Pnina. "The Biotheoretical Gathering, Trans-disciplinary Authority and the Incipient Legitimation of Molecular Biology in the 1930s: New Perspective on the Historical Sociology of Science." *History of Science* 25 (1987): 1–70.

———. "The Discourse of Physical Power and Biological Knowledge in the 1930s: A Reappraisal of the Rockefeller Foundation's 'Policy' in Molecular Biology." *Social Studies of Sciences* 12, no. 3 (1987): 341–82.

Abraham, T. "From Theory to Data: Representing Neurons in the 1940s." *Biology and Philosophy* 18 no. 3 (2003): 415–26.

Achelis, J. D. "Kritische Bemerkungen Zur Chronaxiebestimmung Am Menschen." *Zeitschrift Für Neurologie* 130, nos. 5–6 (1933): 227–47.

Adrian, E. D. *The Basis of Sensation: The Action of the Sense Organs*. London: Hafner, 1928.

———. *The Mechanism of Nervous Action: Electrical Studies of the Neurone*. Philadelphia: Pennsylvania University Press, 1932.

Albright, D. A., T. M. Jessel, and Eric R. Kandel. "Neural Science: A Century of Progress and the Mysteries That Remain." *Neuron* 25 (2000): 1–55.

American Psychiatric Association. *DSM-5*. Washington, DC: Americal Psychiatric Publishing, 2013.

Amsterdamska, Olga. "Demarcating Epidemiology." *Science, Technology, & Human Values* 30 (2005): 17–51.

Anctil, Michel. *Dawn of the Neuron: The Early Struggles to Trace the Origin of Nervous Systems*. Montreal: McGill-Queen's University Press, 2015.

Angrist, B. M., and S. Gershon. "Amphetamine Abuse in New York City—1966 to 1968." *Seminars in Psychiatry* 1, no. 2 (1969): 195–207.

———. "Amphetamine Induced Schizophreniform Psychosis." In *Schizophrenia: Current Concepts and Research*, edited by D. V. S. Sankar, 508–24. Hicksville, NY: PJD Publications, 1969.

———. "The Phenomenology of Experimentally Induced Amphetamine Psychosis: Preliminary Observations." *Biological Psychiatry* 2 (1970): 95–107.

———. "Psychiatric Sequelae of Medical Drugs." In *Psychiatric Complications of Medical Drugs*, edited by R. I. Shader, 175–99. New York: Raven Press, 1972.

Angrist, B. M., B. Shopsin, and S. Gershon. "Comparative Psychotomimetic Effects of Stereoisomers of Amphetamine." *Nature* 234 (1971): 152–53.

Angrist, B. M., H. K. Lee, and S. Gershon. "The Antagonism of Amphetamine-Induced Symptomatology by a Neuroleptic." *American Journal of Psychiatry* 131 (1974): 817–19.

Anonymous. "In Memoriam. Martin Silberberg. 1895–1969." *Gerontologia* 16 no. 4 (1970)): 199–200.

Armitage, David. "What's the Big Idea? Intellectual History and the Longue Durée." *History of European Ideas* 38, no. 4 (2012): 493–507.

Armstrong, Charles. "Postvaccinal Encephalitis." *Public Health Reports* 44 (1929): 2041–44.

Ash, Mitchell G. *Gestalt Psychology in German Culture, 1890–1967: Holism and the Quest for Objectivity.* Cambridge: Cambridge University Press, 1995.

Ash, Mitchell, and Alfons Soellner, eds. *Forced Migration and Scientific Change: Émigré German-Speaking Scientists after 1933.* Cambridge: Cambridge University Press, 1996.

Association for Research in Nervous and Mental Disease. *Acute Epidemic Encephalitis (Lethargic Encephalitis): An Investigation by the Association for Research in Nervous and Mental Diseases.* New York: Paul B. Hoeber, 1921.

Atkinson, Harriet. *The Festival of Britain: A Land and Its People.* London: I. B. Tauris, 2012.

Barbara, Jean-Gaël. "Interplay between Scientific Theories and Researches on the Diseases of the Nervous System in the Nineteenth Century, Paris." *Medicine Studies* 1, no. 4 (2009): 339–52.

———. "The Physiological Construction of the Neurone Concept (1891–1952)." *Comptes Rendus Biologies* 329, nos. 5–6 (2006): 437–49.

Barber, Charles. *Comfortably Numb: How Psychiatry Is Medicating a Nation.* New York: Pantheon Books, 2008.

Barberis, Daniela S. "Changing Practices of Commemoration in Neurology: Comparing Charcot's 1925 and 1993 Centennials." *Osiris* 14 (1999): 102–17.

Barchas, Jack D., Glen R Elliott, Philip A. Berger, Patricia R. Barchas et al. "The Ultimate Stigma: Inadequate Funding for Research on Mental Illness and Addictive Disorders." *American Journal of Psychiatry* 142 (1985): 838–39.

Barnes, Deborah M. "Biological Issues in Schizophrenia." *Science* 235, no. 4787 (January 23, 1987): 430–33.

Bateman, J. B. "Mitogenetic Radiation." *Biological Reviews and Biological Proceedings of the Cambridge Philosophical Society* 10, no. 1 (1935): 42–71.

Baumeister, Alan, and Mike Hawkins. "The Serotonin Hypothesis of Schizophrenia." *Journal of the History of the Neurosciences* 13, no. 3 (2004): 277–91.

Bear, R. S., F. O. Schmitt, and J. Z. Young. "The Sheath Components of the Giant Nerve Fibres of the Squid." *Proceedings of the Royal Society of London*, series B, 123, no. 833 (1937): 496–504.

Bechtel, W. *Mental Mechanisms: Philosophical Perspectives on Cognitive Neuroscience.* New York: Taylor and Francis, 2008.

Bell, D. S. "Comparison of Amphetamine Psychosis and Schizophrenia." *British Journal of Psychiatry* 111 (1965): 701–7.

Bennett, Max R. *A History of the Synapse.* London: Taylor and Francis, 2001.

Berg, Marc, and Paul Harterink. "Embodying the Patient: Records and Bodies in Early 20th-Century US Medical Practice." *Body & Society* 10 (2004): 13–41.

Berge, Ann La. "The History of Science and the History of Microscopy." *Perspectives on Science* 7, no. 1 (1999): 111–42.

Bergmann, Ernst von. *Die Chirurgische Behandlung von Hirnkrankheiten*. Vol. 2. Berlin: Hirschwald, 1889.

———. "Die Gruppierung der Wundkrankheiten." *Berliner klinische Wochenschrift* 19 (1882): 677–79, 701–3.

Berkowitz, Edward. *To Improve Human Health: A History of the Institute of Medicine*. Washington, DC, 1998. http://www.nap.edu/books/0309061881/html .

Bernard, Claude. *Introduction à l'étude de la médecine expérimentale*. Paris: J.-B. Baillière, 1865.

———. *Introduction to the Study of Experimental Medicine*. Translated by Henry Copley Greene. New York: Dover, 1957.

Bhattacharya, Sanjoy. *Expunging Variola: The Control and Eradication of Smallpox in India, 1947–1977*. London: Orient Blackswan, 2006.

Billroth, Theodor. *Die allgemeine chirurgische Pathologie und Therapie in fünfzig Vorlesungen: ein Handbuch für Studierende und Aerzte*. Berlin: Reimer, 1869.

Binger, Carl A. L., and Ronald V. Christie. "An Experimental Study of Diathermy." *Journal of Experimental Medicine* 46, no. 4 (1927): 571–72.

Bleuler, E. *Dementia Praecox or the Group of Schizophrenias*. New York: International Universities Press, 1950.

Bliss, Michael. *Harvey Cushing: A Life in Surgery*. New York: Oxford University Press, 2005.

Board on Mental Health and Behavioral Medicine, Institute of Medicine. *Research on Mental Illness and Addictive Discorders: Progress and Prospects*. Washington, DC: National Academy Press, 1984.

Boodman, Sandra G. "A Horrible Place & A Wonderful Place." *Washington Post Magazine*, October 8, 1989, W18.

Borck, Cornelius. "Between Local Cultures and National Styles: Units of Analysis in the History of Electroencephalography." *Comptes Rendus Biologies* 329, nos. 5–6 (2006): 450–59.

———. "Communicating the Modern Body: Fritz Kahn's Popular Images of Human Physiology as an Industrialized World." *Canadian Journal of Communication* 32, no. 3 (2007): 495–520.

———. "Electricity as a Medium of Psychic Life. Electrotechnological Adventures into Psychodiagnosis in Weimar Germany." *Science in Context* 14, no. 1 (2001): 565–90.

———. "Electrifying the Brain in the 1920s: Electrical Technology as a Mediator in Brain Research." In *Electric Bodies: Episodes in the History of Medical Electricity*, edited by Paolo Bertucci and Giuliano Pancaldi, 239–64. Bologna: Centro Internazionale per la Storia delleUniversita e della Scenza, 2001.

———. *Hirnströme: eine Kulturgeschichte der Elektroenzephalographie*. Göttingen: Wallstein, 2005.

———. "Recording the Brain at Work: The Visible, the Readable, and the Invisible in Electroencephalography." *Journal of the History of the Neurosciences* 17 (2008): 367–79.

———. "Urban Gehirne: Zum Bilduberschuss medientechnischer Hirnwelten der 1920er Jahre." *Archive Fur Mediengeschichte* 2 (2002): 261–67.

Borck, Cornelius, and Michael Hagner, 2001. "Mindful Practices. On the Neurosciences in the Twentieth Century." *Science in Context*, 14, no. 4 (2001): 507–10.

Borell, Merriley E. "Origins of the Hormone Concept: Internal Secretions and Physiological Research, 1889–1905." PhD diss., Yale University, 1976.

Borowy, Iris. *Coming to Terms with International Health: The League of Nations Health Organization, 1921–1946.* Frankfurt am Main: Peter Lang, 2009.

Bowler, Peter J. *Science for All: The Popularization of Science in Early Twentieth-Century Britain.* Chicago: University of Chicago Press, 2009.

Bozler, E., and K. S Cole. "The Electric Impedance and Phase Angle of Muscle in Rigor." *Journal of Cellular and Comparative Physiology* 6, no. 2 (1935): 229–41.

Bracegirdle, Brian. "The History of Histology: A Brief Survey of Sources." *History of Science* 15 (1977): 77–101.

Bradley, J. K., E. M. Tansey, and J. K. Bradley. "The Coming of the Electronic Age to the Cambridge Physiological Laboratory: E. D. Adrian's Valve Amplifier in 1921." *Records of the Royal Society* 50, no. 2 (1996): 217–28.

Braun, Marta. *Picturing Time: The Work of Étienne-Jules Marey (1830–1904).* Chicago: University of Chicago Press, 1992.

Bray, Francesca. "Science, Technique, Technology: Passages between Matter and Knowledge in Imperial Chinese Agriculture." *British Journal for the History of Science* 41, no. 3 (2008): 319–44.

Breggin, Peter. *Toxic Psychiatry: Why Therapy, Empathy, and Love Must Replace the Drugs, Electroshock, and Biochemical Theories of the "New Psychiatry."* New York: St. Martin's Press, 1994.

Breidbach, Olaf. *Die Materialisierung des Ichs: Zur Geschichte der Hirnforschung im 19. und 20. Jahrhundert.* Frankfurt am Main: Suhrkamp Verlag, 1997.

Bresalier, Michael. "Neutralizing Flu: 'Immunological Devices' and the Making of a Virus Disease." In *Crafting Immunity: Working Histories of Clinical Immunology,* edited by Michael Kroker, Kenton Bresalier, J. Keelan, and P. M. H. Mazumdar, 107–44. Aldershot, UK: Ashgate, 2008.

———. "Uses of a Pandemic: Forging the Identities of Influenza and Virus Research in Interwar Britain." *Social History of Medicine* 25 (2008): 400–24.

Breslau, Daniel. Review of "The Selling of DSM: The Rhetoric of Science in Psychiatry by Stuart A. Kirk and Herb Kutchins." *Contemporary Sociology* 22, no. 4 (1993): 607.

Brieger, Gert H. "From Conservative to Radical Surgery in Late Nineteenth-Century America." In *Medical Theory, Surgical Practice: Studies in the History of Surgery,* edited by Christopher Lawrence, 216–31. London: Routledge, 1992.

Broadman, Estella. *The Development of Medical Bibliography.* Baltimore: Waverly Press, 1954.

Brock, D. Heward, and Ann Harward. *The Culture of Biomedicine.* Newark, DE: University of Delaware Press, 1984.

Bronowski, Jacob. *Guide to the Exhibition of Architecture, Town-Planning and Building Research.* Edited by Harding McGregor Dunnett. London: H. M. Stationery Office, 1951.

Brook, L. G., J. S. Coombs, and J. C. Eccles. "The Recording of Potentials from Motorneurons with an Intracellular Electrode." *Journal of Physiology* 117 (1952): 431–60.

Brown, Bertram. "Life of Psychiatry." *American Journal of Psychiatry* 133, no. 5 (1976): 489–95.

Brunner, Jose, and Orna Ophir. "'In Good Times and in Bad': Boundary Relations of Psychoanalysis in Post-war USA." *History of Psychiatry* 22, no. 2 (2011): 215–31.

Buchanan, George S. "An Address on International Organization and Public Health." *British Medical Journal* 1, no. 3140 (1921): 331–35.

Buklijas, Tatjana. "Surgery and National Identity in Late Nineteenth-Century Vienna." *Studies in History and Philosophy of Biology and Biomedical Sciences* 38 (2007): 756–74.

Burckhardt Jr., Richard W. "Constructing the Zoo: Science, Society, and Animal Nature at the Paris Menagerie, 1794–1838." In *Animals in Human Histories: The Mirror of Nature and Culture*, edited by Mary Henniger-Voss, 231–57. Rochester, NY: University of Rochester Press, 2002.

Burdon-Sanderson, John. "An Address on the Relation of Science to Experience in Medicine." *British Medical Journal* 2 (1899): 1333–35.

Burnham, John C. *Accident Prone: A History of Technology, Psychology, and Misfits of the Machine Age*. Chicago: University of Chicago Press, 2009.

Bynum, William F. *Science and the Practice of Medicine in the Nineteenth Century*. Cambridge: Cambridge University Press, 1994.

Caldwell, O. H. "The Electron Tube . . . A Universal Tool in Industry." *Electronics* 1 (1930): 10–11.

Cameron, H. A., C. S. Woolley, B. S. McEwen, and Elizabeth Gould. "Differentiation of Newly Born Neurons and Glia in the Dentate Gyrus of the Adult Rat." *Neuroscience* 56 (1993): 337–44.

Canguilhem, Georges. "The Object of the History of Science." In *Continental Philosophy of Science*, edited by G. Gutting. Oxford: Blackwell, 2005.

Carlson, W. Bernard. *Tesla: Inventor of the Electrical Age*. Princeton, NJ: Princeton University Press, 2013.

Carlsson, Arvid. "The Dopamine Hypothesis of Schizophrenia 20 Years Later." In *Search for the Cause of Schizophrenia*, edited by H. Häffler, W. F. Gattaz and W. Janzarik, 223–35. Berlin: Springer-Verlag, 1987.

———. "Historical Perspective of the Chemistry and Pharmacological Treatment of Schizophrenia." Vol. 2 of *Handbook of Schizophrenia*, edited by F. A. Herm and L. E. DeLisi, 1–15. Elsevier Science, 1987.

Carpenter, C. M., and A. B. Page. "The Production of Fever in Man by Short Radio Waves." *Science* 71, no. 1844 (1930): 450–52.

Carter, B. Noland. "The Fruition of Halsted's Concept of Surgical Training." *Surgery* 32 (1952): 518–27.

Casper, Stephen T. "An Integrative Legacy: History and Neuroscience." *Isis* 105, no. 1 (2014): 123–32.

———. *The Neurologists: A History of a Medical Specialty in Britain, 1789–2000*. Manchester, UK: Manchester University Press, 2014.

———. Review of "Neuro: The New Brain Sciences and the Management of the Mind," by Nikolas S. Rose and Joelle M. Abi-Rached. *Journal of the History of the Behavioral Sciences* 51, no. 1 (2015): 95–98.

Chadarevian, Soraya de. *Designs for Life: Molecular Biology after World War II*. New York: Cambridge University Press, 2002.

———. "Graphical Method and Discipline: Self-Recording Instruments in Nineteenth-Century Physiology." *Studies in History and Philosophy of Science* 24, no. 2 (1993): 267–91.

Changeux, Jean-Pierre. *Neuronal Man: The Biology of Mind.* New York: Pantheon Books, 1985.

Choudhury, Suparna, and Jan Slaby. *Critical Neuroscience: A Handbook of the Social and Cultural Contexts of Neuroscience.* Chichester, UK: Wiley-Blackwell, 2012.

Clarke, Edwin, and Kenneth Dewhurst. *An Illustrated History of Brain Function.* Oxford: Sandhorst, 1972.

Clarke, Edwin, and L. Stephen Jacyna. *Nineteenth Century of Origins of Neuroscientific Concepts.* Berkeley: University of California Press, 1987.

Cole, K. S. *Electric Conductance of Biological Systems.* Vol. 1 of *Cold Spring Harbor Symposia in Quantitative Biology,* 107–16. 1933. Reprint, New York: Johnson Reprints, 1961.

———. *Membranes, Ions, and Impulses: A Chapter of Classical Biophysics.* Berkeley: University of California Press, 1968.

Cole, K. S., and A. L. Hodgkin. "Membrane and Protoplasm Resistance in the Squid Giant Axon." *Journal of General Physiology* 22 (1939): 671–87.

Cole, K. S., and H. J. Curtis. "Electric Impedance of the Squid Giant Axon during Activity." *Journal of General Physiology* 22 (1939): 649–70.

Colgrove, James. *State of Immunity: The Politics of Vaccination in Twentieth-Century America.* Berkeley: University of California Press, 2006.

Committee on Vaccination. "Request to Medical Practitioners." *British Medical Journal* 1 (1926): 748.

Conekin, Becky. *The Autobiography of a Nation: The 1951 Festival of Britain.* Manchester, UK: Manchester University Press, 2003.

Connell, P. H. "Amphetamine Psychosis." *British Medical Journal* 1 no. 5018 (1957): 582.

———. *Amphetamine Psychosis.* London: Chapman and Hall, 1958.

Conners, P. *White Hand Society: The Psychedelic Partnership of Timothy Leary and Allen Ginsberg.* San Francisco: City Lights Bookstore, 2010.

Cook, Walter. "Hitler is My Best Friend (ca. 1935)." In *In Meaning in the Visual Arts,* edited by Erwin Panowsky, 380–81. New York: Penguin, 1970.

Cooper, Astley. "Surgical Lecture." *The Lancet* 1 (1923): 3–10.

Cooter, Roger. "Neural Veils and the Will to Historical Critique: Why Historians of Science Need to Take the Neuro-Turn Seriously." *Isis* 105, no. 1 (2014): 145–54.

———. *Surgery and Society in Peace and War: Orthopaedics and the Organization of Modern Medicine, 1880–1948.* Basingstoke, UK: Macmillan, 1993.

Cooter, Roger, and Claudia Stein. "The New Poverty of Theory: Material Turns in a Latourian World." In *Writing History in the Age of Biomedicine.* New Haven, CT: Yale University Press, 2013.

Cowan, W. Maxwell, and Eric R Kandel. "A Brief History of Synapses and Synaptic Transmission." In *Synapses,* edited by W. Maxwell Cowan, Thomas Südhuf, and Charles F. Stevens. Baltimore: Johns Hopkins University Press, 2001.

Cremer, M. *Erregungsgesetze Des Nerven.* Vol. 9 of *Handbuch Der Normalen Und Pathologischen Physiologie,* edited by A. Bethe. Berlin: Springer, 1929.

Crile, George. *A Bipolar Theory of Living Processes.* New York: Macmillan, 1926.

——. *An Experimental Research into Surgical Shock: An Essay Awarded the Cartwright Prize for 1897*. Philadelphia: J. B. Lippincott, 1899.

——. *A Mechanistic View of War and Peace*. New York: Macmillan, 1915.

Crile, Grace, ed. *George Crile: An Autobiography*. Philadelphia: J. B. Lippincott, 1947.

Crookshank, Francis Graham. *Epidemiological Essays*. London: K. Paul, Trench, & Trubner, 1930.

Crowe, Samuel James. *Halsted of Johns Hopkins: The Man and His Men*. Springfield, IL: Charles C. Thomas, 1957.

Cubitt, Geoffrey, and Allen Warren. *Heroic Reputations and Exemplary Lives*. Manchester, UK: Manchester University Press, 2000.

Cumberbatch, E. P. *Diathermy; Its Production and Uses in Medicine and Surgery*. St. Louis: C. V. Mosby, 1928.

——. "Uses of Diathermy in Medicine and Surgery." *The Lancet* 217 no. 5606 (1931): 281–85.

Cunningham, Andrew. *The Anatomist Anatomis'd: An Experimental Discipline in Enlightenment Europe*. Farnham, UK: Ashgate, 2010.

Cushing, Harvey. "The Special Field of Neurological Surgery after Another Interval." *Archives of Neurology and Psychiatry* 4, no. 6 (1920): 603–37.

Cuvier, Fréderic. "De la sociabilité des animaux." *Mémoires du Muséum* 13 (1825): 1–27.

——. "Essai sur la domesticité des mammifères." *Mémoires du Muséum* 13 (1825): 406–55.

Dagognet, François. *Etienne-Jules Marey: A Passion for the Trace*. Translated by Robert Galeta and Jeanine Herman. New York: Zone, 1992.

Dahlgren, Ulric, and William A. Kepner. *A Text-Book of the Principles of Animal Histology*. New York: Macmillan, 1908.

Damasio, Antonio R. *Descartes' Error: Emotion, Reason, and the Human Brain*. New York: G. P. Putnam's Sons, 1994.

Daston, Lorraine, and Peter Galison. *Objectivity*. New York: Zone, 2007.

Davis, F., and L. Munoz. "Heads and Freaks: Patterns and Meanings of Drug Use among Hippies." *Journal of Health and Social Behavior* 9 (1968): 154–64.

Davis, H., and A. Forbes. "Chronaxie." *Physiological Reviews* 16 (1936): 407–41.

de la Mettrie, Julien Offray. *L'homme machine*. Leyden: Elie Luzac, 1748.

de Sio, Fabio. "Leviathan and the Soft Animal: Medical Humanism and the Invertebrate Models for Higher Nervous Functions, 1950s–90s." *Medical History* 55, no. 3 (2011): 369–74.

Debru, Claude, Jean-Gaëlle Barbara, and Céline Cherici. *Essor des neurosciences en France dans le contexte international (1945–1975)*. Paris: Hermann, 2008.

DeFelipe, Javier. "Brain Plasticity and Mental Processes: Cajal Again." *Nature Reviews Neuroscience* 7 (2006): 811–17.

——. *Cajal's Butterflies of the Soul: Science and Art*. Oxford: Oxford University Press, 2009.

Deichmann, Ute. "Emigration, Isolation and the Slow Start of Molecular Biology in Germany." *Studies in History and Philosophy of Biological and Biomedical Sciences* 33, no. 3 (2002): 449–71.

Dierig, Sven. "Engines for Experiment: Laboratory Revolution and Industrial Labor in the Nineteenth-Century City." *Osiris* 18 (2003): 116–34.

————. *Wissenschaft in der Maschinerstadt: Emil Du Bois-Reymond und seine Laboratorien in Berlin.* Gottingen: Wallstein-Verlag, 2006.

Dierig, Sven, Jens Lachmund, and J. Andrew Mendelsohn. "Introduction: Toward an Urban History of Science." *Osiris* 18 (2003): 1–19.

Dowlatow, Sergeij Donatowitsch. *The Suitcase: A Novel.* Translated by Antonia W. Bouis. Berkeley, CA: Counterpoint, 1990.

Dror, Otneil E. "Techniques of the Brain and the Paradox of Emotions, 1880–1930." *Science in Context,* 14, no. 4 (2001): 643–60.

Dubin, Martin David. "The League of Nations Health Organization." In *International Organizations and Health Movements, 1918–39,* edited by Paul Weindling, 56–80. Cambridge: Cambridge University Press, 1995.

Dumit, Joseph. *Picturing Personhood: Brain Scans and Biomedical Identity.* Princeton, NJ: Princeton University Press, 2004.

Duncan, Kristi. "Is Sleeping Sickness Linked to Spanish Flu of 1918?" *Toronto Star,* January 3, 2006, 15.

Dwyer, Ellen. *Homes for the Mad: Life inside Two Nineteenth-Century Asylums.* New Brunswick, NJ: Rutgers University Press, 1987.

————. "Neurological Patients as Experimental Subjects: Epilepsy Studies in the United States." In *The Neurological Patient in History,* edited by L. Stephen Jacyna and Stephen T. Casper. Rochester, NY: University of Rochester Press, 2012.

————. "Toward New Narratives of Twentieth-Century Medicine." *Bulletin of the History of Medicine* 74, no. 4 (Winter 2000): 786–93.

Dyck, E. *Psychedelic Psychiatry: LSD from Clinic to Campus.* Baltimore: Johns Hopkins University Press, 2008.

Eccles, John. "Conduct and Synaptic Transmission in the Nervous System." *Annual Reviews in Physiology* 10 (1948): 93–116.

Eccles, W. H. "The New Acoustics." *Proceedings of the Physical Society* 41 (1929): 232–33.

Eichler, Walter. "Ueber Die Abhaengigkeit Der Chronaxie Des Nerven Vom Auesseren Widerstande." *Zeitschrift Fuer Biologie* 91 (1931): 475.

Eiselsberg, Anton Freiherr von. "Zur Behandlung der Tetania parathyreopriva." *Archiv für klinische Chirurgie* 118 (1921): 387–410.

————. "Zur Frage der dauernden Einheilung verpflanzter Schilddrüsen und Nebenschilddrüsen." *Verhandlungen der Deutschen Gesellschaft für Chirurgie* 43 (1914): 655–69.

Ellenberger, Henri F. "The Mental Hospital and the Zoological Garden 1965." *University of Florida College of Liberal Arts and Sciences.* Accessed May 23, 2013. http://www.clas.ufl.edu/users/burt/spliceoflife/ellenberger.pdf.

English, Peter. *Shock, Physiological Surgery, and George Washington Crile: Innovation in the Progressive Era.* Westport, CT: Greenwood Press, 1980.

Erichsen, John Eric. "An Address Delivered at the Opening of the Section of Surgery." *British Medical Journal* 2 (1886): 314–16.

————. "Mr. Erichsen's Introductory Address." *The Lancet* 102 (1873): 489–90.

Eyal, Gil, Brendan Hart, Emine Onculer, Neta Oren et al. *The Autism Matrix: The Social Origins of the Autism Epidemic.* Cambridge: Polity, 2010.

Eysenck, H. J. "The Effects of Psychotherapy: An Evaluation." *Journal of Consulting Psychology* 16 (1952): 319–24.

Fantini, Bernardino. "Les organisations sanitaires internationales face à l'émergence de maladies infectieuses nouvelles." *History and Philosophy of the Life Sciences* 15 (1993): 435–57.

Farahany, Nita A. *The Impact of Behavioral Sciences on Criminal Law.* New York: Oxford University Press, 2009.

Farde, L., F. A. Stone-Elander, S. Wiesel, C. Halldin et al. A. "D2 Dopamine Receptors in Neuroleptic-naïve Schiozophrenic Patients: A Positron Emission Tomography Study with [11C]raclopride." *Archives of General Psychiatry* 47 (1990): 213–19.

Fatt, Paul, and Bernhard Katz. "An Analysis of the End-plate Potential Recorded with an Intra-Cellular Electrode." *Journal of Physiology* 115 (1951): 320–70.

Fawcett, John. "Networks, Linkages and Migration Systems." *International Migration* 23, no. 6 (1989): 638–70.

Feighner, John P, Eli Robins, Samuel B. Guze Jr., Robert A. Woodruff et al. "Diagnostic Criteria for Use in Psychiatric Research." *Archives of General Psychiatry* 26, no 1 (1972): 57–63.

Feindel, William. "History of the Surgical Treatment of Epilepsy." In *A History of Neurosurgery in Its Scientific and Professional Contexts,* edited by T Forcht Dagi, Mel H. Epstein, and Samuel H. Greenblatt. Park Ridge, IL: American Association of Neurological Surgeons, 1997.

———. "The Physiologist and the Neurosurgeon: The Enduring Influence of Charles Sherrington on the Career of Wilder Penfield." *Brain* 130, no. 11 (2007): 2758–65.

Feldberg, Wilhelm, and Alfred Fessard. "The Cholinergic Nature of the Nerves of the Electric Organ of the Torpedo (Torpedo Marmorata)." *Journal of Physiology* 101 (1942): 200–215.

Felsch, Philipp. *Laborlandschaften: Physiologen Über Der Baumgrenze 1800–1900.* Goettingen: Wallstein, 2007.

Fermi, Laura. *Illustrious Immigrants: The Intellectual Migration from Europe, 1930–41.* Chicago: University of Chicago, 1971.

Festival of Britain. *The Arts in the Festival of Britain, 1951.* London: Arts Council of Great Britain, 1951.

———. *Catalogue of Activities throughout the Country.* London: The Festival of Britain, 1951.

———. *Exhibition of Science, South Kensington: A Guide to the Story it Tells.* London: H.M. S.O., 1951.

———. *The Story of the Festival of Britain, 1951.* London: HMSO, 1952.

Fiddle, S. "Circles beyond the Circumference: Some Hunches about Amphetamine Abuse." In *Amphetamine Abuse,* edited by J. R. Russo, 66–87. Springfield, IL: Charles C Thomas, 1968.

Finger, Stanley. *Minds Behind the Brain: A History of the Pioneers and their Discoveries.* New York: Oxford University Press, 2000.

———. *Origins of Neuroscience.* Oxford: Oxford University Press, 2001.

Fischer, Georg. *Billroth, Theodor.* 1902. Accessed June 15, 2014. http://www.deutsche-biographie.de/sfz4491.html.

Fischer, Klaus. "Identification of Emigration-Induced Scientific Change." In *Forced Migration and Scientific Change: Émigré German-Speaking Scientists and Scholars after 1933*, edited by Mitchell G. Ash and Alfons Soellner, 23–47. Cambridge: Cambridge University Press, 1996.

Fissell, Mary E. "Making Meaning from the Margins: The New Cultural History of Medicine." In *Locating Medical History: The Stories and Their Meanings*, 364–90. Baltimore: Johns Hopkins University Press, n.d.

Fleck, Christian. "Emigration of Social Scientists' Schools from Austria." In *Forced Migration and Scientific Change: Émigré German-Speaking Scientists and Scholars after 1933*, edited by Mitchell G Ash and Alfons Soellner, 198–223. Cambridge: Cambridge University Press, 1996.

Flexner, Simon. "Postvaccinal Encephalitis." *Transactions of the Association of American Physicians* 44 (1929): 181–82.

Flourens, Pierre. *De l'instinct et de l'intelligence des animaux.* 3rd ed. Paris: L. Hachette, 1851.

———. *Examen de la phrenologie.* Paris: Paulin, 1842.

Focke, Wenda. *Begegnung: Herta Seidemann; Psychiatrin-Neurologin 1900–1984.* Konstanz: Hartung-Gorre, 1986.

Foege, William H. *House on Fire: The Fight to Eradicate Smallpox.* Berkeley: University of California Press, 2011.

Foerster, O., and Wilder Penfield. "The Structural Basis of Traumatic Epilepsy and Results of Radical Operation." *Brain* 53, no. 2 (1930): 99–119.

Foley, Paul. "The Encephalitis Lethargica Patient as a Window on the Soul." In *The Neurological Patient in History*, edited by L. Stephen Jacyna and Stephen T. Casper, 184–211. Rochester, NY: University of Rochester Press, 2012.

Forgan, Sophie. "Festivals of Science and the Two Cultures: Science, Design, and Display in the Festival of Britain, 1951." *British Journal for the History of Science* 31, no. 2 (1998): 217–40.

Foucault, Michel. *The Order of Things: An Archaeology of the Human Sciences*, translated by Richard Howard. London: Pantheon Books, 1970.

Foucault, Michel, Luther H. Martin, Huck Gutman, and Patrick H. Hutton. *Technologies of the Self: A Seminar with Michel Foucault.* Amherst: University of Massachusetts Press, 1988.

Frampton, Sally. "'The Most Startling Innovation': Ovarian Surgery in Britain, c. 1740–1939." PhD diss., University College London, 2013.

Frank, Fenner, D. A. Henderson, I. Arita, Z. Ježek et al. *Smallpox and Its Eradication.* Geneva: World Health Organization, 1988.

Frank, Jerome D. *Persuasion and Healing: A Comparative Study of Psychotherapy.* Baltimore: Johns Hopkins University Press, 1961.

Frank, Robert G. "Instruments, Nerve Action, and the All-or-None Principle." *Osiris* 9 (1994): 208–35.

Franklin, Allan. *The Neglect of Experiment.* Cambridge: Cambridge University Press, 1989.

Fricke, H. *The Electric Impedance of Suspensions of Biological Cells.* Vol. 1, in *Cold Spring Harbor Symposia in Quantitative Biology*, 117–24. 1933. Reprint, New York: Johnson Reprint Company, 1961.

Fricke, H., and S. Morse. "The Electric Capacity of Tumors of the Breast." *Journal of Cancer Research* 16 (1926): 340–76.

Fuhr, Ferdinand. "Die Exstirpation der Schilddrüse: Eine Experimentelle Studie." *Archiv für experimentelle Pathologie und Pharmakologie* 21 (1886): 387–460.

Fuller, Steve. "Neuroscience, Neurohistory, and the History of Science: A Tale of Two Brain Images." *Isis* 105, no. 1 (2014): 100–109.

———. *Preparing for Life in Humanity 2.0.* Houndmills, UK: Palgrave Macmillan, 2013.

Gabbard, Glen O. "A Neurobiologically Informed Perspective on Psychotherapy." *British Journal of Psychiatry* 177 (2000): 117–22.

Gaddum, J. H. "Drugs Antagonistic to 5-Hydroxytryptamine." In *Ciba Foundation Symposium on Hypertension: Humoral and Neurogenic Factors,* edited by G. E. W. Wolstenholme and M. P. Cameron, 75–77, 85–90. Boston: Little, Brown, 1954.

Galison, Peter, Stephen R. Graubard, and Everett Medelsohn. *Science in Culture.* New Brunswick, NJ: Transaction Publishers, 2001.

Gant, F. J. "What Has Pathological Anatomy Done for Medicine and Surgery." *The Lancet* 70 (November 7, 1857): 461–85.

Garcia-Segura, L. M. "Cajal and Glial Cells." *Progress in Brain Research* 136 (2002): 255–60.

Gardner, R. "Psychotomimetic Effects of Central Stimulants." In *Abuse of Central Stimulants,* edited by F. Sjöqvist and M. Tottie, 113–39. New York: Raven Press, 1969.

Garrison, Fielding. "The Uses of Medical Bibliography and Medical History in the Medical Curriculum." *Journal of the American Medical Association* 66 (1916): 319–24.

Gasser, Herbert S. "Axon Action Potentials in Nerve." In *Cold Spring Harbor Symposia in Quantitative Biology,* 138–45. New York: Johnson Reprint Corporation, n.d.

Gasser, Jacques. *Aux origines du cerveau moderne: Localisations, langage et mémoire dans l'oeuvre de Charcot.* Paris: Fayard, 1995.

Gavrus, Delia. "Men of Dreams and Men of Action: Neurologists, Neurosurgeons, and the Performance of Professional Identity, 1920–1950." *Bulletin of the History of Medicine* 85 (2011): 57–92.

———. "Men of Strong Opinions: Identity, Self-Representation and the Performance of Neurosurgery." PhD diss., University of Toronto, 2011.

———. "Mind over Matter: Sherrington, Penfield, Eccles, Walshe and the Dualist Movement in Neuroscience." In *Comparative Program on Health and Society Lupina Foundation Working Paper Series 2005–2006.* Toronto: Munk Centre for International Studies, University of Toronto, 2006.

———. "Skill, Judgement and Conduct for the First Generation of Neurosurgeons, 1900–1930." *Medical History* 59, no. 3 (July 2015): 361–78.

Gisthovel, Alexa, and Alexa Knoch. *Orte de Moderne: Erfahrungswelten des 19. und 20. Jahrhunderts.* Frankfurt: Campus Verlag, 2005.

Gluck, Th. "Referat über die durch das modern chirurgische Experiment gewonnenen positiven Resultate, betreffend die Naht und den Ersatz von Defecten höherer Gewebe, sowie über die Verwerthung resorbirbarer und lebendinger Tampons in der Chirurgie." *Archiv für klinische Chirurgie* 41 (1891): 187–239.

Goffman, Erving. *Asylums: Essays on the Social Situation of Mental Patients and other Inmates.* Garden City, NY: Anchor Books, 1961.

Goldstein, Jan. *Console and Classify: The French Psychiatric Profession in the Nineteenth Century.* Cambridge: Cambridge University Press, 1990.

Goodden, Henrietta. *The Lion and the Unicorn: Symbolic Architecture for the Festival of Britain, 1951.* London: Unicorn Press, 2011.

Gould, E., B. S. McEwen, P. Tanapat, L. A. Galea et al. "Neurogenesis in the Dentate Gyrus of the Adult Tree Shrew Is Regulated by Psychosocial Stress and NMDA Receptor Activation." *Journal of Neuroscience* 17 (1997): 2492–98.

Gould, E., H. A. Cameron, and B. S. McEwen. "Blockade of NMDA Receptors Increases Cell Death and Birth in the Developing Rat Dentate Gyrus." *Journal of Comparative Neurology* 340 no. 4 (1994): 551–65.

Gould, E., P. Tanapat, and H. A. Cameron. "Adrenal Steroids Suppress Granule Cell Death in the Developing Dentate Gyrus through an NMDA Receptor-Dependent Mechanism." *Developments in Brain Research* 103 (1997): 91–93.

Grace, A. A. "Gating of Information Flow within the Limbic System and the Pathophysiology of Schizophrenia." *Brain Research Reviews* 31 (2000): 330–41.

Gradmann, Christoper. "Locating Therapeutic Vaccines in Nineteenth-Century History." *Science in Context* 21 (2008): 145–60.

Gradmann, Christopher, and Johnathan Simon. *Evaluating and Standardizing Therapeutic Agents, 1890–1950.* Basingstoke, UK: Palgrave Macmillan, 2010.

Graybiel, Ann M., and Kyle S. Smith. "Good Habits, Bad Habits." *Scientific American* 310 no. 6 (2014): 39–40.

Greenberg, Gary. *The Book of Woe: The DSM and the Unmaking of Psychiatry.* New York: Blue Rider Press, 2013.

Greenblatt, Samuel H. "Harvey Cushing's Paradigmatic Contribution to Neurosurgery and the Evolution of His Thoughts About Specialization." *Bulletin of the History of Medicine* 77, no. 4 (2003): 789–92.

———. "Inclusiveness and Coherency in the History of the Neurosciences." *Journal of the History of the Neurosciences* 11, no. 2 (2002): 185–93.

Greenblatt, Samuel H., and Dale Smith. "The Emergence of Cushing's Leadership: 1901–1920." In *A History of Neurosurgery in Its Scientific and Professional Contexts,* edited by T. Forcht Dagi, Mel H. Epstein, and Samuel H. Greenblatt. Park Ridge, IL: American Association of Neurological Surgeons, 1997.

Greenland, C. "At the Crichton Royal with William Mayer-Gross." *History of Psychiatry* 13 (2002): 467–74.

Greenspan, Kenneth, Joseph Schildkraut, Edna Gordon, Bernard Levy et al. "Catecholamine Metabolism in Affective Disorders." *Archives of General Psychiatry* 21, no. 6 (1969): 710–16.

Greenwood, Major. "Sir George S. Buchanan, C.B., M.D., F.R.C.P." *British Medical Journal* 2, no. 3954 (1936): 788–89.

Griffith, J. D. "Psychiatric Implication of Amphetamine Abuse." In *Amphetamine Abuse,* edited by M. Russo, 15–31. Springfield, IL: Charles C Thomas, 1968.

Griffith, J. D., J. H. Cavanaugh, J. Held, and J. A. Oates. "Experimental Psychosis Induced by the Administration of d-amphetamine." In *Amphetamines and Related Compounds,* by E. E. Costa and S. Garattini, 897–904. New York: Raven Press, 1970.

Grinspoon, L., and P. Hedblom. *Speed Culture: Amphetamine Use and Abuse in America.* Cambridge, MA: Harvard University Press, 1975.

Grob, Gerald. *From Asylum to Community: Mental Health Policy in Modern America.* Princeton, NJ: Princeton University Press, 1991.

Gross, Alan. *The Rhetoric of Science.* Cambridge: Cambridge University Press, 1996.

Gross, Charles G. *Brain, Vision, Memory: Tales in the History of Neuroscience.* Cambridge, MA: MIT Press, 1998.

———. *A Hole in the Head: More Tales in the History of Neuroscience.* Cambridge, MA: MIT Press, 2009.

———. "Neurogenesis in the Adult Brain: Death of a Dogma." *Nature Reviews Neuroscience* 1 (2000): 67–73.

Grover, Burton Baker. *High Frequency Practice for Practitioners and Students.* Kansas City, MO: The Electron Press, 1925.

Guenther, Katja. "Exercises in Therapy—Neurological Gymnastics between Kurort and Hospital Medicine, 1880–1945." *Bulletin of the History of Medicine* 88, no. 1 (Spring 2014): 102–31.

———. *Localization and Its Discontents: A Genealogy of Psychoanalysis and the Neuro Disciplines.* Chicago: University of Chicago Press, 2015.

Guenther, Katja, and Volker Hess. "Soul Catchers: The Material Culture of the Mind Sciences." *Medical History* 60, no. 3 (July 2016): 301–7.

Guldi, Jo, and David Armitage. *The History Manifesto.* Cambridge: Cambridge University Press, 2014.

Gurwitsch, Aron. "La Science biologique d'après K. Goldstein." *Revue Philosophique* 129, no. 3 (1940): 244–65.

Guttmann, E. "Artificial Psychoses Produced by Mescaline." *British Journal of Psychiatry* 82 (1936): 203–21.

Hacking, Ian. "Telepathy: Origins of Randomization in Experimental Design." *Isis* 79 (1988): 427–51.

Hagner, Michael. *Der Geist bei de Arbeit: historische Untersuchungen zur Hirnforschung.* Göttingen: Wallstein, 2006.

———. *Geniale Gehirne.* Göttingen: Wallstein Verlag, 2004.

———. *Homo Cerebralis: Der Wandel vom Seelenorgan zum Gehirn.* Berlin: Verlag, 1997.

Hale, Piers J. *Political Descent: Malthus, Mutualism, and the Politics of Evolution in Victorian England.* Chicago: University of Chicago Press, 2014.

Halsted, William S. *Surgical Papers.* Baltimore: Johns Hopkins Press, 1924.

Hamilton, David. *The Monkey Gland Affair.* London: Chatto & Windus, 1986.

Haring, Kristen. *Ham Radio's Technical Culture.* Cambridge, MA: MIT Press, 2006.

Harrington, Anne. *The Cure Within: A History of Mind-Body Medicine.* New York: W. W. Norton, 2008.

———. *Medicine, Mind and the Double Brain: A Study in 19th Century Thought.* Princeton, NJ: Princeton University Press, 1989.

———. *Reenchanted Science: Holism in German Culture from Wilhelm II to Hitler.* Princeton, NJ: Princeton University Press, 1996.

———. *Towards a History of the Brain and Behavioral Sciences: Themes and Provocations.* Vol. 6, *The Cambridge History of Science,* edited by Peter J. Bowler and John V. Pickstone, 504–23. Cambridge: Cambridge University Press, 2008.

Hart, E. J. "Hugo Fricke, 1892–1972." *Radiation Research* 52, no. 3 (1972): 642–46.

Harvey, Joy. "L'autre Côté Du Miroir (The Other Side of the Mirror): French Neuro-physiology and English Interpretations." In *Les Sciences Biologiques Ed Médicales En France 1920–1950*, edited by Claude Debru, Jean Gayon, and Jean-Francois Picard, 71–81. Paris: CNRS Editions, 1994.

Harwood, Jonathan. *Styles of Scientific Thought: The German Genetics Community, 1900–1933*. Chicago: University of Chicago Press, 1993.

Healy, David. *The Antidepressant Era*. Cambridge, MA: Harvard University Press, 1999.

———. *The Creation of Psychopharmacology*. Cambridge, MA: Harvard University Press, 2002.

Hedgecoe, Adam. "Schizophrenia and the Narrative of Enlightened Geneticization." *Social Studies of Science* 31, no. 6 (2001): 875–911.

Heinrichs, R. W. *In Search of Madness: Schizophrenia and Neuroscience*. Oxford: Oxford University Press, 2001.

Hemingway, A., and J. F. McClendon. "The High Frequency Resistance of Human Tissue." *American Journal of Physiology* 102 (1932): 56–59.

Henseler, H., and E. Fritsch. *Einführung in Die Diathermie Vom Medizinischen U. Technischen Standpunkt*. Berlin: Radionta-Verlag, 1929.

Hess, Volker, and J. Andrew Mendelsohn. "Case and Series: Medical Knowledge and Paper Technology, 1600–1900." *History of Science* 48 (2010): 287–314.

Hildebrandt, Gerhard, Martin Nikolas Stienen, and Werner Surbeck. "Von Bergmann, Kocher, and Krönlein: A Triumvirat of Pioneers with a Common Neurosurgical Concept." *Acta Neurochirurgica* 155 (2013): 1787–99.

Hildebrandt, Gerhard, Werner Surbeck, and Martin N. Stienen. "Emil Theodor Kocher: The First Swiss Neurosurgeon." *Acta Neurochirurgica* 154 (2012): 1105–15.

Hill, A. V. "Repetitive Stimulation by Commutator and Condenser." *Journal of Physiology* 82, no. 4 (1934): 423–31.

Hobsbawm, Eric. "Introduction: Inventing Traditions." In *The Invention of Tradition*, edited by Eric Hobsbawm and Terrance Ranger. London: Cambridge University Press, 1983.

Hodgkin, A. L. *Chance and Design: Reminiscences of Science in Peace and War*. Cambridge: Cambridge University Press, 1992.

Hodgkin, A. L., and A. F. Huxley. "Action Potentials Recorded from Inside a Nerve Fibre." *Nature* 144 (1939): 710–11.

———. "Potassium Leakage from an Active Nerve Fibre." *Journal of Physiology* 106 (1947): 341–67.

———. "Resting and Action Potentials in Single Neurons." *Journal of Physiology* 104 (1945): 176–95.

Hoffmann, Thomas, and Frank W. Stahnisch. "Einleitung." In *Kurt Goldstein—Der Aufbau des Organismus: Einfuehrung in die Biologie unter besonderer Beruecksichtigung der Erfahrungen am kranken Menschen*, edited by Thomas Hoffmann and Frank W. Stahnisch. Munich: Fink, 2014.

Holden, Constance. "A Top Priority at NIMH." *Science* 235, no. 4787 (1987): 431.

Holdorff, Bernd. "Founding Years of Clinical Neurology in Berlin until 1933." *Journal of the History of the Neurosciences* 13, no. 3 (2004): 223–38.

Holmes, F. L., and K. M. Olesko. "The Images of Precision: Helmholtz and the Graphical Method in Physiology." In *The Values of Precision*, edited by M. Norton Wise. Princeton, NJ: Princeton University Press, 1995.

Holzer, Wolfgang. "Modelltheorie Über Die Stromdichte Im Körper von Lebewesen Bei Galvanischer Durchströmung in Flüssigkeit." *Pflüger's Archiv* 232, no. 1 (1933): 821–34.

Holzer, Wolfgang, and Eugen Weissenberg. *Foundations of Short-Wave Therapy: Physics-Technics-Indications.* London: Hutchinson, 1935.

Horsley, Victor. "The Brown Lectures on Pathology." *British Medical Journal* 2 (1885): 111–15, 211–13.

———. "Remarks on the Function of the Thyroid Gland: A Critical and Historical Review." *British Medical Journal* 1 (1892): 215–19, 265–68.

Howell, Joel D. *Technology in the Hospital: Transforming Patient Care in the Early wentieth Century.* Baltimore: Johns Hopkins University Press, 1995.

Hughes, J. "Plasticine and Valves: Industry, Instrumentation and the Emergence of Nuclear Physics." In *The Invisible Industrialist: Manufactures and the Production of Scientific Knowledge*, edited by Jean-Paul Gaudillière and Illana Löwy, 58–101. London: Macmillan, 1998.

Hunt, Linda. *Secret Agenda: The United States Government, Nazi Scientists, and Project Paperclip, 1945 to 1990.* New York: St. Martin's Press, 1991.

Igo, Sarah E. *The Averaged American: Surveys, Citizens, and the Making of a Mass Public.* Cambridge, MA: Harvard University Press, 2008.

Irwin, Alan, and Brian Wynne. *Misunderstanding Science? The Public Reconstruction of Science and Technology.* Cambridge: Cambridge University Press, 1996.

Israel, Giorgio. "Science and the Jewish Question in the Twentieth Century: The Case of Italy and What it Shows." *Aleph: Historical Studies in Science and Judaism* 2, no. 1 (2004): 191–261.

Jacobs, B. L., H. van Praag, and F. Gage. "Adult Brain Neurogenesis and Psychiatry: A Novel Theory of Depression." *Molecular Psychiatry* 5 (2000): 262–69.

Jacyna, L. Stephen. "'A Host of Experienced Microscopists': The Establishment of Histology in Nineteenth-Century Edinburgh." *Bulletin of the History of Medicine* 75, no. 2 (2001): 225–53.

———. "The Laboratory and the Clinic: the Impact of Pathology on Surgical Diagnosis in the Glasgow Western Infirmary, 1875–1910." *Bulletin of the History of Medicine* 62 (1988): 384–406.

———. *Lost Words: Narratives of Language and the Brain, 1825–1926.* Princeton, NJ: Princeton University Press, 2000.

———. *Medicine in Transformation.* Vol. 2 of *The Western Medical Tradition 1800–2000*, edited by W. F. Bynum and Anne Hardy, 11–110. Cambridge: Cambridge University Press, 2006.

Jeannerod, Marc. *The Brain Machine: The Development of Neurophysiological Thought.* Cambridge, MA: Harvard University Press, 1985.

Jones, Caroline, and Peter Galison. *Picturing Science, Producing Art.* New York: Routledge, 1998.

Jones, Edward G., and Lorne M. Mendell. "Assessing the Decade of the Brain." *Science* 284, no. 5415 (1999): 739.

Jönsson, L. E., and L. M. Gunne. "Clinical Studies of Amphetamine Psychosis." In *Amphetamines and Related Compounds*, edited by E. Costa and S. Garattini, 929–36. New York: Raven Press, 1970.

Jordanova, Ludmilla. *Defining Features: Scientific and Medical Portraits 1660–2000*. London: Reakton Books, 2000.

Jorge, Ricardo. "Post-Vaccinal Encephalitis: Its Association with Vaccination and with Post-Infectious and Acute Disseminated Encephalitis." *The Lancet* 1 (1932): 215–19.

Kandel, Eric R. *The Age of Insight: The Quest to Understand the Unconscious in Art, Mind, and Brain, from Vienna 1900 to the Present*. New York: Random House, 2012.

———. *In Search of Memory: The Emergence of a New Science of Mind*. London: W. W. Norton, 2006.

Katz, Bernard. *Electric Excitation of Nerve: A Review*. London: Oxford University Press, 1939.

———. "The Electric Properties of the Muscle Fibre Membrane." *Proceedings of the Royal Society of London*, series B, 135, no. 881 (1948): 506–34.

Kay, L. E. "From Logical Neurons to Poetic Embodiments of Mind: Warren S. McCulloch's Project in Neuroscience." *Science in Context*, 14, no. 4 (2001): 591–614.

———. *The Molecular Vision of Life*. Oxford: Oxford University Press, 1993.

Keelan, Jennifer. "Risk, Efficacy, and Viral Attenuation in Debates over Smallpox Vaccination in Montreal, 1870–1877." In *Crafting Immunity: Working Histories of Clinical Immunology*, edited by Kenton Kroker, J. Keelan and P. Mazumdar, 29–54. Aldergate: Ashgate, 2008.

Keen, W. W. "Address in Surgery." *Journal of the American Medical Association* 28 (1897): 1102–10.

———. "Transactions of the Section on General Surgery of the College of Physicians of Philadelphia." *Annals of Surgery* 27 (1898): 209–27.

Kempermann, Gerd. *Adult Neurogenesis*. Oxford: Oxford University Press, 2006.

———. *Adult Neurogenesis II*. Oxford: Oxford University Press, 2011.

Kendler, K. S., and K. F. Schaffner. "The Dopamine Hypothesis of Schizophrenia: An Historical and Philosophical Analysis." *Philosophy, Psychiatry, and Psychology* 18 (2011): 41–63.

Kern, Ernst, ed. *Theodor Billroth, 1829–1894: Biographie anhand von Selbstzeugnissen*. Munich: Urban & Schwarzenberg, 1994.

Kettenmann, H., and A. Verkhratsky. "Neuroglia: The 150 Years After." *Trends in Neurosciences* 31, no. 12 (2008): 653–59.

Kety, Seymour S. "Biochemical Theories of Schizophrenia." *Science* 129, nos. 3362–63 (1959): 1528–32, 1590–96.

———. "The Biological Substrates of Mental Illness." *Western Journal of Medicine* 125, no. 6 (1976): 491–93.

———. "A Biologist Examines the Mind and Behavior." *Science* 132, no. 3443 (December 23, 1960): 1861–70.

———. "Disorders of the Human Brain." *Scientific American* 241, no. 3 (1979): 202–14.

———. "The Heuristic Aspect of Psychiatry." *American Journal of Psychiatry* 118 (1961): 385–97.

———. "It's Not All in Your Head." *Saturday Review*, February 21, 1976, 28–32.

———. "The Syndrome of Schizophrenia: Unresolved Questions and Opportunities for Research." *British Journal of Psychiatry* 136 (1980): 421–36.

———. "The Theory and Applications of the Exchange of Inert Gas at the Lungs and Tissues." *Pharmacology Review* 3 (1951): 1–41.

Kety, S. S., D. Rosentha, P. H. Wender, and F. Schulsin. "Mental Illness in the Biological and Adoptive Families of Adopted Schizophrenics." *American Journal of Psychiatry* 128 no. 3 (1971): 302–6.

Kety, S. S., R. B. Woodford, M. H. Freyhan, F. A. Harmel et al. "Cerebral Blood Flow and Metabolism in Schizophrenia: The Effects of Barbiturate Semi-narcosis, Insulin Coma and Electroshock." *American Journal of Psychiatry* 104 (1948): 765–67.

Killen, Andreas. *Berlin Electropolis: Shock, Nerves, and German Modernity.* Berkeley: University of California Press, 2006.

King, Nicholas B. "The Scale Politics of Emerging Disease." *Osiris* 19 (2004): 62–76.

Kirk, Stuart A., and Herb Kutchins. *The Selling of DSM: The Rhetoric of Science in Psychiatry.* New York: Aldine De Gruyter, 1992.

Kirk, Stuart, and Susan Einbinder. *Controversial Issues in Mental Health.* Boston: Allyn and Bacon, 1994.

Knevitt, Charles. *Dome: Ralph Tubbs and the Festival of Britain.* London: Chelsea Space, 2012.

Koch, Eric. *Deemed Suspect: A Wartime Blunder.* Toronto: Methuen, 1980.

Kocher, Theodor. "Concerning Pathological Manifestations in Low-Grade Thyroid Diseases." In *Nobel Lectures: Physiology or Medicine 1901–1921.* Amsterdam: Elsevier, 1967.

———. "Die Pathologie der Schilddrüse: Zweites Referat." In *Verhandlungen des Kongresses für Innere Medizin, Dreiundzwanzigster Kongress Gehalten zu München, vom 23.–26. April 1906,* edited by E. von Leyden and Pfeiffer Emil, 59–98 (Wiesbaden: Verlag von J. F. Bergmann, 1906).

Kowarschik, Josef. *Die Diathermie.* 1913. 7th ed. Vienna: Springer, 1930.

Kozuschek, W., and C. Waleczek. "Die Entwicklung der Magenchirurgie im 19. Jahrhundert." In *Theodor Billroth: Ein Leben für die Chirurgie,* edited by W Kozuschek, D. Lorenz, and H. Thomas, 28–51. Basel, Switzerland: Karger, 1992.

Kremer, Richard L. "Institutes for Physiology in Prussia, 1836–1846: Contexts, Interests and Rhetoric." In *The Laboratory Revolution in Medicine,* edited by Andrew Cunningham and Perry Williams, 72–109. Cambridge: Cambridge University Press, n.d.

Kroener, Hans-Peter. "Die Emigration deutschsprachiger Mediziner im Nationalsozialismus." *Berichte zur Wissenschaftsgeschichte* 12, no. 1 (1989): 1–35.

Krohn, Claus-Dieter. *Vereinigte Staaten von Amerika.* Vol. 3 of *Handbuch der deutschsprachigen Emigration, 1933–1945,* edited by Claus-Dieter Krohn, 284–97, 446–66. Darmstadt: Wissenschaftliche Verlagsbuchhandlung, 1998.

Kroker, Kenton. "Creatures of Reason? Picturing Viruses at the Pasteur Institute during the 1920s." In *Crafting Immunity: Working Histories of Clinical Immunology,* edited by Kenton Kroker, J. J. Keelan and P. M. H. Mazumdar, 107–44. Aldershot: Ashgate, 2008.

———. "Epidemic Encephalitis and American Neurology, 1919–1940." *Bulletin of the History of Medicine* 78, no. 1 (2004): 18–147.

————. "Immunity and Its Other: The Anaphylactic Selves of Charles Richet." *Studies in the History and Philosophy of Science: Part C* 30 (1999): 273–96.

————. *The Sleep of Others and the Transformations of Sleep Research.* Toronto: University of Toronto Press, 2007.

Kuhn, Thomas S. *The Structure of Scientific Revolutions.* Chicago: University of Chicago Press, 1962.

Lacasse, Jeffrey, and Tomi Gomory. "Is Graduate Social Work Education Promoting a Critical Approach to Mental Health Practice?" *Journal of Social Work Education* 39 (2003): 383–409.

Lakhovsky, G. "Curing Cancer With Ultra Radio Frequencies." *Radio News Magazine,* February 1925.

————. *The Secret of Life.* London: Heinemann, 1939.

Lakoff, Andrew. "Diagnostic Liquidity: Mental Illness and the Global Trade in DNA." *Theory and Society* 34 (2005): 63–92.

Langenbuch, Carl. "Aus den Sectionssitzungen des VII. Internationalen medicinischen Congresses zu London." *Berliner klinische Wochenschrift* 19 (1882): 31–32.

Langlitz, Nicolas. *Neurospychedelia: The Revival of Hallucinogen Research since the Decade of the Brain.* Berkeley: University of California Press, 2013.

Lapicque, L. "Recherches quantitatives sur l'excitation électrique des nerfs traitée comme une polarisation." *Journal de Physiologie et de Pathologie Générale* 9 (1907): 620–35.

Laslett, T. P. R. *The Physical Basis of Mind: A Series of Broadcast Talks.* Edited by P. Laslett. Oxford: Basil Blackwell, 1950.

Latour, Bruno. "On Technical Mediation—Philosophy, Sociology, Genealogy." *Common Knowledge* 3, no. 2 (1994): 29–64.

————. *Science in Action: How to Follow Scientists and Engineers through Society.* Cambridge, MA: Harvard University Press, 1987.

————. "Visualisation and Cognition: Thinking with Eyes and Hands." *Knowledge and Society: Studies in the Sociology of Culture* 6 (1988): 1–40.

Lawrence, Christopher. "Democratic, Divine and Heroic: The History and Historiography of Surgery." In *Medical History and Surgical Practice: Studies in the History of Surgery,* edited by Christopher Lawrence, 1–47. London: Routledge, 1992.

————. "Incommunicable Knowledge: Science, Technology and the Clinical Art in Britain 1850–1914." *Journal of Contemporary History* 20 (1985): 503–20.

————. "The Nervous System and Society in the Scottish Enlightenment." In *Natural Order: Historical Studies of Scientific Culture,* edited by B. Barnes and S. Shapin. Beverly Hills, CA: Sage Publications, 1979), 19–40.

Lederer, Susan E. *Subjected to Science: Human Experimentation in America before the Second World War.* Baltimore: Johns Hopkins University Press, 1995.

Lenoir, Timothy. "Laboratories, Medicine and Public Life in Germany 1830–1849." In *The Laboratory Revolution in Medicine,* edited by Andrew Cunningham and Perry Williams. Cambridge: Cambridge University Press, 1992.

————. "Models and Instruments in the Development of Electrophysiology, 1845–1912." *Historical Studies in the Physical Sciences* 17, no. 1 (1986): 1–54.

————. *The Strategy of Life: Teleology and Mechanics in Nineteenth-Century German Biology.* Chicago: University of Chicago Press, 1982.

Leo, Jonathan, and Jeffrey Lacasse. "Serotonin and Depression: A Disconnect between the Advertisements and the Scientific Literature." *PLoS Medicine* 2, no. 12 (2005): e392. doi:10.1371/journal.pmed.0020392.

Leriche, René. *Souvenirs de ma vie morte.* Paris: Éditions du Seuil, 1956.

Lesch, John E. *Science and Medicine in France: The Emergence of Experimental Physiology, 1790–1844.* Cambridge, MA: Harvard University Press, 1984.

Leuret, François, and Pierre Gratiolet. *Anatomie comparée du système nerveux considéré dans ses rapports avec l'intelligence.* 2 vols. Paris: J.-B. Baillière, 1839, 1857.

Lewis, Jefferson. *Something Hidden: A Biography of Wilder Penfield.* Toronto: Doubleday Canada, 1981.

Lewy, F. H. "Bericht: Die Chronaxie." *Deutsche Zeitschrift Fuer Nervenheilkunde* 129, nos. 5–6 (1933): 185–95.

Leys, Ruth. "The Turn to Affect: A Critique." *Critical Inquiry* 37 (2011): 434–72.

Link, Bruce G, Jo C. Phelan, Michaeline Bresnahan, Ann Stueve et al. "Public Conceptions of Mental Illness: Labels, Causes, Dangerousness, and Social Distance." *American Journal of Public Health* 89, no. 9 (1999): 1328–33.

Lock, Margaret. *Encounters with Aging: Mythologies of Menopause in Japan and North America.* London: University of California Press, 1993.

Loewi, Otto. "The Excitement of a Life in Science." In *A Dozen Doctors: Autobiographical Sketches,* edited by Dwight J. Ingle, 109–26. Chicago: University of Chicago Press, 1963.

Lombard, H.-Cl. "Sur les fonctions du corps thyroïde d'après des documents récents." *Revue Médicale de la Suisse Romande* 3 (1883): 594–604.

Longerich, Peter. *Holocaust: The Nazi Persecution and Murder of the Jews.* New York: Oxford University Press, 2010.

Luhrmann, T. M. *Of Two Minds: The Growing Disorder in American Psychiatry.* New York: Alfred Knopf, 2010.

Luyet, B. "Variations of the Electric Resistance of Plant Tissues for Alternating Currents of Different Frequencies during Death." *Journal of General Physiology* 15, no. 3 (1932): 283–87.

MacArthur Mental Health Module. "Americans' View of Mental Health and Illness at Century's End: Continuity and Change." 1996ff. http://www.indiana.edu/~icmhsr/docs/Americans'%20Views%20of%20Mental%20Health.pdf.

MacCallum, W. G. *William Stewart Halsted, Surgeon.* Baltimore: Johns Hopkins Press, 1930.

Macdonald, Sharon. *Behind the Scenes at the Science Museum.* Oxford; New York; and Berg, Germany: Oxford University Press, 2002.

Magoun, Horace Winchell. *American Neuroscience in the Twentieth Century: Confluence of the Neural, Behavioral, and Communicative Streams.* Edited by Louise H. Marshall. Lisse, The Netherlands: A. A. Balkema, 2002.

Manriz, C. P. "Influenza Caused Epidemic Encephalitis: The Circumstantial Evidence and a Challenge to the Nay-Sayers." *Medical Hypothesis* 28 (1989): 139–42.

Marchand, F. *Der Process der Wundheilung mit Einschluss der Transplantation.* Stuttgart: Enke, 1901.

Marks, Harry M. *The Progress of Experiment: Science and Therapeutic Reform in the United States, 1900–1990.* Cambridge: Cambridge University Press, 1997.

———. "Trust and Mistrust in the Marketplace: Statistics and Clinical Research, 1945–1960." *History of Science* 38, no. 3 (2000): 343–55.

———. "'Until the Sun of Science . . . the True Apollo of Medicine Has Risen': Collective Investigation in Britain and America, 1880–1910." *Medical History* 50 (2006): 147–66.

Marley, E. "Response to Some Stimulant and Depressant Drugs of the Central Nervous System." *British Journal of Psychiatry* 106 (1960): 76–92.

Matheson Commission. *Epidemic Encephalitis: Etiology, Epidemiology, Treatment; Report of a Survey by the Matheson Commission.* New York: Columbia University Press, 1929.

Mathey, Emily K., Ariel Arthur, and Patricia J. Armati. "Cns Oligarchs; the Rise of the Oligodendrocyte in a Neuron-Centric Culture." In *The Biology of Oligodendrocytes*, edited by Patricia J. Armati and Emily K. Mathey. Cambridge: Cambridge University Press, 2010.

Maulitz, Russell C. *Morbid Appearances: The Anatomy of Pathology in the Early Nineteenth Century.* Cambridge: Cambridge University Press, 1987.

Mayer-Gross, W. "Experimental Psychoses and Other Mental Abnormalities Produced by Drugs." *British Medical Journal* 1 (1951): 317–21.

Mayes, Rick, and Allan Horwitz. "DSM III and the Revolution in the Classification of Mental Illness." *Journal of the History of Behavioral Sciences* 41, no. 3 (2005): 249–67.

Mazumdar, Pauline M. H. "Antitoxin and Anatoxine: The League of Nations and the Institut Pasteur, 1920–1939." In *Crafting Immunity: Working Histories of Clinical Immunology*, edited by Kenton Kroker, J. Keelan, and P. M. H. Mazumdar, 177–97. Aldergate, UK: Ashgate, 2008.

McCall, Sherman, James M. Henry, Ann H. Reid, and Jeffery K Taubenberger. "Influenza RNA Not Detected in Archival Brain Tissues from Acute Encephalitis Lethargica Cases or in Postencephalitic Parkinson Cases." *Journal of Neuropathology and Experimental Neurology* 60, no. 7 (2001): 696–704.

McClendon, J. F. "Polarization-Capacity as Measured with a Wheatstone Bridge with Sine-Wave Alternating Currents of High and Low Frequency." *American Journal of Physiology* 91, no. 1 (1929): 83–93.

McClure, Lucretia W. "A Student of History: Perspectives on the Contributions of Estelle Brodman." *Journal of the Medical Library Association* 96 (2008): 255–61.

McConnell, W. B. "Amphetamine Substances in Mental Illnesses in Northern Ireland." *British Journal of Psychiatry* 109 (1963): 218–24.

McGlashan, Thomas H. "The Chestnut Lodge Follow-up Study I: Follow-up Methodology and Study Sample." *Archives of General Psychiatry* 41 (1984): 573–601.

McNally, Richard. *What Is Mental Illness?* Cambridge, MA: Belknap Press, 2011.

Medawar, Jean, and David Pyke. *Hitler's Gift: The True Story of the Scientists Expelled by the Nazi Regime.* New York: Arkade Publishing, 2001.

Meltzer, H. Y., and S. M. Stahl. "The Dopamine Hypothesis of Schizophrenia." *Schizophrenia Bulletin* 2 (1976): 19–76.

Mendelsohn, J. Andrew. "From Eradication to Equilibrium: How Epidemics Became Complex after World War I." In *Greater Than the Parts: Holism in Biomedicine, 1920–1950*, edited by Christopher Lawrence and George Weisz, 303–31. New York: Oxford University Press, 1998.

Micale, Mark S. "The Ten Most Important Changes in Psychiatry since World War II." *History of Psychiatry* 25, no. 4 (2014): 485–91.

Michler, Markwart. *Langenbeck, Bernhard von.* 1982. Accessed June 15, 2014. http://www.deutsche-biographie.de/pnd11887490X.html.

Miller, Gregory, and Jennifer Jennifer Keller. "Psychology and Neuroscience: Making Peace." *Current Directions in Psychological Science* 9, no. 6 (2000): 212–15.

Millet, David. "Wiring the Brain: From the Excitable Cortex to the EEG, 1870–1940." PhD diss., University of Chicago, 2001.

Moncrieff, Joanna. "The Creation of the Concept of an Antidepressant: An Historical Analysis." *Social Science and Medicine* 66 (2008): 2346–55.

Monroe, R. R., and H. J. Drell. "Oral Use of Stimulants Obtained from Inhalers." *Journal of the American Medical Association* 135 (1947): 909–15.

Morris, Robert T. *Dawn of the Fourth Era in Surgery.* Philadelphia: W. B. Saunders, 1910.

Mortimer, P. P. "Historical Review: Was Encephalitis Lethargica a Post-Influenzal or Some Other Phenomenon? Time to Re-Examine the Problem." *Epidemiology and Infection* 137 (2009): 449–55.

Mosher, Loren. "The Center for Studies of Schizophrenia." *Schizophrenia Bulletin* 1, no. 1 (1969): 4.

Murard, Lion. "La santé publique et ses instruments de mesure: Des barèmes évaluatifs américains aux indices numériques de la Société des Nations, 1915–1955." In *Body Counts: Medical Quantification in Historical and Sociological Perspective,* edited by G. Jorland, A. Opinel, and George Weisz, 266–308. Montreal: McGill-Queen's University Press, 2005.

Muséum national d'histoire naturelle (Paris). *Notice des animaux vivans de la Ménagerie du Muséum d'histoire naturelle (Levrault, Schoell et Comp., 1804).* Paris: Schoell et Comp, 1804.

Musselman, Elizabeth Green. *Nervous Conditions: Science and the Body Politic in Early Industrial Britain.* Albany: State University of New York, 2006.

Nagelschmidt, Franz. *Lehrbuch Der Diathermie Für Ärzte Und Studierende.* 2nd ed. Berlin: Springer, 1921.

National Advisory Mental Health Council's Workgroup on Basic Sciences. "Setting Priorities for Basic Brain and Behavioral Science Research at NIMH." 2004. https://www.nimh.nih.gov/about/advisory-boards-and-groups/namhc/reports/bbbs-research_42531.pdf.

Nernst, W. "Zur Theorie Des Elektrischen Reizes." *Pflügers Archiv* 122 (1908): 275–314.

New York Times. "'Flu' the Precursor of Sleeping Sickness." March 18, 1923, 4.

———. "New Clues Found to Life Process." February 27, 1938, 35.

Olch, Peter D. "Evarts A. Graham, the American College of Surgeons, and the American Board of Surgery." *Journal of the History of Medicine and Allied Sciences* 27 (1972): 247–61.

Olfson, Mark, and Steven C. Marcus. "National Trends in Outpatient Psychotherapy." *American Journal of Psychiatry* 167, no. 12 (2010): 1456–63.

Oppenheim, G. "Die Schallplatte Im Dienste Der Elektro-Medizin." *Klinische Wochenschrift* 11, no. 14 (1932): 595–97.

Otis, Laura. "The Metaphoric Circuit: Organic and Technological Communication in the Nineteenth Century." *Journal of the History of Ideas* 63, no. 1 (2002): 105–28.

Outram, Dorinda. *Georges Cuvier: Vocation, Science and Authority in Post-Revolutionary France.* Manchester, UK: Manchester University Press, 1984.

Owen, F. *No Speed Limit: The Highs and Lows of Meth.* New York: St. Martin's Griffin, 2007.

Paget, Stephen. *Sir Victor Horsley: A Study of His Life and Work.* New York: Harcourt, Brace and Howe, 1920.

Parpura, V., and A. Verkhratsky. "Neuroglia at the Crossroads of Homoeostasis, Metabolism and Signalling: Evolution of the Concept." *ASN Neuro* 4, no. 4 (2012). doi:10.1042/AN20120019.

Parsons, Allan C., A. Salusbury Macnalty, and J. R. Perdrau. *Report on Epidemic Encephalitis.* Reports on Public Health and Medical Subjects, Ministry of Health. London: HSMO, 1922.

Payr, E. *Die physiologisch-biologische Richtung der modernen Chirurgie: Antrittsvorlesung gehalten am 11. Dezember 1912 in der Aula der Universität Leipzig.* Leipzig: S. Hirzel, 1913.

Pearce, J. M. S. "Louis Pierre Gratiolet (1815–1865)." *European Neurology* 56 (2006): 262–64.

Pearle, Kathleen M. "Aerzteemigration nach 1933 in die USA: Der Fall New York." *Medizinhistorisches Journal* 19, no. 1 (1984): 112–37.

Pedersen, Susan. "Back to the League of Nations." *American Historical Review* 112 (2007): 1091–17.

Peña, C. Thomas de la. *The Body Electric: How Strange Machines Built the Modern American.* New York: New York University Press, 2003.

Penfield, Wilder. "Alterations of the Golgi Apparatus in Nerve Cells." *Brain* 43, no. 3 (1920): 290–305.

———, ed. *Cytology and Cellular Pathology of the Nervous System.* New York: Paul B. Hoeber, 1932.

———. "Epilepsy and Surgical Therapy." *Archives of Neurology and Psychiatry* 36, no. 3 (1936): 449–84.

———. "The Evidence for a Cerebral Vascular Mechanism in Epilepsy." *Annals of Internal Medicine* 7 (1933): 303–10.

———. "Intracerebral Vascular Nerves." *Archives of Neurology and Psychiatry* 27 (1932): 30–44.

———. "The Mechanism of Cicatricial Contraction in the Brain." *Brain* 50, nos. 3–4 (1927): 499–517.

———. *No Man Alone: A Neurosurgeon's Life.* Boston: Little, Brown, 1977.

Penfield, Wilder, and Richard C. Buckley. "Punctures of the Brain: The Factors Concerned in Gliosis and in Cicatricial Contraction." *Archives of Neurology and Psychiatry* 20 (1928): 1–13.

Penfield, Wilder, and William Cone. "Neuroglia and Microglia (the Metallic Methods)." In *Handbook of Microscopical Technique for Workers in Both Animal and Plant Tissues,* edited by Clarence Erwin McClung. New York: P. B. Hoeber, 1926.

Peter, Kernahan. "Franklin Martin and the Standardization of American Surgery, 1890–1940." PhD diss., University of Minnesota, 2010.

Peters, Uwe-Hendrik. "Emigration deutscher Psychiater nach England. (Teil 1)." *Fortschritte der Neurologie und Psychiatrie* 64, no. 5 (1996): 161–67.

Pickersgill, Martin. "From Psyche to Soma? Changing Accounts of Antisocial Personality Disorders in the American Journal of Psychiatry." *History of Psychiatry* 21 (2010): 294–311.

Pickersgill, Martin, and Ira van Keulen. *Sociological Reflections on the Neurosciences.* Bingley, UK: Emerald Group, 2011.

Pickstone, John V. "Objects and Objectives: Notes on the Material Cultures of Medicine." In *Technologies of Modern Medicine*, edited by Ghislaine Lawrence, 13–24. London: Science Museum, 1994.

———. "Ways of Knowing: Towards a Historical Sociology of Science, Technology and Medicine." *British Journal for the History of Science* 26 (1993): 433–58.

Pletscher, Alfred, Parkhurst Shore, and Bernard B. Brodie. "Serotonin Release as a Possible Mechanism of Reserpine Action." *Science* 122, no. 3165 (1955): 374–75.

Pliszka, S. R. *Neuroscience for the Mental Health Clinician.* New York: Guilford Press, 2003.

Pollin, W., and J. R. Stabenau. "Biological, Psychological and Historical Differences in a Series of Monozygotic Twins Discordant for Schizophrenia." In *The Transmission of Schizophrenia*, translated by D. Rosenthal and S. S. Kety, 317–32. New York: Pergamon Press, 1968.

Polyak, H., ed. *The History and Philosophy of Knowledge of the Brain and Its Functions.* Oxford: Blackwell, 1957.

Porter, Theodore M. "How Science Became Technical." *Isis* 100, no. 3 (2009): 292–309.

———. *The Rise of Statistical Thinking, 1820–1900.* Princeton, NJ: Princeton University Press, 1988.

Pressman, Jack. *Last Resort: Psychosurgery and the Limits of Medicine.* Cambridge: Cambridge University Press, 1998.

Prüll, Cay-Rüdiger. "Pathology and Surgery in London and Berlin 1800–1930: Pathological Theory and Clinical Practice." In *Pathology in the 19th and 20th Centuries: The Relationship between Theory and Practice*, edited by Cay-Rüdiger Prüll, 71–99. Sheffield, UK: EAHMH, 1998.

Rajewsky, B., and H. Lampert. *Erforschung Und Praxis Der Wärmebehandlung in Der Medizin Einschliesslich Diathermie Und Kurzwellentherapie.* Dresden: Steinkopff, 1937.

Randrup, A., and I. Munkvad. "Biochemical, Anatomical and Psychological Investigations of Stereotyped Behavior Induced by Amephtamines." In *Amphetamines and Related Compounds*, edited by E. Costa and S. Garattini, 695–713. New York: Raven Press, 1970.

———. "Evidence Indicating an Association between Schizophrenia and Dopaminergic Hyperactivity in the Brain." *Orthomolecular Psychiatry* 1 (1972): 2–7.

———. "Stereotyped Activites Produced by Amphetamine in Several Animal Species and Man." *Psychopharmacologia* 11 (1967): 300–310.

Ranke, O. F. "Philipp Broemser." *Ergebnisse Der Physiologie* 44, no. 1 (1941): 1–2.

Rapport, Richard. *Nerve Endings: The Discovery of the Synapse.* New York: W. W. Norton, 2005.

Rasmussen, Nicolas. "The Mid-Century Biophysics Bubble: Hiroshima and the Biological Revolution in America, Revisited." *History of Science* 35, no. 1 (1997): 245–93.

———. *On Speed: The Many Lives of Amphetamines*. New York: New York University Press, 2008.

———. "What Moves When Scientific Instruments Migrate? Software and Hardware in the Transfer of Biological Electron Microscopy to Postwar Australia." *Technology and Culture* 40, no. 1 (1999): 47–73.

Rauch, Renate. "Richard Wagner, Habseligkeiten. Roman, Berlin: Akademie Verlag, 2004." *Berliner Zeitung*, October 28, 2004, 36.

"Raw Materials, Costs—in Tube Manufacture." *Electronics* (1930): 366.

Rawlin, J. W. "Amphetamine Abuse." In *Amphetamine Abuse*, edited by J. R. Russo, 51–65. Springfield, IL: Charles C Thomas, 1968.

Raz, Mical. *The Lobotomy Letters: The Making of American Psychosurgery*. Rochester, NY: University of Rochester Press, 2013.

Rees, Tobias. "Being Neurologically Human Today: Life, Science, and Adult Cerebral Plasticity (An Ethical Analysis)." *American Ethnologist* 37, no. 1 (2010): 150–66.

"Register of Biophysical Assistants." *The Lancet* 215, no. 5570 (May 31, 1930): 1195–96.

Remington, Roe E. "The High Frequency Wheatstone Bridge as a Tool in Cytological Studies; with Some Observations on the Resistance and Capacity of the Cells of the Beet Root." *Protoplasma* 5, no. 1 (1928): 338–99.

Richards, Robert J. *Darwin and the Emergence of Evolutionary Theories of Mind and Behavior*. Chicago: University of Chicago Press, 1989.

Riese, Walther. *A History of Neurology*. New York: MD Publications, 1959.

Robertson, Brian. "An Interview with Eric Kandel." *Journal of Physiology* 588, no. 5 (2010): 743–45.

Robinson, Joseph D. *Mechanisms of Synaptic Transmission: Bridging the Gaps (1890–1990)*. Oxford: Oxford University Press, 2001.

Roleff, Tamara L., and Laura K. Egendof, eds. *Mental Illness: Opposing Viewpoints*. New York: Greenhaven Press, 2000.

Rose, Nikolas. "Medicine, History and the Present." In *Reassessing Foucault: Power, Medicine, and the Body*, edited by Colin Jones and Roy Porter, 48–72. London: Routledge, 1994.

———. "The Neurochemical Self and its Anomalies." In *Risk and Morality*, edited by R. Ericson, 407–37. Toronto: University of Toronto Press, 2003.

———. *The Politics of Life Itself: Biomedicine, Power, and Subjectivity in the Twenty-First Century*. Princeton, NJ: Princeton University Press, 2007.

Rose, Nikolas, and Joelle Abi-Rached. *Neuro: The New Brain Sciences and the Management of the Mind*. Princeton, NJ: Princeton University Press, 2013.

Rosenberg, H. "Untersuchungen Über Nervenaktionsströme." *Pflüger's Archiv* 223, no. 1 (1930): 120–21.

Rosenfeld, A. "Drugs That Even Scare Hippies." *Life*, October 27, 1967, 81–82 .

Rosenhan, D. L. "On Being Sane in Insane Places." *Science* 179 (1973): 250–58.

Rousseau, G. S. *Nervous Acts: Essays on Literature, Culture and Sensibility*. New York: Palgrave Macmillan, 2004.

Rowland, Lewis P. *The Legacy of Tracy J. Putnam and H. Houston Merritt: Modern Neurology in the United States*. Oxford: Oxford University Press, 2008.

Ravenholt, R. T., and W. H. Foege. "Influenza, Encephalitis Lethargica, Parkinsonism." *Lancet* 2 (1982): 860–64.

Rubin, Robert. "Review of Brain Imaging in Clinical Psychiatry, edited K Ranga Rama Krishnan and P Murali Doraiswamy." *American Journal of Psychiatry* 155, no. 8 (1998): 1125–26.

Rubin, Ronald P. "A Brief History of Great Discoveries in Pharmacology: In Celebration of the Centennial Anniversary of the Founding of the American Society of Pharmacology and Experimental Therapeutics." *Pharmacological Reviews* 59, no. 4 (2007): 289–359.

Rubinstein, Nina. *In Search of Exile, 1880–2000.* New York: Bard College, 1989.

Rushton, W. A. H. "A Physical Analysis of the Relation between Threshold and Interpolar Length in the Electric Excitation of Medullated Nerve." *Journal of Physiology* 82, no. 3 (1934): 483.

Rutkow, Ira M. "William Halsted and Theodor Kocher: 'An Exquisite Friendship.'" *Annals of Surgery* 188 (1978): 630–37.

Rutty, Christopher. "Canadian Vaccine Research, Production and International Regulation: Connaught Laboratories and Smallpox Vaccines, 1962–1980." In *Crafting Immunity: Working Histories of Clinical Immunology,* edited by K. Kroker, J. Keelan, and P. Mazumdar, 273–300. Aldergate, UK: Ashgate, 2008.

Rylander, G. "Addiction to Preludin Intravenously Injected." *Proceedings of the Fourth World Congress of Psychiatry.* Amsterdam: Excerpta Medica Foundation, 1966.

———. "Clinical and Medico-Criminological Aspects of Addiction to Central Stimulating Drugs." In *Abuse of Central Stimulants: Symposium Arranged by the Swedish Committee on International Health Relations, Stockholm, November 25–27, 1968,* edited by F. Sjöqvist and M. Tottie, 251–73. New York: Raven Press, 1969.

Sachar, Howard M. *A History of the Jews in America.* New York: Knopf, 1992.

Sachs, Leslie. "Advice from the Midwest." In *Hitler's Exiles: Personal Stories of the Fight from Nazi Germany to America,* edited by Mark M. Anderson, 229–32. New York: The New Press, 1998.

Saint-Hilaire, Étienne Geoffroy, and Frédéric Cuvier. *Histoire naturelle des mammifères.* Vol. 1. Paris: A. Belin, 1833.

Sakmann, Bernd. "Sir Bernard Katz: 26 March 1911–20 April 2003." *Biographical Memoires of the Fellows of the Royal Society* 53, no. 1 (2007): 185–202.

Sapir, Philip, Julius Segal, and Marcus S. Goldstein. "Anthropology and the Research Grant and Fellowship Programs of the National Institute of Mental Health." *American Anthropologist,* n.s., 65, no. 1 (February 1963): 117–32.

Schaefer, Hans. *Elektrophysiologie. I. Band: Allgemeine Elektrophysiologie.* Vienna: Franz Deuticke, 1940.

———. "Neuere Untersuchungen Ueber Den Nervenaktionsstrom." *Ergebnisse Der Physiologie* 36, no. 1 (1934): 151–248.

Scheminzky, F. "Über Einige Anwendungen Der Elektronenröhren in Widerstandsschaltung Und Der Glimmlampen Für Die Physiologie." *Pflüger's Archiv* 213, no. 1 (1926): 126–27.

Schiller, Francis. *Paul Broca: Founder of French Anthropology, Explorer of the Brain.* New York: Oxford University Press, 1991.

Schimmelbusch, Curt. *Anleitung zur Aseptischen Wundbehandlung.* Berlin: Hirschwald, 1892.

Schlich, Thomas. "Asepsis and Bacteriology: A Realignment of Surgery and Laboratory Science." *Medical History* 56 (2012): 308–43.

———. "Changing Disease Identities: Cretinism, Politics and Surgery (1844–1892)." *Medical History* 38 (1994): 421–43.

———. "Farmer to Industrialist: Lister's Antisepsis and the Making of Modern Surgery in Germany." *Notes and Records of the Royal Society* 67 (2013): 245–60.

———. *The Origins of Organ Transplantation: Surgery and Laboratory Science, 1880s–1930s.* Rochester, NY: University of Rochester Press, 2010.

———. *Surgery, Science and Industry: A Revolution in Fracture Care, 1950s–1990s.* Basingstoke, UK: Palgrave, 2002.

———. "Surgery, Science and Modernity: Operating Rooms and Laboratories as Spaces of Control." *History of Science* 45 (2007): 231–56.

Schliephake, E. "Die Biologische Wärmewirkung Im Elektrischen Hochfrequenzfeld." *Verhandlungen Der Deutschen Gesellschaft Für Innere Medizin* 4 (1928): 307–10.

Schmidgen, Henning. *Die Helmholtz-Kurven: Auf Der Spur Der Verlorenen Zeit.* Berlin: Merve, 2009.

Schmidgen, Henning, Peter Geimer, and Sven Dierig. *Kultur im Experiment.* Berlin: Cadmos, 2004.

Schmitt, Francis O. *The Never-Ceasing Search.* Philadelphia: American Philosophical Society, 1990.

Schmitt, F. O., and O. H. A. Schmitt. "A Universal Precision Stimulator." *Science* 76, no. 1971 (1932): 328–30.

Schoenfeld, Robert L. *Exploring the Nervous System: With Electronic Tools, an Institutional Base, a Network of Scientists.* Boca Raton, FL: Universal Publishers, 2006.

Schönbauer, Leopold. "Billroth, Christian Albert Theodor." In *Neue Deutsche Biographie.* Vol. 2. Berlin: Duncker & Humblot, 1955. http://www.deutsche-biographie.de/pnd118510916.html.

Scull, Andrew. "The Mental Health Sector and the Social Sciences in Post–World War II USA Part 1: Total War and Its Aftermath." *History of Psychiatry* 22, no. 1 (2011): 3–19.

———. "The Mental Health Sector and the Social Sciences in Post–World War II USA Part 2: The Impact of Federal Research Funding and the Drugs Research." *History of Psychiatry* 22, no. 3 (2011): 268–84.

"Seymour S. Kety, 25 August 1915–25 May 2000." *Proceedings of the American Philosophical Society* 146, no. 1 (2002): 101–10.

Shapin, Steven. "The Invisible Technician." *American Scientist* 77, no. 6 (1989): 554–63.

———. *Social History of Truth: Civility and Science in Seventeenth-Century England.* Chicago: University of Chicago Press, 1994.

Sheehan, John. "The Role and Rewards of Asylum Attendants in Victorian England." *International History of Nursing Journal* 3, no. 4 (Summer 1998): 25–33.

Shepherd, Gordon. *Creating Modern Neuroscience: The Revolutionary 1950s.* Oxford: Oxford University Press, 2010.

———. *Foundations of the Neuron Doctrine.* Oxford: Oxford University Press, 1991.

———. *The Synaptic Organization of the Brain.* Oxford: Oxford University Press, 2004.

Shick, J. F. E., D. E. Smith, and F. H. Meyers. "Patterns of Drug Use in the Haight-Ashbury Neighborhood." *Clinical Toxicology* 3, no. 1 (1970): 19–56.

Shinohara, Mami, Beth Dollinger, Gwen Brown, Stanley Rapoport et al. "Cerebral Glucose Utilization: Local Changes During and After Recovery from Spreading Cortical Depression." *Science* 203, no. 4376 (1979): 188–90.

Shorter, Edward. *A History of Psychiatry: From the Era of the Asylum to the Age of Prozac.* New York: John Wiley, 1997.

Shorvon, S. "The Evolution of Epilepsy Theory and Practice at the National Hospital for the Relief and Cure of Epilepsy, Queen Square between 1860 and 1910." *Epilepsy & Behavior* 31 (2014): 228–42.

Simmer, Hans H. "Innere Sekretion der Ovarien als Ursache der Menstruation: Halbans Falsifikation der Pflügerschen Hypothese." In *Festschrift für Erna Lesky zum 70. Geburtstag*, edited by Kurt Ganzinger, Hans H. Simmer, Manfred Skopec, and Helmut Wyklicky, 123–48. Vienna: Brüder Hollin, 1981.

———. "Robert Tuttle Morris (1857–1945): A Pioneer in Ovarian Transplants." *Obstetrics and Gynecology* 35 (1970): 314–28.

Simmons, Ian G. "Environments, Ecologies, and Cultures across Space and Time." In *A Companion to World History*, edited by Douglas Northrop, 143–55. Oxford: Wiley-Blackwell, 2012.

Slater, E. "*Amphetamine Psychosis,*" *British Medical Journal* 1, no. 5120 (1959): 488.

Smail, Daniel Lord. "Neurohistory in Action: Hoarding and the Human Past." *Isis* 105, no.

1 (2014): 110–22.

———. *On Deep History and the Brain.* Berkeley: University of California Press, 2008.

Smith, D. "Speed Freaks vs. Acid Heads: Conflict Between Drug Subcultures." *Clinical Pediatrics* 8 (1969): 185–92.

Smith, D., and C. M. Fischer. "An Analysis of 310 Cases of Acute High-Dose Methamphetamine Toxicity in Haight-Ashbury." *Clinical Toxicology* 3, no. 1 (1970): 117–24.

Smith, R. C. "The World of the Haight-Ashbury Speed Freak." *Journal of Psychoactive Drugs* 2 (1969): 77–83.

Smith, Roger. *Inhibition: History and Meaning in the Sciences of Mind and Brain.* Berkeley: University of California Press, 1992.

Snow, Stephanie J. *Operations without Pain: The Practice and Science of Anaesthesia in Victorian Britain.* Basingstoke, UK: Palgrave Macmillan, 2006.

Snyder, S. H. "Amphetamine Psychosis: A 'Model' Schizophrenia Mediated by Catecholamines." *American Journal of Psychiatry* 130, no. 1 (1973): 61–67.

———. "Catecholamines in the Brain as Mediators of Amphetamine Psychosis." *Archives of General Psychiatry* 27 (1972): 169–79.

———. "The Dopamine Hypothesis of Schizophrenia: Focus on the Dopamine Receptor." *American Journal of Psychiatry* 133, no. 2 (1976): 197–202.

Snyder, S. H., E. Richelson, H. Weingartner, and L. A. Faillace. "Psychotropic Methoxyamphetamines: Structure and Activity in Man." In *Amphetamines and Related Compounds*, edited by E. Costa and S. Garattini, 905–28. New York: Raven Press, 1970.

Snyder, Solomon. *Madness and the Brain.* New York: McGraw-Hill, 1974.

Söderqvist, Thomas. "Neurobiographies: Writing Lives in the History of Neurology and Neuroscience." *Journal of the History of Neurosciences* 11, no. 1 (2002): 38–48.

Sokoloff, Louis. "Mapping Cerebral Activity with Deoxyglucose." *Journal of the American Medical Association* 244, no. 14 (1980): 1612.

Specter, Michael. "Rethinking the Brain." *New Yorker*, July 23, 2001.

Spitzer, R. L., and J. Endicott. "Medical and Mental Disorder: Proposed Definition and Criteria." In *Critical Issues in Psychiatric Diagnosis*, edited by R. L. Spitzer and D. F. Klein, 15–39. New York: Raven Press, 1978.

Squire, Larry, and Eric Kandel. *Memory: From Mind to Molecule.* San Francisco: W. H. Freeman, 1999.

Stabenau, James B., and William Pollin. "Comparative Life History Differences of Families of Schizophrenics, Delinquents and 'Normals.'" *American Journal of Psychiatry* 124, no. 11 (1968): 1526–34.

Stadler, Max. "Assembling Life: Models, the Cell, and the Reformations of Biological Science, 1920–1960." PhD diss., Imperial College London, 2009.

Stafford, J. "Radio Waves Cause Fever in Patients to Cure Dreaded Paresis." *Science News-Letter* 18, no. 484 (1930): 36.

Stahnisch, Frank W. "German-Speaking Émigré Neuroscientists in North America after 1933: Critical Reflections on Emigration-Induced Scientific Change." *Oesterreichische Zeitschrift fuer Geschichtswissenschaften* 21, no. 3 (2010): 36–68.

———. "Transforming the Lab: Technological and Societal Concerns in the Pursuit of De- and Regeneration in the German Morphological Neurosciences, 1910–1930." *Medicine Studies* 1, no. 1 (2009): 41–54.

———. "Zur Zwangsemigration deutschsprachiger Neurowissenschaftler nach Nordamerika: Der historische Fall des Montreal Neurological Institute." *Schriftenreihe der Deutschen Gesellschaft fuer Geschichte der Nervenheilkunde* 14, no. 1 (2008): 414–42.

Stahnisch, Frank W., and Peter J. Koehler. "Three 20th Century Multi-authored Handbooks Serving as Vital Catalyzers of an Emerging Specialization—A Case Study from the History of Neurology and Psychiatry." *Journal of Mental and Nervous Diseases* 200, no. 12 (2012): 1067–75.

Stahnisch, Frank W., and Thomas Hoffman. "Kurt Goldstein and the Neurology of Movement during the Interwar Years—Physiological Experimentation, Clinical Psychology and Early Rehabilitation." In *Was bewegt uns? Menschen im Spannungsfeld zwischen Mobilitaet und Beschleunigung*, edited by Christian Hoffstadt, Franz Peschke, and Andreas Schulz-Buchta, 283–311. Bochum, Germany: Projektverlag, 2010.

Star, Susan Leigh. *Regions of the Mind: Brain Research and the Quest for Scientific Certainty.* Stanford, CA: Stanford University Press, 1989.

Stiles, Anne. *Neurology and Literature, 1860–1920.* Basingstoke, UK: Palgrave Macmillan, 2007.

———. *Popular Fiction and Brain Science in the Late Nineteenth Century.* Cambridge: Cambridge University Press, 2011.

Stoerk, Oskar, and Hans v. Haberer. "Ueber das anatomische Verhalten intrarenal eingepflanzten Nebennierengewebes." *Verhandlungen der Deutschen Gesellschaft für Chirurgie* 37 (1908): 692–729.

Strand, Michael. "Where Do Classifications Come From? The DSM-III, the Transformation of American Psychiatry, and the Problem of Origins in the Sociology of Knowledge." *Theoretical Sociology* 40 (2011): 273–313.

Strickhausen, Waltraud. *Kanada.* Vol. 3 of *Handbuch der deutschsprachigen Emigration 1933–1945,* edited by Krohn Claus-Dieter, 293–95. Darmstadt: Wissenschaftliche Verlagsbuchhandlung, 1998.

Sturdy, Steve, and Roger Cooter. "Science, Scientific Management, and the Transformation of Britain c. 1870–1950." *History of Science* 36 (1998): 421–66.

Sturges, C. S. *Dr. Dave: A Profile of David E. Smith, M.D., Founder of the Haight Ashbury Free Clinics.* Walnut Creek, CA: Devil Mountain, 1993.

Swazey, Judith. *Chlorpromazine in Psychiatry.* Cambridge, MA: MIT Press, 1974.

Taylor, John Russell. *Strangers in Paradise: The Hollywood Émigrés, 1933–1950.* New York: Holt Rinehart and Winston, 1983.

Temkin, Owsei. "The Role of Surgery in the Rise of Modern Medical Thought." *Bulletin of the History of Medicine* 25 (1951): 248–59.

Teuber, Hans L. "Kurt Goldstein's Role in the Development of Neuropsychology." *Neuropsychologia* 4, no. 4 (1966): 299–310.

Thase, Michael E., Joel B. Greenhouse, Ellen Frank, Charles F. Reynolds III et al. "Treatment of Major Depression with Psychotherapy or Psychotherapy-Pharmacotherapy Combinations." *Archives of General Psychiatry* 54 (1997): 1009–15.

Thompson, E. *The Soundscape of Modernity: Architectural Acoustics and the Culture of Listening in America, 1900–1933.* Cambridge: MIT Press, 2002.

Thompson, Mathew. "Disability, Psychiatry, and Eugenics." In *The Oxford Handbook of the History of Eugenics,* edited by Alison Bashford and Philippa Levine, 116–33. Oxford: Oxford University Press, 2010.

———. *Psychological Subjects: Identity, Culture, and Health in Twentieth-Century Britain.* New York: Oxford University Press, 2006.

Thornton, Davi Johnson. *Brain Culture: Neuroscience and Popular Media.* New Brunswick, NJ: Rutgers University Press, 2011.

Tonkin, Bill, and George Simner. *Post Cards and Related Collectibles of the Festival of Britain.* West Wickham, UK: Exhibition Study Group, 2001.

Tröhler, Ulrich. *Mikulicz-Radecki, Johannes von.* Vol. 4 of *Dictionary of Medical Biography,* edited by William F. Bynum and Helen Bynum, 877–78. Westport, CT: Greenwood Press, 2006.

———. *Der Nobelpreisträger Theodor Kocher 1841–1917: Auf dem Weg zur Physiologischen Chirurgie.* Basel, Switzerland: Birkhäuser, 1984.

———. "Surgery (Modern)." In *Companion Encyclopedia of the History of Medicine,* edited by William F. Bynum and Roy Porter, 2:984–1028. London: Routledge, 1993.

———. "Theodor Kocher: Chirurgie und Ethik." *Gesnerus* 49 (1992): 119–35.

———. "Die Wechselwirkung von Anatomie, Physiologie und Chirurgie im Werk Kochers und einiger Zeitgenossen." In *Theodor Kocher 1841–1917,* edited by Urs Boschung, 53–71. Bern, Switzerland: Huber, 1991.

Trotter, Robert J. "Psychiatry for the 80's." *Science* 119, no. 22 (1981): 348–49.

Turnbull, H. M., and J. McIntosh. "Encephalo-myelitis following vaccination." *British Journal of Experimental Pathology* 7 (1926): 181–222.

Twohig, Peter L. *Labour in the Laboratory Medical Laboratory Workers in the Maritimes, 1900–1950*. Montreal: McGill-Queen's University Press, 2005.

Ullmann, Emerich. "Experimentelle Nierentransplantation: Vorläufige Mittheilung." *Wiener klinische Wochenschrift* 15 (1902): 281–82.

Unger, Ernst. "Nierentransplantationen." *Berliner klinische Wochenschrift* 47 (1910): 573–78.

Untangling the Mind: The Legacy of Dr. Heinz Lehmann. Produced by Inc. Filmaker's Library. 1999.

US Department of Health and Human Services. *Mental Health: A Report of the Surgeon General*. Rockville, MD: US Department of Health and Human Services, Substance Abuse and Mental Health Services Administration, 1999.

"Vaccination and Encephalitis." *British Medical Journal* vol. 1 (1931): 104–5.

van Kammen, D. P., W. B. van Kammen, L. S. Mann, T. Seppala et al. "Dopamine Metabolism in the Cerebrospinal Fluid of Drug-Free Schizophrenic Patients with and without Cortical Atrophy." *Archives of General Psychiatry* 43, no 10 (1986): 978–83.

"Variola Research." *British Medical Journal* 1, no. 3398 (1926): 293–94.

Vidal, Fernando. "Brainhood, Anthropological Figure of Modernity." *History of the Human Sciences* 22, no. 1 (2009): 5–36.

———. "Le Sujet cérébral: Une esquisse historique et conceptuelle." *Psychiatrie, Sciences Humaines, Neurosciences* 3, no. 11 (2005): 37–48.

Vilensky, J. A., and S. Gilman. "Encephalitis Lethargica: Could This Disease Be Recognised If the Epidemic Recurred?" *Nature Clinical Practice Neurology* 6 (2006): 360–67.

Volkov, Sulamit. "Jewish Scientists in Imperial Germany (Parts I and II)." *Aleph: Historical Studies in Science and Judaism* 1, no. 1 (2001): 1–36.

Wagner, Richard. *Habseligkeiten: Roman*. Berlin: Aufbau Verlag, 2004.

Warner, John Harley. "The History of Science and the Sciences of Medicine." *Osiris* 10 (1995): 164–93.

———. "Ideals of Science and Their Discontents in Late Nineteenth-Century American Medicine." *Isis* 82 (1991): 454–78.

———. *The Therapeutic Perspective: Medical Practice, Knowledge, and Identity in America, 1820–1885*. Cambridge, MA: Harvard University Press, 1986.

Weber, Matthias M. "Psychiatric Research and Science Policy in Germany: The History of the Deutsche Forschungsanstalt fuer Psychiatrie." *History of Psychiatry* 11, no. 2 (2000): 235–58.

Wechsler, Lawrence M. *An Émigré Life, Munich, Berlin, Pacific Palisades: Marta Feuchtwanger*. Vol. 3. Los Angeles: University of California, 1976.

Weekly Epidemiological Record. "Epidemic and Other Forms of Encephalitis." December 14, 1939, 542–47.

Weindling, Paul. "The Impact of German Medical Scientists on British Medicine: A Case Study of Oxford, 1933–45." In *Forced Migration and Scientific Change: Emigré German-Speaking Scientists after 1933*, edited by Mitchell Ash and Alfons Soellner, 86–114. Cambridge: Cambridge University Press, 1996.

Weisz, George. *Divide and Conquer: A Comparative History of Medical Specialization*. Oxford: Oxford University Press, 2006.

————. *The Medical Mandarins: The French Academy of Medicine in the Nineteenth and Early Twentieth Centuries.* Oxford: Oxford University Press, 1995.

Whipple, Allan O. "Halsted's New York Period." *Surgery* 32 (1952): 542–50.

Wilson, Mitchell. "DSM-III and the Transformation of American Psychiatry: A History." *American Journal of Psychiatry* 150 (1993): 399–410.

Winner, B., Z. Kohl, and F. H. Gage. "Neurodegenerative disease and adult neurogenesis." *European Journal of Neuroscience* 33, no. 6 (2011): 1139–51.

Winter, Alison. *Memory: Fragments of a Modern History.* Chicago: University of Chicago Press, 2011.

Wise, M. Norton. *Neo-Classical Aesthetics of Art and Science: Hermann Helmholtz and the Frog-Drawing Machine.* Uppsala, Sweden: Hans Rausing Lecture, 2007.

Wittje, Roland. "The Electrical Imagination: Sound Analogies, Equivalent Circuits, and the Rise of Electroacoustics, 1863–1939." *Osiris* 28 (2013): 40–63.

Woolley, D. W., and E. Shaw. "A Biochemical and Pharmacological Suggestion about Certain Mental Disorders." *Science* 119, no. 3096 (1954): 577–78.

Wright, James R. "The 1917 New York Biopsy Controversy: A Question of Surgical Incision and the Promotion of Metastases." *Bulletin of the History of Medicine* 62 (1988): 546–62.

————. "The Development of the Frozen Section Technique, the Evolution of Surgical Biopsy, and the Origins of Surgical Pathology." *Bulletin of the History of Medicine* 59 (1985): 295–326.

Young, D. M., and W. Scoville. "Paranoid Psychosis in Narcolepsy and the Possible Danger of Benzadrine Treatment." *Medical Clinics of North America* 22 (1938): 637–42 .

Young, Robert M. *Mind, Brain and Adaptation in the Nineteenth Century: Cerebral Localization and Its Biological Context from Gall to Ferrier.* Oxford: Clarendon Press, 1970.

Zirkle, R. E. "Howard James Curtis, 1906–1972." *International Journal of Radiation Biology* 23, no. 6 (1972): 530–32.

Zucker, Bat-Ami. "Frances Perkins and the German-Jewish Refugees, 1933–1940." *American Jewish History* 89, no. 1 (2001): 35–59.

Contributors

BRIAN P. CASEY received his PhD from Yale's History of Science and Medicine Program in 2009. Broadly, Brian's work encompasses scientific practices, controversies, and the metaphysical implications of the twentieth-century life sciences. He has been a postdoctoral fellow at the National Institute of Mental Health, and he is a recent graduate of the School of Social Service Administration at the University of Chicago. He is currently a mental health counselor pursuing projects in the history of psychiatry.

STEPHEN T. CASPER is associate professor in the history of science at Clarkson University. After completing an undergraduate degree in biochemistry and neuroscience, he joined the Wellcome Centre for the History of Medicine in London, where he completed his doctoral studies in the history of medicine and science. He has published extensively on the history of the mind and brain sciences, including *The Neurological Patient in History* (Rochester, NY: University of Rochester Press, 2012) and *The Neurologists: A History of a Medical Specialty in Britain, c. 1789–2000* (Manchester, UK: Manchester University Press, 2014).

JUSTIN GARSON is associate professor of philosophy at Hunter College of the City University of New York. His areas of interest include the history and philosophy of biology. He is the author of *The Biological Mind: A Philosophical Introduction* (London: Routledge, 2015), *A Critical Overview of Biological Functions* (Dordrecht: Springer, 2016), and numerous articles.

DELIA GAVRUS is assistant professor in the history of science at the University of Winnipeg in Canada. She has published on the history of neurosurgery, neurology, and anesthesia in the twentieth century, and she is particularly interested in the ways in which professional and personal identity inform medical practice and scientific epistemology.

KATJA GUENTHER is assistant professor of history at Princeton University, working at the intersection of the history of medicine and the human sciences. She is the author of *Localization and Its Discontents: A Genealogy of*

Psychoanalysis and the Neuro Disciplines (Chicago: University of Chicago Press, 2015), and has published articles in journals such as *Medical History, Journal of the History of the Behavioral Sciences*, and *Modern Intellectual History*. She is currently working on a book project on the history of the mirror self-recognition test, examining the conceptualization of human nature in such diverse fields as developmental psychology, cybernetics, psychoanalysis, and neuroscience.

L. STEPHEN JACYNA is reader in the history of medicine at University College London. He has published extensively in the field of history of neuroscience.

KENTON KROKER has published on numerous topics in the history of twentieth-century biomedicine. His first book was *The Sleep of Others and the Transformations of Sleep Research* (Toronto: University of Toronto Press, 2007), and he is currently completing a book-length reconstruction of the history of epidemic encephalitis. He is associate professor in the Department of Science & Technology Studies at York University in Toronto.

THOMAS SCHLICH, MD, is James McGill Professor in the History of Medicine at McGill University in the Department of Social Studies of Medicine. After working as a physician at the University Hospital in Marburg, Germany, he switched to the history of medicine and worked in various research and teaching positions in Cambridge (England), Stuttgart (Germany), and Freiburg (Germany) before moving to McGill University (Montreal) in 2002. He held a Heisenberg Fellowship of the German Research Council (DFG) (2000–2002) and a Canada Research Chair (2002–12). His main research interests are the history of modern medicine and science (eighteenth to twenty-first centuries), in particular the history of surgery, the history of medicine and technology, and body history. His latest monograph is *The Origins of Organ Transplantation: Surgery and Laboratory Science, 1880s–1930s* (Rochester, NY: University of Rochester Press 2010).

MAX STADLER is a postdoctoral researcher at the Federal Institute of Technology, Zurich. As a historian of science and technology, his research interests center on the industrial and postindustrial contexts of the sciences of life, mind, and brain in the twentieth century. His current project, "The Users: Psychology, Machines, Design, 1930–1980," concerns a genealogy of that category—the user—as a model of late modern thinking and doing.

FRANK W. STAHNISCH holds the AMF/Hannah Professorship in the History of Medicine and Health Care at the University of Calgary in Canada. As a historian of medicine and health care, Frank's interests span the development of experimental physiology and laboratory medicine since the late eighteenth century (particularly France and Germany), the historical relationship between neurology/the neurosciences and the philosophy of the mind (with a focus on the German-speaking countries and North America), the relationship between clinical neuroscience and public mental health (particularly in Canada and the United States), the historical epistemology of the life sciences (eighteenth to twenty-first centuries), and the longer history of visualization practices in medicine and health care. His current research as a principle investigator is supported by research grants from SSHRC, CIHR, and AHRF. A recent book publication is *Medicine, Life and Function: Experimental Strategies and Medical Modernity at the Intersection of Pathology and Physiology* (Bochum, Germany: Projektverlag, 2012).

Index

Lightning Source UK Ltd.
Milton Keynes UK
UKHW012250201021
392552UK00001B/24